Positional Release Techniques

Senior Content Strategist: Rita Demetriou-Swanwick
Content Development Specialist: Carole McMurray
Project Manager: Anne Collett
Designer/Design Direction: Miles Hitchen
Illustration Manager: Karen Giacomucci
Illustrator: Suzanne Ghuzzi

Positional Release Techniques

with access to
www.chaitowpositionalrelease.com

FOURTH EDITION

Leon Chaitow ND DO

Registered Osteopathic Practitioner and Honorary Fellow, School of Integrated Health, University of Westminster, London, UK

With contributions by

Julia Brooks MSc DO

Edward Goering DO

Raymond J. Hruby DO MS FAAO (Dist)

Anthony J. Lisi DC

Dylan Morrissey PhD MSc MMACP MCSP

†**Anthony G. Pusey** DO FECert

Christopher Kevin Wong PT PhD MSc

Foreword by

Paolo Tozzi MSc Ost BSc DO PT

ELSEVIER Edinburgh London New York Oxford Philadelphia St Louis Sydney Toronto 2016

ELSEVIER

© 2016 Elsevier Ltd. All rights reserved.

First edition 1996
Second edition 2001
Third edition 2007
Fourth edition 2016

ISBN 978-0-7020-5111-1

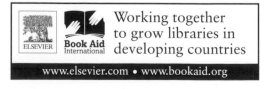

Contents

The website – www.chaitowpositionalrelease.com – accompanying this text includes video sequences of all the techniques indicated in the text. To look at the video for a given technique, click on the relevant icon in the contents list on the website. The website is designed to be used in conjunction with the text and not as a standalone product.

Companion website:
www.chaitowpositionalrelease.com
- video bank
- image bank

Contributors

Julia Brooks MSc DO
A. G. Pusey & Associates, Registered Osteopaths,
Haywards Heath,
West Sussex, UK

Edward Goering DO
Department of Neuromusculoskeletal Medicine/Osteopathic
Manipulative Medicine,
College of Osteopathic Medicine of the Pacific,
Western University of Health Sciences,
Pomona, CA, USA

Raymond J Hruby DO MS FAAO (Dist)
Department of Neuromusculoskeletal Medicine/Osteopathic
Manipulative Medicine,
College of Osteopathic Medicine of the Pacific,
Western University of Health Sciences,
Pomona, CA, USA

Anthony J Lisi DC
Staff Chiropractor,
VA CT Healthcare System,
West Haven, CT, USA

Dylan Morrissey PhD MSc MMACP MCSP
Clinical Reader and Consultant Physiotherapist,
Bart's Health NHS Trust,
Queen Mary University of London,
London, UK

†Anthony G Pusey DO FECert **(Deceased)**
A. G. Pusey & Associates, Registered Osteopaths,
Haywards Heath,
West Sussex, UK

Christopher Kevin Wong PT PhD MSc
Department of Rehabilitation and Regenerative Medicine,
Program in Physical Therapy,
Columbia University,
New York, NY, USA

Foreword

It is my profound privilege to write this foreword to the fourth edition of *Positional Release Techniques*, the latest invaluable contribution to the literature in manual therapy by Leon Chaitow and his team of experts in the field.

This latest edition offers an excellent selection of beautifully illustrated positional release techniques (PRTs), which will provide the reader with well-balanced instruction in the clinical application of this often underestimated manual approach. The authors bring to the profession a fresh, new and improved presentation of both well-known and recent advancements in the field, through easy-to-read palpatory procedures for diagnosis and treatment, supported by colour photographs, videos and illustrations to assist the reader in visualizing these methods.

Since their first effects were described based on the clinical experience of Lawrence Jones, over 60 years ago (Jones 1964), PRTs have offered many practical ways to manage pain and body dysfunctions, by creating the optimal tensional and physiological context to allow a spontaneous tissue release. One of the strengths of this book is that it explores principles and modalities of application of the main different forms of PRTs, from the original strain/counterstrain method to functional technique, from balanced ligamentous tension to various applications in physical therapy, such as McKenzie's exercise protocols, kinesio-taping methods that 'unload' tissues, and more. The book traces these methods from their historical roots up to their current practice, passing through the integration with emerging research and evidence. Although the aforementioned forms of PRTs reflect different ways of achieving a position of comfort, they all aim to gently support the tissues towards a spontaneous beneficial change. In any case, despite the appearance of simplicity, a detailed anatomical knowledge, together with clinical experience and palpatory skills, are strictly necessary to safely and efficiently perform these techniques. For this reason, the reader will find particularly useful a series of detailed, comprehensive, problem-solving clinical descriptions, more than ably supported by illustrations, photos of assessment and treatment methods. In addition, a number of exercises will offer a chance to experiment with PRT methodology, and to become familiar in a 'hands-on' way with the mechanics of their use. Therefore, mechanisms, guidelines and exercises provide a comprehensive foundation for the safe clinical application of this versatile methodology, supported by excellent references to the literature throughout the text.

Eighteen years have passed since publication of the first edition of this text. Despite the time, this book still maintains a balance of information in a straightforward, well-illustrated, and understandable manner that will not only challenge the avid student but also provide a solid reference for practicing therapists wishing to develop or expand their understanding of PRTs.

The emphasis remains the principles, methods of applications and mechanisms of PRTs addressed to different tissues and clinical conditions, with a focus on their advantages in normalizing somatic dysfunctions in many types of patients (as well as to animals), including those who are hospitalized, post-operative and/or bedbound. To achieve this scope, techniques are clearly and concisely written, and follow directly from their illustrative depictions.

Furthermore, while the broad content of previous editions has been updated and polished, this fourth edition attempts to help the reader look beyond the general application of PRTs in order to pursue the 'how many ways' PRTs can be safely applied, as well as 'how' they can be effective. This is accomplished by providing the latest evidence and research that bring traditional concepts within an innovative perspective of a modern practice, offering to the curious reader the opportunity to further explore individual aspects of PRTs and to inform clinical decision-making related to PRTs, in the context of the individual patient.

Finally, new and interesting chapters have been added to this fourth edition:

- a chapter on balanced ligamentous tension techniques by Ray Hruby, DO
- a chapter on counterstrain for visceral conditions by Edward Goering, DO
- a chapter on research evidence supporting PRTs by Christopher Kevin Wong, PT
- the introduction of new concepts, such as the potential for use of PRTs in management of specifically fascia-related conditions.

As for existing chapters, and also in these new chapters, considerable care has been taken to integrate the written and visual components, as well as to offer a balance of interesting synopsis of concepts and clinical-approach models. This material provides the neophyte, as well as the experienced practitioner, with an up-to-date snapshot of the field.

In conclusion, this book is designed to make learning about PRTs easier for teachers, students, and practitioners in manual therapy. It provides an invaluable resource by providing the building blocks necessary to gain the conceptual understanding of PRTs for their safe and effective clinical application to the human and animal body, as well as to increase practitioner awareness of the various modalities of PRTs and their respective mechanisms.

Paolo Tozzi MSc Ost DO PT
Rome, Italy 2015

REFERENCES

Jones, L.H., 1964. Spontaneous release by positioning. Doctor of Osteopathy 4, 109–116.

Preface to the third edition

The ideas that permeate positional release technique (PRT) methodology can be equated with non-invasive, non-interventionist, passive and gentle approaches that 'allow' change to emerge, rather than forcing it do so. Despite the apparently general nature of PRT methods, clinical experience within the osteopathic profession shows that they can be intensely practical and specific.

Two main themes emerge from PRT in its original form. The strain/counterstrain approach derives from the original work of osteopathic physician Lawrence Jones. It uses a pain monitor to find optimal positioning (i.e. when pain is no longer felt at the monitoring point). Functional technique also emerged out of osteopathic medicine; this PRT approach is based on positioning whilst sensing/palpating the tissues involved, so that they achieve their greatest degree of comfort or ease, without using pain as a guide.

In order to gain a sense of the underlying concepts involved in PRT application it is necessary to accept that the self-regulating mechanisms of the body are always the final determinants as to what happens following any form of intervention. For example, a high velocity, low amplitude thrust adjustment (HVLA), or application of a muscle energy technique (MET) or myofascial release (MFR), or almost any other procedure, acts as a catalyst for change. If the treatment is appropriate the body produces an adaptive response that will allow enhanced function and therapeutic benefit. The adaptive response is the key to whether or not benefit follows treatment. Excessive adaptive demands simply load the system more heavily, and symptoms are likely to worsen, while if there is inadequate therapeutic stimulus little value emerges from the exercise. The methods mentioned above (HVLA, MET and MFR) are all 'direct', that is to say, a barrier (or several barriers) will have been identified, and the therapeutic objective will be to push the barrier(s) back, in order to mobilise a restricted joint, or to lengthen shortened myofascial structure (for example).

Consider another way of addressing the restriction problem – an indirect one: reflect on whether, if the barrier is 'disengaged', the inherent tendency towards normality, demonstrated in the natural propensity for dysfunction to normalise (broken bones mend, tissues heal), is capable of restoring functionality to the types of dysfunction to which HVLA MET and MFR (as examples) are being applied.

Is it possible for self-regulating, homeostatic mechanisms to be encouraged to act when the load on dysfunctional tissues is temporarily eased?

- Can a restricted joint release without force?
- Can an excessively tight, muscular condition release spontaneously?
- And can pain sometimes be relieved instantaneously, merely by holding the painful tissues in an 'eased' position?

Clinical PRT evidence shows that all these questions can be answered affirmatively, at times. If restriction – whether of joint or soft tissue – involves hypertonicity and relative circulatory deficit (ischaemia, etc.), then is it possible that an opportunity for spontaneous change may occur by holding these same restricted tissues in a way that reduces the tone and allows (albeit temporarily) enhanced circulation through the tissues, and a chance for neural resetting (involving proprioceptors and nociceptors), to take place?

PRT methodology suggests that this is the case and a number of variations have evolved that incorporate the concept of 'offering an opportunity for change', as distinct from 'forcing a change', as is the case with HVT and MET for example.

There are particular settings and contexts in which PRT is probably the treatment method of first choice – as in extreme pain, recent trauma (for example whiplash, or immediately following a sporting or everyday strain), post surgery, extreme fragility (for example advanced osteoporosis). In addition, PRT is sufficiently versatile, with numerous variations, to be useful as a part of a sequence involving other interventions, for example before or following HVLA application, or as part of a sequence involving MET and neuromuscular technique, in trigger point deactivation, or as a means of easing hypertonicity during a massage therapy treatment.

The ideas that underpin PRT are also to be found in craniosacral methodology, in which disengagement of restrictions, moving away from restriction barriers, is a common approach.

Positional release variations, based on traditional osteopathic methodology are detailed in Chapters 1 through 7 inclusive, and are demonstrated on the accompanying DVD.

Of particular interest in this third edition is the inclusion of chapters that discuss a number of physiotherapy-derived systems, (Mulligan's Mobilisation with Movement, Unloading taping, and McKenzietype exercises) as well as from chiropractic methodology (Sacro-occipital Technique – SOT) that have strong links to the underlying concepts of PRT.

Robert Cooperstein has outlined and illustrated the useful 'positional release' concepts and methods used in sacro-occipital technique (SOT), in Chapter 8. SOT derives from the work of Major deJarnette, whose early work with cranial osteopathic pioneer Sutherland demonstrates how osteopathic and chiropractic ideas and methods that evolved in the early to mid-20th century, had a great deal in common.

Anthony Lisi has presented some of the core McKenzie methods in Chapter 9. The concepts of exercises being employed guided by 'preferred directions of movement', is pure positional release, although used in quite distinctive and original ways.

In Chapter 10 Ed Wilson presents a description of those aspects of the work of Brian Mulligan, the innovative New Zealand physiotherapist, whose mobilisation with movement (MWM) concepts have been so widely adopted in physiotherapy settings. There are specific variations within MWM that have close similarities with PRT ideas and Wilson has performed the invaluable task of moving beyond descriptions of methods to evaluation of underlying mechanisms.

The elegant approach that 'proprioceptively unloads' dysfunctional joints and tissues and then tapes the structures into their 'ease' state, for hours or days, in contrast to the minutes of 'ease' used in osteopathic PRT methodology is described by Dylan Morrissey in Chapter 11.

Finally in Chapter 12 Julia Brooks and Anthony Pusey illustrate the remarkably successful use of osteopathic positional release in treatmernt of animals, including dogs and horses. No clearer examples can be offered of the true breadth of usefulness of these most gentle of methods.

The cross-fertilisation and interdisciplinary possibilities that are exemplified by the coming together of osteopathic, chiropractic and physiotherapeutic methods and ideas, highlight the potential for the future, as barriers and rivalries give way to cooperation, collaboration and ultimately integration, for the benefit of all.

Preface

In preparing to revise and expand this 4th edition my aim was to ensure that, as well as revisiting every line of the text to check for accuracy and clarity, new text, illustrations, videos and chapters would be added, that expanded on the potential and the variety of manual positional release approaches.

All original chapters from the previous edition have been updated and revised, and in some cases combined – where this seemed appropriate.

The content now comprises:

Spontanous Release by Positioning (ch.1) – an introduction to the potentials for therapeutic benefit of easing tissues (and the whole person) into 'positions of ease'.

Somatic Dysfunction and Positional Release (ch.2) expands on these ideas as it explores the processes of adaptation and decompensation that lead to dysfunction and pain – and where positional release methods might fit into clinical care.

This is followed by an excellent chapter (3) by Dr Christopher Kevin Wong on *Strain/counterstrain Research,* that reviews current evidence relating to this most widely used of all positional release methods.

Chapter 4 focuses on the detailed application of *Counterstrain models of Positional Release,* while Chapter 5 provides a review of *Functional and Facilitated Positional Release Approaches, Including Cranial Techniques.*

Chapter 6 offers insights into use of *Positional Release Techniques in Special Situations* – for example when treating a bed-ridden individual.

In response to increasing evidence of interest in this topic, I have compiled a focused chapter (ch.7): *Positional Release and Fascia.*

Raymond Hruby DO (ch.8) has provided a highly illustrated chapter (supported by fine video demonstrations) on *Balanced Ligamentous Tension Techniques.*

Edward Goering DO has contributed a very useful chapter (9): *Visceral Positional Release: the Counterstrain Model.*

Anthony Lisi DC has expanded his chapter: *Overview of the McKenzie Method* (ch.10), as has Dr Dylan Morrissey in his chapter (11) *'Offloading' taping to reduce pain and facilitate movement.*

All chapters – including the fascinating: *Application of positional release techniques in treatment of animals* (ch12) by Julia Brooks DO and the late Anthony Pusey DO, have been revised and improved, and all illustrations have been redrawn, with many new video clips added.

I hope and believe that this new edition offers students and practitioners of manual therapy the clearest and most current information on this most useful of manual approaches to pain and dysfunction.

Leon Chaitow, Corfu, Greece, June 2015

Acknowledgements

My profound thanks to the team of clinician/authors who have contributed chapters to this book: Julia Brooks, Edward Goering, Ray Hruby, Anthony Lisi, Dylan Morrisey, the late Anthony Pusey, Christopher Kevin Wong. The richness of their contributions adds so much to the content.

I also thank the team at Elsevier for their friendly support during the lengthy production process.

To my wonderful wife Alkmini. … my continued thanks for her ability to create a warm and loving environment in which writing becomes a pleasure instead of a task.

Abbreviations

A
AA: atlantoaxial
AIIS: anterior inferior iliac spine
AK: applied kinesiology
ASIS: anterior superior iliac spine

B
BLT: balanced ligamentous tension
BMT: balanced membranous tension

C
CABG: coronary artery bypass graft
CCP: common compensatory pattern
CMP: chronic myofascial pain
CMRT: chiropractic manipulative reflex technique
CNS: central nervous system
CRI: cranial rhythmic impulse
CS: central sensitization
CS: counterstrain
CSRM: cranial-sacral respiratory mechanism
CT: cervicothoracic

D
DTP: dominant tender points

E
EMG: electromyographic
ENOS: endothelial nitrous oxide synthetase

F
FMS: fibromyalgia syndrome
FPR: facilitated positional release
FT: functional technique
FuPR: functional positional release

G
GERD: gastroesophageal reflux disease

H
HVLA: high-velocity low amplitude

I
IL: interleukin
INIT: integrated neuromuscular inhibition technique
ITBFS: iliotibial band friction syndrome

L
LAS: ligamentous articular strain
LS: lumbosacral

M
MET: muscle energy technique
MFR: myofascial release
MIS: medial intramuscular septum
MPS: myofascial pain syndrome
MPT: myofascial trigger points
MRI: magnetic resonance imaging
MWM: mobilization with movement

N
NAGs: natural apophyseal glides
NMT: neuromuscular technique

O
OA: occipitoatlantal
OMT: osteopathic manipulative therapy

P
PFP: patellofemoral pain
PI: posterior, inferior
PNF: proprioceptive neuromuscular facilitation
PPI: proton pump inhibitor
PRT: positional release technique
PSIS: posterior superior iliac spine

Q
QL: quadratus lumborum

R
REST: restricted environmental stimulation technique

Abbreviations

S

SBIS: silicone breast implant syndrome
SCS: strain and counterstrain
SD: somatic dysfunction
SE: scanning evaluation
SIJ: sacroiliac joint
SMWLM: spinal mobilization with limb movement
SNAGs: sustained natural apophyseal glides
SOT: sacro-occipital technique
SRC: static resisted contraction

T

TART: texture, asymmetry, range of motion, tenderness

TARTT: texture, asymmetry, range of motion, tenderness, temperature
TeP: tender point
TFL: tensor fascia lata
TL: thoracolumbar
TMJ: temporomandibular joint
TP: tender point
TPPS: tender point palpation scale
TrP: trigger point

V

VMO: vastus medialis oblique

Chapter | 1 |

Spontaneous release by positioning

POSITIONAL RELEASE TECHNIQUES (PRT)

Positional release techniques (PRT) offer practical ways of managing pain and biomechanical dysfunction. They are also intellectually satisfying because they do not *impose* solutions on dysfunctional tissues; instead they are designed to offer the opportunity for a spontaneous resolution of pain, spasm, hypertonicity and restriction.

One of the major forms of PRT: strain/counterstrain (SCS, or simply counterstrain, CS), was initially known as 'spontaneous release by positioning' (Jones 1964).

The essence of all forms of PRT is to gently support tissues in a position of comfort or 'ease', until a spontaneous beneficial change ('release') occurs. The differences between the various forms of PRT reflect the variety of ways in which 'ease' may be achieved.

SCS, as well as other models of positional release methodology, are fully described later in this book, while in this chapter, a broad descriptive overview is offered, of a variety of ways in which the practical application of positional release methods can be used therapeutically.

The concept behind the techniques is simple, as are some of its protocols, to the extent that some can be taught to patients for self-application (see Chapter 4). However, more often, PRT in clinical practice requires patience, skill and delicacy of touch.

A painful example

If a symptomatic patient presents with tissues that are excessively tense, indurated, hypertonic, shortened or contracted – and most probably painful, therapeutic objectives are likely to include reduction in pain, as

1

well as removal or reduction of barriers to free movement. Of course there are times when hypertonicity or spasm may be appropriately protective – and in such cases (e.g. where there is underlying pathology such as osteoporosis), there should be no attempt to remove such protective support, by means of positional release or anything else.

Many therapeutic approaches, confronted with restricted soft-tissue or joint dysfunction, employ methods of a direct nature – in which barriers are engaged, in one way or another, obliging these to retreat. The soft tissue in question may be stretched, massaged, mobilized or manipulated, using any of dozens of perfectly appropriate techniques, such as 'muscle energy technique' or 'passive stretching' (as examples). However, if the tissues are painful, in spasm, inflamed or have recently been traumatized, or if the direct manual method causes discomfort, then an alternative approach is required.

Take for example a restricted joint where an osteopath, physiotherapist or chiropractor might introduce a high-velocity, low-amplitude (HVLA) thrust, in order to normalize motion. In particular situations, HVLA methods might be considered inappropriate – for any number of reasons, ranging from patient preference, to safety – as in an osteoporotic condition. However, a frequently efficient alternative choice might be the use of a positional release method that involves placing and maintaining (possibly for several minutes), the joint in a pain-free, balanced, unstressed position.

Descriptions as to how and why enhanced pain-free movement of the previously restricted joint might be achieved by positional release methods, will be explained further in later chapters.

Positional release approaches to treatment of hypertonic, contracted soft tissues would not involve lengthening or stretching methods, but would attempt to find a way (depending on which PRT variation was selected) of offering an 'opportunity for change' to those tissues. This would commonly involve disengagement from the barrier, and holding or supporting the hypertonic, contracted tissues in a painless but even more shortened state, 'inviting' a spontaneous change to take place.

The cluster of methods that can be grouped together as *positional release techniques* (PRTs), which this text describes, offer just such possibilities of *encouraging positive* changes in dysfunctional tissues – soft tissue – or joints (see in particular, Chapters 4–6 and 8).

The mechanisms whereby these changes occur seem to involve a combination of the neurological and circulatory changes that take place when a distressed area is placed into its most comfortable, its most 'easy', most pain-free position.

Descriptions of the major variations of PRT methods are given below. Many of these have chapters devoted entirely to exploring their individual methodology.

Some PRT variations

As will become clear, there are a variety of ways of incorporating indirect, extremely gentle, methods into a treatment protocol. Osteopathic medicine has contributed the main positional release approaches – including:

- Strain/counterstrain (SCS) (Jones 1964; Wong et al. 2013) – see Chapters 3 and 4 for details of this powerful therapeutic tool.
- Functional technique (FT) – and its variants – facilitated positional release (FPR) (Johnstone 1997; McPartland & Zigler 1993; Schiowitz 1990) and indirect myofascial release – are all described in Chapter 5.
- Balanced ligamentous tension (BLT) is a variant of PRT that uses skilled palpation to ease dysfunctional joint structures – to a position in which ligamentous tensions are equally balanced, in order to encourage improvement or resolution of underlying dysfunction – see Chapter 8.
- Visceral technique, involves the same principles of disengagement – directed at assisting in improved function of organs – see Chapter 9 for explanations and descriptions.

Physiotherapy has also contributed to this indirect approach to dysfunction.

- The important work of McKenzie, involving as it does rehabilitation methods that encourage movement into comfortable, and not painful positions – for example in management of low back pain – clearly relates to positional release, and is described in Chapter 10.
- Physical therapy has also produced a number of innovative concepts and methods that unload soft tissues and joints, and which then supports them in this unloaded state, by means of taping, as described in Chapter 11.
- A combination of these methods have been successfully applied to animals, most effectively in treatment of horses, and equine positional release methods are discussed in Chapter 12.

As this (growing) list of variations suggests, there are a number of different methods involving the positioning of an area of the body, or the whole body, in such a way as to evoke a therapeutically significant physiological response that – evidence suggests – can assist in resolving musculoskeletal dysfunction. Mounting evidence for the clinical efficacy of SCS is provided in Chapter 3, where proposed mechanisms are also examined. For a summary of these methods and definitions, see Chapter 8, Table 8.1.

Therapeutic benefit of reduced stimulus?

In a different context entirely, reduced environmental stimulus has been shown to have the potential to offer therapeutic benefit.

Use of the effects of being placed into a flotation tank – described as 'restricted environmental stimulation technique' (REST) – has been used in the treatment of anxiety and depression in individuals suffering chronic pain.

Such treatment involves individuals spending time immersed in a tank filled with neutral temperature water (i.e. body heat), of an extremely high salt concentration to increase buoyancy. In one study, 37 patients (14 men and 23 women) suffering from chronic pain, were randomly assigned to either a control group (17 participants) or an experimental group (20 participants). The experimental group received nine flotation – (REST) – treatments, over a 3-week period. The results indicated that the most severely perceived pain intensity was significantly reduced, whereas low perceived pain intensity was not influenced. Flotation-REST treatment elevated the participants' optimism and reduced the degree of anxiety or depression and improved the sleep pattern.

This example of reduced stimulus, leading to spontaneous change, should be kept in mind as we explore the equivalent, when applied (without the flotation tank) to distressed somatic tissues that are carefully placed into comfort/ease positions.

Additional theoretical models that attempt to explain the effects of the various forms of positional release are outlined in Chapters 4–9.

Terminology – 'ease' and 'bind'

As explanations and descriptions are offered for the spontaneous physiological responses that take place when tissues are placed into a balanced state, in this and later chapters (Chapter 3 in particular), the terms 'ease' and 'bind' will frequently be used to describe the extremes of restriction (bind) and freedom of movement (ease).

The term 'dynamic neutral' may be considered as being interchangeable with 'maximal ease'. Hoover (1969), the developer of functional technique (Chapter 5), one of the major methods of spontaneous positional release, used the term, 'dynamic neutral', to describe what is being aimed for, as the tissues associated with a structurally disturbed joint or area are positioned into a state of comfort or 'ease'.

Bowles (1969) has also discussed this phenomenon, stating:

> *Dynamic neutral is a state in which tissues find themselves when the motion of the structures they serve are free, unrestricted and within the range of normal physiological limits …. Dynamic neutral is not a static condition … it is a continuing state of normal, during living motion, during living activity … it is the state and condition to be restored to a dysfunctional area.*

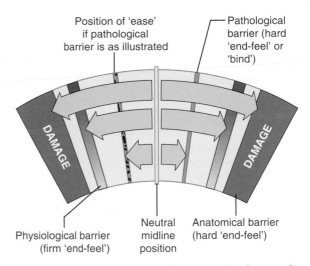

Figure 1.1 label text:
Position of 'ease' if pathological barrier is as illustrated

Pathological barrier (hard 'end-feel' or 'bind')

DAMAGE

DAMAGE

Physiological barrier (firm 'end-feel')

Neutral midline position

Anatomical barrier (hard 'end-feel')

Figure 1.1 Illustrating mid-range between ends of range of motion in dysfunctional tissues.

Finding the 'easy' barrier

In normal tissues there exists, in the mid-range of motion, an area of 'ease' or 'balance', where the tissues are at their least tense. However, when there is a restriction in the normal range of motion of tissues, whether of osseous or of soft-tissue origin, the now limited range will almost always still have a position, a moment, a point of maximum comfort or ease, lying somewhere between the new restriction barrier in one direction, and the physiological barrier in the other.

Finding this 'balance point' is a key element in PRT application. And, it is suggested, maintaining such an 'ease' state, for an appropriate length of time (see below), may well offer restrictions a chance to release or normalize (Fig. 1.1).

The process of positioning – by the practitioner – of distressed tissues into a three-dimensional comfort, or 'ease', position creates the environment of reduced proprioceptive stimulus during which time self-regulating changes are invited to occur. The 'treatment' itself can therefore be seen to be self-generated by tissues, as they respond to being supported in their ease position. Inevitably, some degree of neurological – proprioceptive – feedback, as well as circulatory, and possibly mechanotransduction (see Chapter 7) related changes, are likely to be involved in the responses to the positioning process. Jones's original name for what became known as strain/counterstrain, was 'spontaneous release by positioning' (Greenman 1996).

Jones's contribution

The impetus towards the use of this most basic and non-invasive of treatment approaches, in a coherent, rather than a hit-and-miss manner, lies in the work of Lawrence Jones DO, who developed an approach to somatic dysfunction (Jones 1981) that he termed 'strain and counterstrain' (SCS) (described in detail in Chapters 3 and 4).

Walther (1988) describes the moment of discovery in these words:

> Jones's initial observation of the efficacy of counterstrain was with a patient who was unresponsive to treatment. The patient had been unable to sleep because of pain. Jones attempted to find a comfortable position for the patient to aid him in sleeping. After 20 minutes of trial and error, a position was finally achieved in which the patient's pain was relieved. Leaving the patient in this position for a short time, Jones was astonished when the patient came out of the position and was able to stand comfortably erect. The relief of pain was lasting and the patient made an uneventful recovery.

The position of 'ease' that Jones identified for this patient was an exaggeration of the position in which spasm was holding him, and this provided Jones with an insight into the possible mechanisms involved.

Over the years since Jones first made the observation, that a position which exaggerated a patient's distortion could provide the opportunity for a release of spasm and hypertonicity, many variations on this basic theme have emerged, some building logically on that first insight, with others moving in new directions.

Upledger & Vredevoogd (1983) offered a practical explanation of indirect methods of treatment, especially as related to cranial therapy (see Chapter 5). The idea of moving a restricted area into its directions of ease is, they say, 'a sort of "unlatching" principle. Often in order to open a latch we must first exaggerate its closure'.

Most of the variations on the theme of PRT, described briefly in this chapter, are discussed in greater detail later in the book.

What are 'tender points'?

Jones (1981) described localized areas, associated with distressed and dysfunctional tissues, as 'tender points'. A possibility exists for confusion when identifying areas of unusual tenderness during examination or palpation. The characteristics of tender points, as used in positional release, as well as those used in the diagnosis of fibromyalgia, and the similarities and differences between these and myofascial trigger points are discussed in Box 1.1.

Common basis

The positional release methods summarized later in this chapter are as comprehensive as possible at the time of writing; however, new variants are regularly appearing, and the author acknowledges that it has been impossible to exhaustively detail all versions.

The need for the existence of variations of PRT should be obvious, as different clinical settings require the availability of a variety of therapeutic approaches – ranging (as examples) from those suitable during a clinical office appointment, to someone who is bedridden – possibly hospitalized, to an athlete lying at the trackside after injury.

Although PRT approaches have a broad commonality, in that they involve passive movement of the patient, or the affected tissues, away from any restricted, uncomfortable, resistance barriers ('bind'), and towards positions of increased comfort and 'ease' – subtle differences allow their use in distinctly contrasting settings.

Examples of positional release methods that are described in more detail in later chapters, include outlines of methods used in the care of severely ill, pre- and post-operative, bedridden (see Chapter 6) patients, treated for their current pain and discomfort, without leaving their beds. In such settings, no rigid application of procedures can be adhered to, and flexibility can best be achieved by the practitioner/therapist having available a set of skills for achieving the same ends – enhanced function and diminished pain (Schwartz 1986; O-Yurvati et al. 2005).

The use of a selection of indirect and direct modalities during one treatment session is common to all forms of manual therapy – including massage, physiotherapy, chiropractic and osteopathy. It is obvious that in real-life clinical settings, when a selection of different treatment approaches are used during one treatment session, it becomes impossible to say which of the methods had any particular effect. Indeed, it may be that maximum benefit would only be experienced when a combination of methods are being employed.

What if patients cannot communicate verbally?

The form of PRT that has been most widely researched is SCS – and much of the evidence for its value is described in Chapter 3. SCS requires verbal feedback from the patient as to the degree of sensitivity of a 'tender' point, which is being used as a monitor, and which the practitioner/therapist is palpating while attempting to find a position of ease, where tissue-tension reduces and reported discomfort is minimized. Where pain provocation is deliberately being avoided – or where the individual is unable to report to the practitioner changes in pain levels – the palpated sense of tension in the tissues can be used to identify the position of maximum comfort/ease.

It is possible to imagine such situations, for example, in the case of someone who had lost the ability to communicate verbally; or who does not speak the same language as the therapist; or who is too young or too ill to offer

Box 1.1 'Tender points' in the context of positional release – and other conditions

As tissues adapt and modify due to the effects of age, overuse, misuse, disuse, etc. (see Chapter 2 for discussion of the evolution of soft-tissue dysfunction), localized areas of ischaemic, sensitized tissues emerge.

A variety of biomechanical, biochemical, neurological, circulatory and psychological influences are associated with such changes, which gradually evolve from sensitivity to discomfort, and eventually pain (Mense & Simons 2001).

A general term that can be applied to such tissues, whatever level of the spectrum of dysfunction happens to be operating, is 'hyperalgesia'. Lewit (1999) described the phenomenon as a 'hyperalgesic skin zone'. A simpler, more user-friendly word, is 'tender point' (Jones 1964).

Whether such localized areas ('points') are in their early embryonic formative stages, or have reached a state where they display the characteristics of active myofascial trigger points (see Chapter 2), they will undoubtedly be sensitive or 'tender', and this is the term given to them in SCS methodology, in which they are used as a major feature of the protocol of assessment and treatment (see Chapter 4).

Myofascial trigger points are, by definition, localized, tender areas that are painful when compressed and, when active, display the significant characteristic of being able to radiate or refer pain, as well as other sensations, to adjacent or even distant tissues – reproducing symptoms that are familiar to the patient.

A potential for confusion lies in the use of the term 'tender points' in the diagnostic procedures involved in assessment of individuals suspected of having fibromyalgia.

In 1990, the American College of Rheumatology issued criteria for the diagnosis of fibromyalgia that included identification of tenderness in at least 11 out of 18 prescribed palpated sites (Wolfe et al. 1990). These tender areas may simply be tender, and may not display the 'spreading' characteristics of myofascial trigger points. However, this distinction may not be easily made, since, because fibromyalgia involves widespread diffuse pain, pressure on tender points in someone with fibromyalgia may easily reproduce pain familiar to that individual.

In other words *tender points* may also be active *trigger points*, and trigger points will always be tender. However, in the context of PRT in general, and strain/counterstrain in particular, tender points are more usually described as simply tender, without the ability to refer or radiate symptoms.

Another major distinction is that while trigger points become a target for treatment, manually or via needling or laser treatment – the 'tender points' in fibromyalgia assessment are used purely for diagnostic purposes, as compared with those in PRT that are used as key elements in guiding the practitioner towards identification of 'positions of ease'.

Nevertheless, as will become clear in later chapters, all tender or painful areas may be used when following SCS treatment protocols – whether or not they are active trigger points, and whether or not they are 'tender points' identified during a fibromyalgia assessment.

verbal feedback; or in the case of animals (see Chapter 12). In such cases, a need would be apparent for a method that allows the practitioner/therapist to achieve the same objective – of achieving an 'ease' position – without verbal communication.

This is possible, as will be demonstrated, using either 'functional' methods or facilitated positional release approaches, that involve the practitioner/therapist identifying a position of maximum ease by means of palpation alone, assessing for a state of 'ease' in the tissues. See Chapter 5 for more detail of this approach, which epitomizes some of the methodology of an SCS derivative, Ortho-Bionomy, which is briefly described later in this chapter.

Outcomes in different clinical settings

It is important to note that if PRT methods are being applied to chronically indurated or fibrosed tissues, the results may well be expected to produce a reduction in hypertonicity, but would not result in any reduction in structural changes in the tissues, such as fibrosis.

Pain relief or improved mobility may therefore be only temporary or partial in such cases. This does not nullify the usefulness of PRT in chronic settings, but emphasizes the need to use such methods as part of an integrated approach.

Integrated methods will be seen to be of particular value in deactivation of myofascial trigger points, using a combination of manual methods in a sequence known as integrated neuromuscular inhibition technique – INIT (see below, and in more detail in Chapter 5).

Clinical considerations

Exaggeration of distortion

The concept of exaggerating an existing degree of distortion is a common aspect of clinical reasoning in PRT/SCS methodology. Take the example of an individual bent forward in psoas spasm/lumbago. This would involve someone in considerable discomfort or pain, who is posturally distorted – bent forward into flexion, together with rotation and side-bending. Any attempt by the person (or the practitioner) to straighten the individual towards a more physiologically normal posture would be met by increased pain and a great deal of resistance. Movement toward, or engagement of, the resistance barrier would therefore not be an ideal first option.

However, moving the area *away from* the restriction barrier in such a situation is not usually a problem. Clinical experience has shown that the position required to find the position of 'ease' for someone in this state normally involves painlessly, and usually passively, increasing the degree of distortion displayed, placing the person (in the example given) into some variation based on forward bending (possibly supine or while side-lying, rather than weight-bearing – see examples in Chapter 4) until pain is found to reduce or resolve.

After 60–90 seconds in this 'position of ease', a slow return to neutral would be carried out and – theoretically, and commonly in practice – the patient would be somewhat or completely relieved of pain and spasm.

Replication of position of strain

This is another feature of PRT/SCS clinical reasoning. Take for example that someone describes the onset of their problem as starting when bending to lift a load, during which process an emergency stabilization was required – as the load shifted (see notes on the mechanisms involved in SCS, in Chapter 4). The patient was then locked in a position of 'lumbago-like' antalgic spasm and distortion, as described in the previous few paragraphs.

If, as PRT in general, and SCS in particular, suggests, the position of ease commonly equals the position of strain – then the patient needs to be taken back into flexion – in supported, passive, slow-motion – until tenderness vanishes from the monitored tender point, and/or a sense of ease is perceived in the previously hypertonic shortened tissues. Adding small 'fine-tuning' positioning to the initial position of ease – achieved by flexion – usually achieves a situation in which just such a maximum reduction in pain is possible.

This position would be held for 60–90 seconds before slowly returning the patient to neutral, at which time, as in the example above, a partial or total resolution of hypertonicity, spasm and pain may result.

It should be obvious that the position of strain, as just described, is probably going to be a duplication of the position of exaggeration of distortion.

These two elements of SCS – 'exaggeration of existing distortion' and 'replication of the position of strain' – are described as examples only, since patients can rarely describe precisely the way in which their symptoms developed. Nor is obvious spasm, such as torticollis or acute antalgic spasm ('lumbago'), the norm, however it is strongly recommended that attention be paid to chronic distortion patterns, where adaptive shortening and crowding may have occurred over a period of years. PRT applied

to chronic holding patterns can be a valuable approach in patient management. The evolution of such patterns is a feature discussed in Chapter 2.

The methods of McKenzie (Chapter 10), in which movement in directions that are free and easy (relatively) rather than in directions that are restricted or painful, carries echoes of the positions that emerge when incorporating 'exaggeration' or 'strain replication' into management of dysfunction. An addition of supportive taping to hold tissues in 'easy' exaggerated distortion (Chapter 11) can be seen to be an amplification of the approach offered manually in SCS or functional technique, as described below.

POSITIONAL RELEASE VARIATIONS

(see also Chapter 8, Table 8.1)

1. Functional positional release (FuPR)

(Bowles 1981; Hoover 1969)

Osteopathic functional technique ignores pain as its guide to the position of ease, and relies instead on a reduction in palpated tone in stressed (hypertonic, spasmed, restricted) tissues, as the body (or part) is being positioned, or fine-tuned, towards three-dimensional 'ease' involving use of different vectors of force.

A position of palpated ease is achieved using what is known as a 'stacking' sequence, explained and described in more detail in Chapter 5.

One hand palpates the affected tissues without invasive pressure. This is described as the 'listening' hand, since it assesses changes in tone as the practitioner/therapist guides the patient (or part) through a sequence of positions that are aimed at enhancing ease and reducing bind.

A sequence of evaluations are carried out, involving different directions/vectors of movement (flexion/extension, rotation right and left, side-bending right and left, distraction, compression, etc.), with each new movement starting at the point of maximum ease established during the previous evaluation; or combined position of ease involving a number of previous evaluations. In this way, one position of ease is 'stacked' onto another, until all directions of movement have been assessed for ease, and their combined positions incorporated into the final 'position of ease'.

Functional low back approach

If an individual with a low back problem, as previously described, was being treated using the functional technique, the tense tissues in the low back, would be the ones palpated.

With the patient seated or side-lying, following a sequence of supported passive movements involving flexion/extension, side-bending and rotation, in each direction, translation right and left, translation anterior and posterior and compression/distraction (so involving all available directions of movement of the area) – a position of maximum ease would be arrived at. This 'stacked' position of ease would then be held for 30–90 seconds, so that a release of hypertonicity and/or a reduction in pain, might result.

The precise sequence in which the various directions of motion are evaluated seems to be irrelevant, as long as all possibilities are included.

Theoretically (and usually, in practice) the position of palpated maximum ease (reduced tone) in the distressed tissues should correspond with the position that would have been identified if pain was being used as a guide, or if the more basic 'exaggeration of distortion' or 'replication of position of strain' were being used as guides to positioning.

Functional 'diaphragm release'

For a simple functional exercise – using only one direction of 'ease' (Noll et al. 2008), see Figure 1.2.

1. The patient lies supine.
2. One of the operator's hands is placed under the patient's back, at the level of the thoracolumbar junction.
3. The other hand is placed on the abdominal epigastric area.

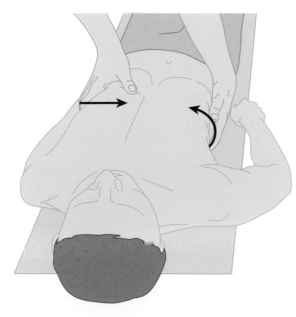

Figure 1.2 Functional treatment of the lower thorax/diaphragm area.

4. The operator rotates the tissues to one side and then the other to determine the direction of greatest freedom of movement.
5. The tissues are then rotated towards the direction of greatest freedom, to a point of 'balance' – where minimal tension is noted – and held there until a release is palpated, allowing a more symmetrical rotation in both directions.
6. As this position is held, the patient may be requested to produce a full cycle of breathing, and the patient should be asked to maintain (for as long as is comfortable) the position where – in that cycle – the operator determines the tissues to be even more 'relaxed'.

The maintenance of an 'ease' stage of the breathing cycle is thought to have a potentially facilitating influence on the release process.

More complex 'stacking' procedures to determine maximum ease – in use of functional technique – are described in Chapter 7.

A functional technique variation: integrated neuromuscular release

(Danto 2003)

Integrated neuromuscular release is a form of FuPR involving a segmental, antero-posterior approach that aims to correct muscular, fascial and neural imbalances. 'Osteopathic manipulative treatment has been concerned, purposefully or not, with manipulation of the fascia' (Danto 2003).

- With the patient seated, the practitioner's hands are placed anteriorly and posteriorly, where – independently – they perform evaluations of tissue direction preferences (Fig. 1.3).
- Each direction sequence is asking the same question – in which direction do the tissues move most freely – with each change in direction commencing from the position(s) of ease previously identified?
- Superior/inferior?
- Lateral to the left/lateral to the right?
- Clockwise/anticlockwise?
- In this way, the palpated tissues are taken into their preferred directions of motion, towards a combined 'ease' position, at which time compression is added. This is held for 60–90 seconds – or longer if changes in the tissues are being sensed – pulsation, rhythmic motion, etc. – before a slow release.

2. Facilitated positional release (FPR)

(Schiowitz 1990)

This variation on the theme of functional methods involves the positioning of the distressed area into the direction of

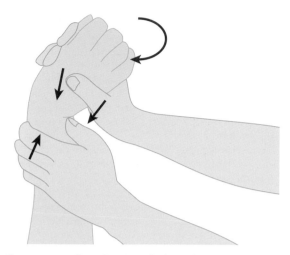

Figure 1.4 Facilitated positional release for hypertonic medial wrist musculature.

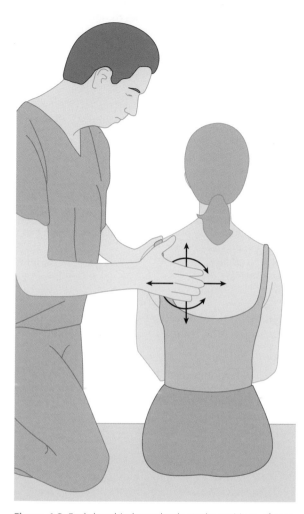

Figure 1.3 Each hand independently stacks positions of ease onto each other as all directions are assessed for 'ease'. The final combined position of ease is held for 90 seconds, during which circulatory, proprioceptive and viscoelastic effects are thought to start a self-regulating process.

its greatest freedom of movement, starting from a position of 'neutral' in terms of the overall body position.

To start with, the seated patient's sagittal posture might be modified to take the body or the part (neck, for example) into a more 'neutral' position – a balance between flexion and extension – following which, an application of a facilitating force (usually a crowding of the tissues) would be introduced. No pain monitor is used in FPR but rather a palpating/listening hand is applied (as in functional technique), which senses for changes in ease and bind in distressed tissues as the body/part is carefully positioned and repositioned.

The final 'crowding' of the tissues, to encourage a 'slackening' of local tension, is the facilitating aspect of the

process, according to its developers. This 'crowding' might involve compression applied through the long axis of a limb, or directly downwards through the spine via cranially applied pressure, or some such variation.

Once a facilitating force is added to positioning into 'ease', the length of time the position of ease is held is usually suggested to be around ≤5 seconds. It is claimed that altered tissue texture, either surface or deep, can be successfully treated in this way (Schiowitz 1990).

FPR is evaluated and discussed in greater detail in Chapter 5. It can also be employed as part of SCS methodology (where it more closely resembles 'Ortho-Bionomy', see item 6 below).

Facilitated positional release exercise: hypertonic medial right wrist muscles:

1. The practitioner holds the patient's hand with his right hand (Fig. 1.4).
2. The practitioner's left hand holds the patient's wrist while the thumb of that hand palpates the degree of hypertonicity.
3. The practitioner 'crowds' the wrist by approximating his hands, as he assesses the reduction in tone of the palpated tissues.
4. When an optimal degree of relaxation is perceived, the wrist is taken into radial deviation and slightly pronated – until further reduction in tone is perceived.
5. This should be held for up to 5 seconds before releasing and re-evaluating.
6. *Note*: Different aspects of the wrist musculature would require variations of wrist deviation, rotation and degree of compression – always seeking maximal reduction in tone.

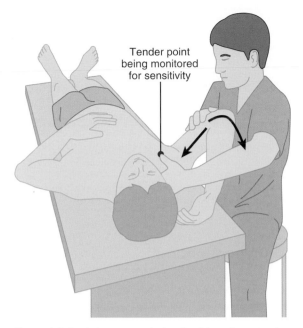

Figure 1.5 Strain/counterstrain for shoulder using a tender point on anterior aspect, as the arm is positioned into 'ease', to reduce sensitivity.

Tender point being monitored for sensitivity

3. Strain/counterstrain (SCS): using Jones's tender points as monitors

(Jones 1981)

Over many years of clinical experience, Jones compiled charts and lists of specific tender point areas, relating to every imaginable strain, involving most of the joints and muscles of the body (Fig. 1.5).

These are his 'proven' (by clinical experience) points. The tender points that he described are usually found in tissues that were in a shortened state at the time of strain (or are chronically shortened), rather than those that were stretched, and in tissues that have become chronically shortened over time.

New points – outside of Jones's lists and charts – have been periodically reported in the literature; for example, a group of sacral foramen points relating to sacroiliac strains were identified and described by Ramirez et al (1989); see Chapter 4.

Jones and his followers provided strict guidelines for achieving ease in any tender points being palpated (the position of ease usually involving a 'folding' or 'crowding' of the tissues in which the tender point lies), which neatly incorporates the concept of 'exaggeration of distortion', discussed earlier – since it makes what is already short, shorter.

This method is described in detail in Chapter 4 and involves maintaining pressure on the monitored tender point, or periodically probing it, as a position is achieved in which:

- there is no additional pain in whatever area is symptomatic
- pain in the monitored point reduces by at least 70%.

This ease-position is then held for an appropriate length of time, which is 90 seconds, according to Jones; however, there are marked variations in the suggested length of time that tissues need to be held in the position of ease, as will become apparent in the discussions of the many variables available in positional release methodology.

In the example of the person with acute low back pain – locked in flexion – tender points will usually be located on the anterior surface of the abdomen, in the muscle structures that were shortened at the time of strain (when the patient was in flexion), and the position that removes tenderness from such a tender point will, as in previous examples, usually require flexion and possibly some fine-tuning involving rotation and/or side-bending.

4. Goodheart's approach to SCS: avoiding formulaic and prescriptive approaches

(Goodheart 1985; Walther 1988)

If there is a problem with Jones's formulaic approach, it is that, while he is frequently correct as to the position of ease recommended for particular points, he is sometimes wrong. Or, to put it differently, the mechanics of the particular strain with which the practitioner/therapist is confronted may not coincide with Jones's guidelines.

A practitioner/therapist who relies solely on Jones's 'menus' or formulae, could find difficulty in handling a situation in which use of the prescribed tender points, and accompanying prescribed direction to achieve 'ease', fails to produce the desired results. Reliance on Jones's menu of points and positions can therefore lead to the practitioner/therapist becoming dependent on them, and it is suggested that the use of palpation skills, and other variations on Jones's original observations, offers a more rounded approach to dealing with strain and pain.

Fortunately, Goodheart and others have offered less rigid frameworks within which to work using positional release mechanisms – avoiding prescriptions. Goodheart (1985) has described an almost universally applicable formula that relies more on the individual features displayed by the patient, and less on rigid formulae, as used in Jones's approach.

Goodheart suggests that a suitable tender point be sought in tissues *antagonistic* to those that are active when pain or restriction is noted. For example, if pain or restriction is reported, or is apparent, on any given movement, the *antagonist* muscles to those operating at the time that pain is noted will be those that house the tender point(s).

Thus, for example, pain (*wherever it is experienced*) that occurs when the neck is being turned to the left, will require that a tender point be located in the muscles that would turn the head to the right – and there may well be a number of such locally sensitive areas – all equally appropriate for use as monitors.

In the earlier example of a person locked in forward bending with acute pain and spasm, if the Goodheart's approach was being used, pain and restriction would be experienced as the person attempted to straighten up (i.e. moving into extension) from the position of enforced anteflexion.

The action of straightening up would almost certainly cause pain, probably in the back, however, *irrespective of where the pain is noted*, the tender point would be sought in the muscles *antagonistic to those working when pain was experienced*, i.e. it would lie in the flexor muscles – such as psoas or rectus abdominis – in this example. Once identified, it would be used as a monitor during treatment, as in all SCS protocols.

Note: It is important to emphasize that tender points that are going to be used as 'monitors' during the positioning phase of treatment are not searched for in the muscles opposite those where pain is experienced, but in the muscles antagonistic to those that are actively involved in moving the patient or body part, when pain or restriction is noted.

5.   Any painful point as a starting place for SCS

(McPartland & Zigler 1993)

All areas that palpate as painful are responding to, or are associated with, some degree of imbalance, dysfunction or reflexive activity that may well involve acute strain or chronic adaptation. However, it may not always be possible to identify the complex strain pattern that is responsible for the dysfunction.

The Jones's approach identifies the likely position of tender points relating to particular strain patterns (everted ankle, lumbar flexion strain, torticollis, etc.).

However, it makes just as much sense to consider that any painful point identified during soft-tissue evaluation, massage or palpation (including a search for trigger points) can be treated by positional release, *whether we know what strain produced it or not, and whether the problem is acute or chronic*.

Experience, and simple logic, tells us that the response to positional release of a chronically fibrosed area will be less dramatic than that from tissues that are in spasm or are hypertonic. Nevertheless, even in chronic settings, a degree of release and ease can commonly be produced, allowing for easier access to deeper fibrosis.

This approach, of being able to treat any painful tissue using positional release, is valid whether the pain is being monitored via feedback from the patient (using reducing levels of pain in the palpated point as a guide, i.e. strain/counterstrain) or whether the functional technique concept of assessing a reduction in tone in the tissues by palpation is being used.

A period of 60–90 seconds is recommended as the time for holding the position of maximum ease – although some (such as Schiowitz (1990); see discussion of FPR, above, and notes on Ortho-Bionomy, below), suggest that a very much reduced holding time may be just as efficient at times.

6.   Ortho-Bionomy

British osteopath Arthur Pauls modified Jones's SCS approach by adding facilitating forces to the ease position that was identified using a 'tender point' as a monitor during positioning. He called the method 'Ortho-Bionomy'.

The addition of crowding or distraction is similar to the approach formalized in facilitated positional release (FPR), as developed by Schiowitz – described above – where such additional forces are added to positioning into ease achieved functionally (see discussion of functional technique above).

Figure 1.3, illustrating SCS involving an anterior shoulder tender point, can be seen to involve long-axis compression of the humerus – and so can be seen to match the Ortho-Bionomy as well as the facilitated positional release (FPR) protocol.

Ortho-Bionomy is not explored further in this text, and those interested should read Pauls' 2002 book on the subject.

7.   Integrated neuromuscular inhibition technique (INIT)

INIT (Chaitow 1994) uses a 'position of ease' involving tissues housing a trigger point, as part of a sequence for its deactivation ('trigger point release') (Mense & Simons 2001).

Note: A detailed INIT protocol is given in Chapter 6, and the outline below describes the basic framework.

- The sequence commences with the identification of a tender/pain/trigger point.
- This is followed by application of ischaemic compression (this is optional and is avoided if pain is too intense or the patient too fragile or sensitive).
- Following the period of intermittent or constant pressure, a positional release of the tissues is

introduced (as in the SCS methodology described above).

- After an appropriate length of time, during which the tissues are held in 'ease', the patient is asked to introduce an isometric contraction into the affected tissues (muscle energy technique) for approximately 5 seconds.
- After the contraction, the local tissues surrounding the trigger point are stretched for up to 30 seconds.
- An isometric contraction and stretch involving the whole muscle is then performed – again for up to 30 seconds.
- Methods to facilitate activation of the antagonists to the muscles involved are then introduced.

A number of studies have validated the INIT method, for example Nagrale et al. (2010).

8. Proprioceptive taping

A quite different approach (the practical aspects of which will be outlined in Chapter 11) is 'unloading' taping; a physiotherapy variant of PRT (Fig. 1.6).

This is a method that incorporates many of the principles associated with PRT.

In recent years, for example, physiotherapists have treated specific conditions, commonly involving knee and/or shoulder dysfunction, by applying supportive

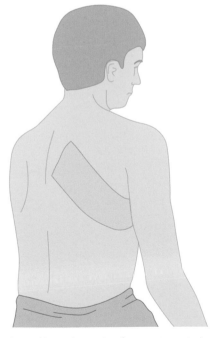

Figure 1.6 Proprioceptive taping for serratus anterior facilitation and inferior scapula angle abduction.

taping to 'unload' the affected joints (spinal unloading is also used at times). Morrissey (2000) explains:

Proprioception is a critical component of co-ordinated shoulder movement with significant deficits having been identified in pathological and fatigued shoulders (Carpenter 1998). It is an integral part of rehabilitation programs to attempt to minimize or reverse these proprioceptive deficits. Taping is a useful adjunct to a patient-specific integrated treatment approach aiming to restore full pain-free movement to the shoulder girdle. Taping is particularly useful in addressing movement faults at the scapulo-thoracic, gleno-humeral and acromio-clavicular joints. The exact mechanisms by which shoulder taping is effective is not yet clear but the suggestion is that the effects are both proprioceptive and mechanical.

It is interesting to note that some of the methods used in taping deliberately place distressed joints and tissues into ease positions for hours, or even days, with marked benefit. Additional information regarding this approach can be found in Chapter 11.

9. McKenzie's method

By careful assessment of the effects of different movements and positions, on existing pain (commonly involving extension of the spine), the McKenzie method attempts to identify those that effectively centralize pain (Fig. 1.7).

Those movements or positions that centralize peripheral or extremity symptoms are prescribed as self-treatment (McKenzie 1990). For example, in a patient with sciatica (referred symptoms in the leg coming from the spinal S1 nerve root), movements or positions are explored in the hope of finding those that 'centralize' symptoms towards the low back. Symptom centralization is seen to be a positive prognostic sign (Timm 1994).

The McKenzie concept is fully described in Chapter 10.

10. Sacro-occipital 'blocking' technique (SOT)

In 1964, DeJarnette (1967) introduced the use of pelvic wedges (padded blocks, made from foam or wood) to allow gentle repositioning of the pelvis or spine. This method is largely used in the chiropractic profession.

The reclining patient (supine or prone – decided based on establishment of 'categories' of the dysfunction being treated) is positioned and supported by blocks or wedges to allow changes to take place spontaneously and to assess changes in symptoms (Fig. 1.8).

DeJarnette is reported as saying: 'the tableboard provided the foundation for the blocks, so that when the patient

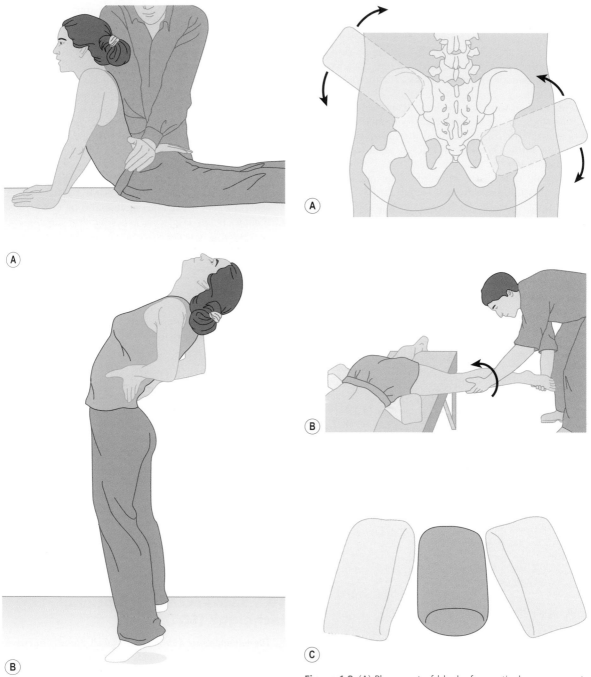

Figure 1.7 (A) McKenzie extension position with practitioner adding overpressure. (B) Patient self-application of extension.

Figure 1.8 (A) Placement of blocks for particular assessment. (B) Treatment or assessment while positionally blocked. (C) Various typically shaped solid and 'air' blocks.

breathes this energy can be transmitted to motion for correction of the subluxation dysfunction' (Heese 1991).

Cooperstein (2000) has described the use of padded wedges for what he terms 'provocation testing'. One procedure involves identifying a tender or painful monitoring point – for example in the low back, and then placing the patient on the blocks in various positions that act as fulcrums, to evaluate the influence of different force vectors, by noting changes in reported pain or tenderness.

A simpler approach has also been described by Cooperstein (2007), which he suggests is more conducive to clinical practice. Instead of evaluating reported changes in a tender or painful monitoring point, the patient is asked to decide which position is more comfortable, which is preferred to the other and when different patterns of blocking are used – diagonal or sagittal, for example. SOT methods are not described more fully in this text.

11. Balanced ligamentous tension (BLT)

Tozzi (2014) has described balanced ligamentous tension (BLT) as follows:

> BLT is a non-invasive, safe and fairly common technique in the osteopathic profession (Sleszynski and Glonek, 2005). According to BLT principles, all joints in the body are balanced ligamentous articular mechanisms that may be altered after injury, infection or mechanical stress. Therefore BLT was originally conceived as an indirect technique to address articular strains. This initially required a disengagement of tissues from their guarding position, then an exaggeration of the dysfunctional pattern into the direction of ease, up to the point when a ligamentous tensional compromise is achieved – where a tensional ligamentous balance is achieved, and a release is felt. Although specifically proposed for articular disturbances, the same principles have been applied to membranous, body fluid flow, fascial and visceral dysfunctions.

Balanced ligamentous tension is fully described in Chapter 8.

12. Visceral techniques

(see Chapter 9)

Just as in treatment of somatic dysfunction – involving joint, muscle and fascial structures – there are indirect positional release methods that are applicable to organ/visceral dysfunction. Both functional and FPR-like approaches are used, where tone and tissue tensions are evaluated or where a 'tender' area is used as a monitor.

Visceral techniques are fully described in Chapter 9.

Visceral techniques are fully described in Chapter 8, from a counterstrain perspective.

OTHER APPROACHES

There are a variety of methods involving positional release that do not quite fit into any of the categories listed above. These range from an effective rib-release technique devised by the founder of cranial osteopathy, W. G. Sutherland and described by P. E. Kimberley (1980), to various cranial techniques described by Upledger & Vredevoogd (1983) and others, as well as fascial restriction techniques described by Dickey (1989) and variations of myofascial release methodology, modified by George Goodheart (Walther 1988) and others.

Reducing the time the position of ease is held

Goodheart (Walther 1988) has suggested that it is possible to reduce the length of time during which a 'position of ease' is maintained, without losing the therapeutic benefits potentially offered by that position being maintained for 90 seconds, or more.

There are two elements to Goodheart's suggested approach:

1. When the position of ease has been located, a 'respiration assist' is added. The nature of the respiratory strategy used depends upon the location of the tender point: if it lies on the anterior surface of the body, inhalation is used, and if on the posterior aspect, exhalation is used. This phase of breathing is held for as long as is comfortable, during which time the practitioner adds the following element.
2. A stretching of the tissues being palpated (the tender point) is introduced by means of the practitioner's fingers being spread over the tissues (Fig. 1.9).

Walther explains this approach as follows:

> The patient takes a deep breath [the inhalation or exhalation phase being held, depending on anterior or posterior location of point] and holds it while the physician spreads his fingers over the previously tender point. The patient is maintained in the 'fine-tuned' position-of-ease with the practitioner's fingers spreading the point and respiration assist for 30 seconds, as opposed to 90 seconds required without the assisting factors. On completion the patient is slowly and passively returned to a neutral position.

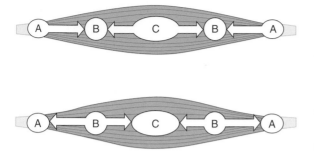

Figure 1.9 Proprioceptive manipulation of muscles. Upper: Pressure directed towards the belly of a muscle (B) from the region of the Golgi tendon organs (A) produces a toning effect, i.e. 'strengthens' it. Pressure from the spindle (C) towards the belly (B) also 'strengthens' it. Lower: Pressure directed from the belly of a muscle (B) towards the Golgi tendon organs (A) produces relaxation of the muscle. Pressure towards the muscle spindle (C) from the belly of the muscle (B) also weakens the muscle.

Is Goodheart's 'respiration assist' instruction too simplistic?

It is necessary to look a little beyond the fact that clinical experience often supports Goodheart's breathing guidelines in application of counterstrain methods, in order to gain an understanding of what might be happening physiologically.

Cummings & Howell (1990) have demonstrated the effects of respiration on myofascial tension, showing that there is a mechanical effect of respiration on resting myofascial tissue (using the elbow flexors as the tissue being evaluated). They quote the work of Kisselkova & Georgiev (1976), who reported that resting EMG activity of the biceps brachii, quadriceps femoris and gastrocnemius muscles, for example 'cycled with respiration following bicycle ergometer exercise, thus demonstrating that non-respiratory muscles receive input from the respiratory centres'.

The conclusion was that:

These studies document both a mechanically and a neurologically mediated influence on the tension produced by myofascial tissues, which gives objective verification of the clinically observed influence of respiration on the musculoskeletal system and validation of its potential role in manipulative therapy.

But what is that role?

Lewit (1999) has helped to create subdivisions in the simplistic picture of 'inhalation enhances effort' and 'exhalation enhances movement'.

Among the relationships Lewit has identified are:

- movement into flexion of the lumbar and cervical spines is assisted by exhalation, and
- movement into extension of the lumbar and cervical spine is assisted by inhalation, whereas
- movement into extension of the thoracic spine is assisted by exhalation, while
- thoracic flexion is enhanced by inhalation.

The influences of breathing on the tone of extensor and flexor muscles would therefore seem to be somewhat more complex than Goodheart's suggestions indicate, with an increase in tone being evident in the extensors of the thoracic spine during exhalation, while, at the same time, the flexors of the cervical and lumbar spine are also toned.

Similarly, inhalation increases tone in the flexors of the thoracic spine and the extensors of the cervical and lumbar regions.

Goodheart's proposed pattern of breathing during application of SCS would therefore increase tone in some of the tissues being treated, while inhibiting their antagonists.

Since the 'finger spread', which he also advocates during SCS, increases strength/tone in the tissues being treated, the use of a held breath would seem to require more discrimination than the simple injunction to hold the breath during inhalation when treating flexor muscles, and during exhalation when treating extensors.

What does the finger spread do?

SCS methods act upon the muscle spindles that lie throughout the muscle, with greatest concentration in the centre, around the belly (Gowitzke & Milner 1980).

There are many more spindles found in muscles with an active (phasic) function than are found in those with a stabilizing, postural (tonic) function.

The role of spindles (based on the complex interplay between intra- and extrafusal fibres) is as a length comparator, as well as a means for supplying the central nervous system with information as to the rate of change (Fig. 1.10). Spindles also exert an effect on the strength displayed by the muscle, a phenomenon used in applied kinesiology (AK) and which Goodheart has incorporated into his version of counterstrain methodology.

Spindle density is not uniform; for example, muscles in the cervical region contain a high density of muscle spindles, especially the deep suboccipital muscles.

Peck et al. (1984) report that:

- Rectus capitis posterior minor muscles are rich in proprioceptors, containing an average of 36 spindles/g muscle.
- Rectus capitis posterior major muscles average 30.5 spindles/g muscle.

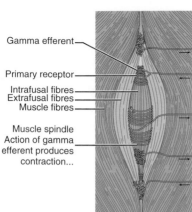

Gamma efferent

Primary receptor

Intrafusal fibres
Extrafusal fibres
Muscle fibres

Muscle spindle
Action of gamma
efferent produces
contraction...

Reporting station
Golgi tendon body...

Conveys information
to muscle...
Gamma efferent

Reporting station
Annulospiral fibres...

Reporting station
Flower spray fibres...

Conveys information
to muscle
Alpha efferent

Figure 1.10 Illustration of muscle spindles, showing Golgi tendon organs and neural pathways to and from these reporting stations.

- In contrast, the splenius capitis contains 7.6 spindles/g muscle.
- Gluteus maximus contains only 0.8 spindles/g muscle.

'Manipulating' the spindles

If the practitioner's thumbs are placed about 5 cm apart over the belly of the muscle, where spindles are most densely sited, and pressure is exerted by the thumbs pushing towards each other – parallel with the fibres of the muscle in question – a weakening effect will be noted if the muscle has been previously tested and is now tested again (Fig. 1.9).

The explanation lies in the neurology, as Walther (1988) explains:

> *The digital maneuver appears to take pressure off the intrafusal muscle fibers, causing a decrease in the afferent nerve impulse and, in turn, causing temporary [minutes at most] inhibition of the extrafusal fibers.*

This effect of 'weakening' a muscle can be reversed by means of the precisely opposite manipulation of the spindles, in which the thumbs pressing into the tissues are 'pulled' apart. This will only 'strengthen' a hypotonic or inhibited, weak muscle and will not enhance the strength of an already strong one.

The introduction of a spread of the fingers over the spindle cells, during the time when the tissues, in which the spindles lie, are being held in a position of ease, strengthens the muscle and inhibits the antagonist to that muscle; a combination of influences that it is suggested

enhances the process of balancing neuromuscular function and reducing the time required for the spindle to 're-set'.

COMMONALITIES, DIFFERENCES – AND TIMING

Many of the PRT methods have in common an objective of reduction in the tone of distressed tissues associated with the dysfunction being treated.

The means whereby this is achieved vary, some (strain/counterstrain) using reduced pain levels as a guide to the comfort/ease position, and others using variations on palpated change (functional and facilitated positional release methods).

Some methods are entirely passive (SCS, functional, FPR, SOT blocks, taping), while some are active (McKenzie methods) and a few involve a combination of active and passive activity.

Apart from the variations of application, the protocol differences between the various methods often relate to details concerning how long the ease position should be held, including guideline timings such as:

- Under 5 seconds for facilitated positional release (FPR)
- 90 seconds for strain/counterstrain and functional technique
- 3 minutes or more for treatment of neurological conditions (Weiselfish 1993)
- Up to 20 minutes with some aspects of positional release therapy (D'Ambrogio & Roth 1997)
- Hours or days in taping.

Timing in clinical settings is explored in later chapters.

In Chapter 2, an outline is offered of the ways in which dysfunction evolves as a process of (failed or failing) adaptation, and how positional release methods may offer some solutions.

THIS CHAPTER

This chapter has introduced some of the history, and concepts, of 'spontaneous release by positioning', as well as many of the different versions of PRT.

NEXT CHAPTER

An overview is provided of the ways in which local and global dysfunction emerges from a background of failed or failing adaptation – offering therapeutic opportunities for interventions that include PRT.

REFERENCES

Bowles, C., 1969. 'Dynamic neutral' – a bridge. Academy of Applied Osteopathy Yearbook, Colorado Springs, pp. 1–2.

Bowles, C., 1981. Functional technique – a modern perspective. The Journal of the American Osteopathic Association 80, 326–331.

Carpenter, J., 1998. The effects of muscle fatigue on shoulder joint position sense. The American Journal of Sports Medicine 26, 262–265.

Chaitow, L., 1994. Integrated neuromuscular inhibition technique. British Journal of Osteopathy 13, 17–20.

Cooperstein, R., 2000. Padded wedges for lumbopelvic mechanical analysis. Journal of American Chiropractic Association 37, 24–26.

Cooperstein, R., 2007. Sacro-occipital technique. In: Chaitow, L. (Ed.), Positional Release Techniques. Elsevier, Edinburgh.

Cummings, J., Howell, J., 1990. The role of respiration in the tension production of myofascial tissues. The Journal of the American Osteopathic Association 90 (9), 842.

D'Ambrogio, K., Roth, G., 1997. Positional Release Therapy. Mosby, St Louis.

Danto, J.B., 2003. Review of integrated neuromusculoskeletal release and the novel application of a segmental anterior/posterior approach in the thoracic, lumbar, and sacral regions. The Journal of the American Osteopathic Association 103, 583–596.

DeJarnette, M.B., 1967. The Philosophy, Art and Science of Sacral Occipital Technic. Self-published, Nebraska City, NE, p. 72.

Dickey, J., 1989. Postoperative osteopathic manipulative management of median sternotomy patients. The Journal of the American Osteopathic Association 89, 1309–1322.

Goodheart, G., 1985. Applied Kinesiology Workshop Procedure Manual, twenty-first ed. Privately published, Detroit.

Gowitzke, B., Milner, M., 1980. Understanding the Scientific Bases of Human Movement. Williams & Wilkins, Baltimore.

Greenman, P., 1996. Principles of Manual Medicine, second ed. Williams & Wilkins, Baltimore.

Heese, N., 1991. Major Bertrand DeJarnette: six decades of sacro occipital research, 1924–1984. Chiropractic History: The Archives and Journal of the Association for the History of Chiropractic 11, 13–15.

Hoover, H.V., 1969. Collected papers. Academy of Applied Osteopathy Year Book, Colorado Springs.

Johnstone, W.L., 1997. Functional technique. In: Ward, R. (Ed.), Foundations for Osteopathic Medicine. Williams & Wilkins, Baltimore.

Jones, L., 1981. Strain and counterstrain. Academy of Applied Osteopathy, Colorado Springs.

Jones, L.H., 1964. Spontaneous release by positioning. The DO 1, 109–116.

Kimberley, P. (Ed.), 1980. Outline of Osteopathic Manipulative Procedures. Kirksville College of Osteopathic Medicine, Kirksville.

Kisselkova, G., Georgiev, V., 1976. Effects of training on post-exercise limb muscle EMG synchronous to respiration (Jun). Journal of Applied Physiology 46 (6), 1093–1095.

Lewit, K., 1999. Manipulation in Rehabilitation of the Locomotor System. Butterworth Heinemann, London.

McKenzie, R., 1990. The Cervical and Thoracic Spine: Mechanical Diagnosis and Therapy. Spinal Publications, Waikanae, New Zealand.

McPartland, J.H., Zigler, M., 1993. Strain-Counterstrain Course Syllabus, second ed. St Lawrence Institute of Higher Learning, East Lansing.

Mense, S., Simons, D.G., 2001. Muscle Pain. Understanding Its Nature, Diagnosis, and Treatment. Lippincott Williams & Wilkins, Baltimore.

Morrissey, D., 2000. Proprioceptive shoulder taping. Journal of Bodywork and Movement Therapies 4, 189–194.

Nagrale, A.V., Glynn, P., Joshi, A., et al., 2010. Efficacy of an integrated neuromuscular inhibition technique on upper trapezius trigger points in subjects with non-specific neck pain. Journal of Manual and Manipulative Therapy 18, 37–43.

Noll, D.R., Degenhardt, B.F., Johnson, J.C., et al., 2008. Immediate effects of osteopathic manipulative treatment in elderly patients with chronic obstructive pulmonary disease. The Journal of the American Osteopathic Association 108, 251–259.

O-Yurvati, A.H., Carnes, M.S., Clearfield, M.B., et al., 2005. Hemodynamic effects of osteopathic manipulative treatment immediately after coronary artery bypass graft surgery. The Journal of the American Osteopathic Association 105, 475–481.

Pauls, A.L., 2002. The Philosophy and History of Ortho-Bionomy. ALP Publishing, Rossland, Canada.

Peck, D., Buxton, D.F., Nitz, A., 1984. Comparison of spindle concentrations in large and small muscles acting in parallel combinations. Journal of Morphology 180, 243–252.

Ramirez, M.A., Haman, J., Worth, L., 1989. Low back pain – diagnosis by six newly discovered sacral tender points and treatment with counterstrain technique. The Journal of the American Osteopathic Association 89, 905–913.

Schiowitz, S., 1990. Facilitated positional release. The Journal of the American Osteopathic Association 90, 145–156.

Schwartz, H., 1986. The use of counterstrain in an acutely ill in-hospital population. The Journal of the American Osteopathic Association 86, 433–442.

Sleszynski, S.L., Glonek, T., 2005. Outpatient osteopathic SOAP note form: preliminary results in osteopathic outcomes-based research. The Journal of the

American Osteopathic Association 105, 181–205.

Timm, K., 1994. A randomized-control study of active and passive treatments for chronic low back pain following L5 laminectomy. The Journal of Orthopaedic and Sports Physical Therapy 20, 276–286.

Tozzi, P., 2014. Balanced ligamentous tension. In: Chaitow, L. (Ed.), Fascial Dysfunction: Manual Therapy Approaches. Handspring, Edinburgh.

Upledger, J., Vredevoogd, J., 1983. Craniosacral Therapy. Eastland Press, Seattle.

Walther, D., 1988. Applied Kinesiology Synopsis. Systems DC, Pueblo, CO.

Weiselfish, S., 1993. Manual Therapy for Orthopedic and Neurologic Patients. Regional Physical Therapy, Hartford.

Wolfe, F., Smythe, H.A., Yunus, M.B., et al., 1990. The American College of Rheumatology. 1990. Criteria for the classification of fibromyalgia. Report of the Multicenter Criteria Committee. Arthritis and Rheumatism 3333, 160–172.

Wong, C.K., Abraham, T., Karimi, P., et al., 2013. Strain counterstrain technique to decrease tender point palpation pain compared to a control condition: a systematic review with meta-analysis. Journal of Bodywork and Movement Therapies 18, 165–173.

Chapter | 2 |

Somatic dysfunction and positional release

The vast majority of individuals consulting manual therapists do so because of pain and/or musculoskeletal restriction. In the absence of actual pathology a useful nonspecific term that describes the background to such pain and restriction is 'somatic dysfunction'. A major purpose of this chapter is to suggest means of improving or normalizing somatic dysfunction – with the emphasis on positional release techniques (PRT), based on published evidence.

Palpation and assessment methods that help to identify *local dysfunction* – a requirement in some forms of positional release, such as counterstrain (SCS) – are detailed later in this chapter, and elsewhere in this book.

Since problems associated with 'somatic dysfunction' are the target of therapeutic intervention, that term requires definition (Box 2.1).

FAILED OR FAILING ADAPTATION AND SOMATIC DYSFUNCTION

Somatic dysfunction almost always involves failed or failing biomechanical adaptation, possibly involving:

- Overuse, e.g. repetitive strain
- Misuse, e.g. poor posture
- Underuse and disuse, e.g. lack of exercise
- Abuse, e.g. trauma or surgery.

Ageing, inflammation, fibrosis and adhesions, as well as pathologies (e.g. arthritic changes), may all be involved in the evolution and/or maintenance of somatic dysfunctions, as may a variety of biochemical (nutritional, toxic, hormonal, etc.) and psychosocial (chronic depression, anxiety, anger, fear, etc.) factors.

Selye (1956) described both local and general adaptation models that help to inform our understanding of a common feature of all our lives. The 'non-specific response of the body to any demand placed upon it' – was summarized by Selye with the word 'stress'.

Box 2.1 **Somatic dysfunction defined (AACOM 2011)**

Somatic dysfunction involves impaired or altered function of related components of the somatic (body framework) system: skeletal, arthrodial and myofascial structures, and their related vascular, lymphatic and neural elements.

As a rule, when somatic dysfunction is discussed, it is in the absence of pathology. In other words dysfunction is not disease. Rather, it is an altered state of functionality that may result in symptoms, such as restriction, discomfort or pain – in the absence of pathological changes.

Somatic dysfunction, acute or chronic, may therefore be correctable, using manual treatment methods.

- The characteristics of *acute* somatic dysfunction may include tenderness, asymmetry of motion or relative position, reduced range of motion, tissue texture changes and possibly altered temperature (warmer than surrounding tissues if inflamed).

- The characteristics of *chronic* somatic dysfunction may include tenderness, fibrosis, paraesthesias and tissue contraction, restricted motion and possibly altered temperature (cooler than surrounding tissues if ischaemic).

The positional and motion aspects of somatic dysfunction are best described using at least one of three variables:

1. The position of a body part, as determined by palpation, in relation to adjacent defined structures … as, for example, 'the 4th lumbar vertebral segment is rotated left in relation to the 5th lumbar segment'.

2. The directions in which motion is freer … as, for example, in this same situation: 'the 4th lumbar segment demonstrates greater freedom in rotation to the left'.

3. The directions in which motion is more restricted … as, for example, in this same situation: 'the 4th lumbar segment demonstrates greater restriction in rotation to the right'.

These defining features of somatic dysfunction help to identify essential features that might need to be targeted clinically – whether by positional release or other methodologies – in order to restore greater freedom of motion and reduce pain.

- Apart from conditions where instability – excessive motion – may be a factor, most examples of somatic dysfunction – whether soft tissue or joint-related – involve partial or total restriction, a reduction of free motion (Wolf 1970).

- When a barrier exists that cannot painlessly be passed, unless that restriction is a structural obstacle, for example pathological changes in a joint, such as arthritis – it is likely that soft tissues are preventing further movement (see Fig. 1.1).

- Kappler & Jones (2003) have explained that: 'The word "barrier" may be misleading if it is interpreted as a wall or rigid obstacle to be overcome with a push. As a joint reaches a restriction barrier, restraints in the form *of tight muscles and fascia*, serve to inhibit further motion. We are pulling against restraints rather than pushing against some anatomic structure'.

- In the example of the fourth lumbar segment being rotated left in relation to L5 – it is possible that the barrier to free movement towards the right might be intra-articular – for example an actual arthritic change. It is more likely however, that soft-tissue features would be preventing free motion.

It is these restraints to free motion that require releasing, relaxing, modifying – and as the evidence makes clear (see Chapter 3) – PRT/SCS methods are efficiently designed to achieve or assist in achieving just such effects.

Palpation/assessment methods, outlined later in this chapter (see TARTT discussion) have, as one of their major targets, identification of reduced freedom of motion.

The ingredients of 'stress' may include any combination of biomechanical, biochemical and/or psychosocial features – interacting with the individual's unique inherited and acquired features – including the common compensatory pattern (Box 2.2).

Selye demonstrated that stress (anything to which the body is obliged to adapt) results in a pattern of adaptation, unique to each individual.

The results of the repeated postural and traumatic insults of a lifetime, combined with the effects of emotional and psychological distress, as well as the unique inherited and acquired biochemical status of each individual, will often present a confusing pattern of tense, contracted, bunched, fatigued and ultimately fibrous tissue.

Symptoms of restriction and/or pain, may involve features that are acute, subacute, chronic or that relate to acute aggravation of chronic changes.

Within those categories, clinical interventions are likely to require variations of direct and indirect modalities (such as positional release) as well as health education and rehabilitation. Our focus in this text is clearly on indirect options.

Box 2.2 Common compensatory patterns (Zink & Lawson 1979)

Fascial compensation is seen as a useful, beneficial and above all functional (i.e. no obvious symptoms result) response on the part of the musculoskeletal system, for example as a result of anomalies, such as a short leg or overuse.

Decompensation describes the same phenomenon where adaptive changes are seen to be dysfunctional, to produce symptoms, evidencing a failure of homeostatic mechanisms (i.e. adaptation and self-repair).

Zink & Lawson (1979) have described a model of postural patterning resulting from the progression towards fascial decompensation.

By testing the tissue 'preferences' (tight–loose) in different areas, Zink & Lawson maintain that it is possible to classify patterns in clinically useful ways:

- Ideal patterns (resulting in adaptive load being safely transferred to other regions)
- Well compensated patterns, which alternate in the direction of greater movement, from one spinal transition area to the next (e.g. atlanto-occipital–cervicothoracic–thoracolumbar–lumbosacral) – and which are commonly adaptive in nature
- Uncompensated patterns which do not alternate in the direction of greater movement, from one spinal transition area to the next, possibly as a result of trauma, congenital anomalies or failed adaptation.

Zink & Lawson described four transitional crossover sites where fascial tension patterns can most easily be assessed for rotation and side-bending preferences:

1. Occipito-atlantal (OA) – which correlates with the tentorium cerebelli.
2. Cervico-thoracic (CT) – which correlates with the thoracic outlet.
3. Thoracolumbar (TL) – which correlates with the respiratory diaphragm.
4. Lumbosacral (LS) – which correlates with the pelvic floor.

Their research showed that most people display alternating patterns of rotatory preference with about 80% of people showing a common pattern of L-R-L-R (termed the 'common compensatory pattern' or CCP) (Fig. 2.1A).

In their evaluation of over 1000 hospitalized patients Zink & Lawson observed that the 20% of people whose compensatory pattern did not alternate (Fig. 2.1B) had the worst health histories.

Treatment of either CCP, or uncompensated fascial patterns, has the objective of trying, as far as is possible, to create a symmetrical degree of rotatory motion at the key transitional crossover sites. The methods used to achieve symmetrical motion range from direct muscle energy approaches, to indirect positional release techniques.

It has been suggested that the origin of the common fascial compensatory pattern may be the result of fetal

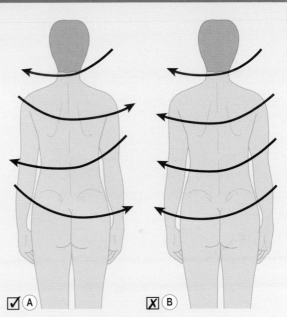

✓(A)   ✗(B)

Figure 2.1 (A,B) Common compensatory pattern (CCP).

stresses, possibly relating to the position in the womb, as well as the birthing process. Pope (2003) notes that 'it is possible to observe the similarity between the fascial bias of the fetus and the common compensatory pattern in the adult'.

Davis et al. (2007) have confirmed the clinical relevance of CCP evaluation in different juvenile populations, for example in children with cerebral palsy as well as otitis media.

Assessment of tissue preference in the Zink & Lawson sequence

Occipito-atlantal area (Fig. 2.2A)

- Patient is supine.
- Practitioner/therapist sits or stands at the head of the table.
- The head is supported at the occiput and the neck is taken into full flexion so that rotation is restricted to C1/C2 only.
- The neck is gently rotated left and right to evaluate the side to which it travels more freely.

Cervico-thoracic area (Fig. 2.2B)

- With the patient supine, the first thoracic segment is examined by the practitioner (who is seated or standing at the head of the table).

Box 2.2 **Continued**

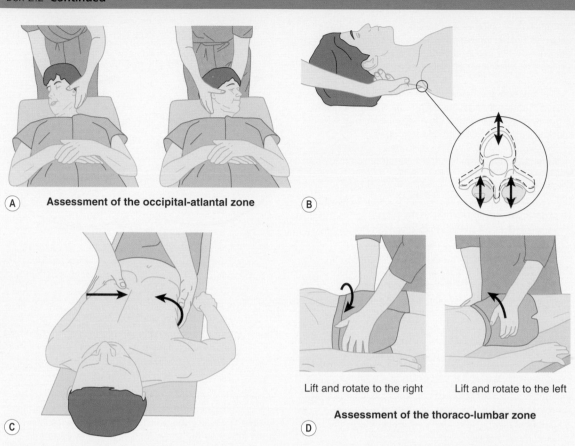

A   **Assessment of the occipital-atlantal zone**   B

C

D

Lift and rotate to the right   Lift and rotate to the left

Assessment of the thoraco-lumbar zone

Figure 2.2 (A) Assessment of the occipital-atlantal zone. (B) Upper thoracic spring test. (C) Thoracolumbar area. (D) Assessment of the lumbo-sacral zone.

- The fingers of one hand are placed so that the upper thoracic transverse processes are lying on the palmer surface of the index and middle fingers of that hand, with the other hand supporting the patient's neck.
- An anterior compressive force is applied to the left and right transverse processes individually (Fig. 2.2B) to assess their responses to the 'springing' – in order to evaluate the preference to rotate more freely to one side or the other?
- An alternative assessment for this area is demonstrated on the accompanying video.

Thoracolumbar area (Fig. 2.2C)

- Patient is supine, practitioner/therapist at waist level faces cephalad and places hands over lower thoracic structures, fingers along lower rib shafts laterally.

- Treating the structure being palpated as a cylinder, the hands test the preference this has to rotate around its central axis, one way and then the other.
- As an additional assessment, once this has been established, the preference to side-bend one way or the other is evaluated, so that combined ('stacked') positions of ease or bind, can be established.
- By holding tissues in their 'loose' or ease positions (or by holding tissues in their 'tight' or 'bind' positions – and introducing isometric contractions, or by just waiting for a release), changes can be encouraged. (See Video 1, Chapter 1: Diaphragm release, to see this assessment used therapeutically.)

Lumbosacral area (Fig. 2.2D)

- Patient is supine, practitioner/therapist stands below waist level facing cephalad and places hands on left and right ilia, using these contacts as a 'steering wheel' to evaluate tissue preference as the pelvis is

---

Box 2.2 Continued

rotated around its central axis seeking information as to its 'tightness–looseness' (see above) preferences.
- Once this has been established, the preference to side-bend one way or the other is evaluated, so that combined ('stacked') positions of ease or bind, can be established.
- By holding tissues in their 'loose' or ease positions (or by holding tissues in their 'tight' or 'bind' positions

– and introducing isometric contractions, or by just waiting for a release) changes can be encouraged.
- These general evaluation approaches, which seek evidence of compensation and of global adaptation patterns involving loose and tight tissues, offer a broad means of commencing rehabilitation, by altering structural features associated with dysfunction.

Why awareness of the patient's CCP status can be useful in considering employment of positional release methodology

As an individual's adaptation potential becomes exhausted, at some point, if stresses (adaptation demands) are constant or increasing, symptoms will emerge. Just as an elastic band will fray then snap when stretched too far.

How is the practitioner to know when an individual, or a particular region, joint or area, has reached its 'elastic' limit?

Overlying adaptation patterns, such as the CCP, together with ageing and whatever unique adaptive changes have been acquired, or are current (overuse, misuse, disuse, trauma), inevitably lead to tissue failure and symptoms – generally or locally.

The potential implication for an individual who demonstrates a decompensated pattern (see Box 2.2 for details of this, particularly Fig. 2.1B) may have direct implications relative for use of indirect – positional release – treatment choices.

Zink and Lawson's findings were partly based on the findings after evaluating the health status of well over 1000 individuals. They were able to correlate poor (i.e. non-alternating) compensation patterns with poor general health. Clinical experience suggests that these are the same individuals who are likely to be poor responders to adaptive demands resulting from manual therapies, in which changes are forcibly induced, for example when high velocity manipulation, or passive stretching methods, are employed.

On the other hand – where indirect modalities are used, as outlined in Chapter 1, Box 1.1 – in which dysfunctional tissues *are not forcibly modified, where responses are invited rather than demanded* – negative adaptive demands appear to be minimized.

Note: The clinical implications are therefore that, where a decompensated pattern exists, positional release methods should be the first choice when attempting to modify somatic dysfunction.

Conclusion and clinical implications

The more dysfunctional the individual, and the greater the adaptive burden, the more appropriate indirect, positional release methods become – since they impose the least additional adaptive demand on the system.

PRT: INVITING CHANGE RATHER THAN DEMANDING IT

It is useful to recognize that all forms of treatment, manual, chemical, psychological, etc., invite responses, some more forcibly than others.

> *In other words all treatment is a form of imposed stress.*

When an individual's self-regulating, homeostatic, functions respond to such therapeutic demands positively, the method used can be seen to have matched the adaptation potential of the individual.

When results are poor, the treatment methods used may have misjudged the degree of remaining resilience in the system – the potential for a positive response – or may simply be inappropriate to the situation.

In manual therapy, indirect positional release methods (see below for discussion of barriers), such as those described in Chapter 1, provide an *opportunity* for a beneficial response – they do not impose change, they offer it. In other words, indirect positional release methods cannot overwhelm remaining local or general adaptation reserves, since they provide an environment ('position of ease') for spontaneous changes and so avoid forcing a response.

In contrast, direct methods, such as high velocity manipulation or muscle energy techniques and passive or active stretching, impose demands – sometimes beneficially, and sometimes not.

This does not make direct methods inappropriate in all situations, however it does make indirect methods less stressful – and frequently successful – in all situations.

The acute/chronic spectrum

Therapeutic interventions need to take account of these variables, since it is obviously undesirable to apply the same manual methods that may be suitable for chronic indurated tissues, to acutely irritated ones.

- 'Acute' can be defined as recently acquired pain, and/or dysfunction, with implications of some degree of inflammation.
- 'Acute' can also relate to aggravation of pre-existing chronic dysfunction.

As will become clear in later chapters, while PRT/SCS methods are potentially clinically useful in both acute and chronic dysfunctional states, there is a great deal of evidence (see Chapter 3 in particular), suggesting that the value of PRT/SCS may be particularly valuable in acute settings.

In summary therefore, PRT variations are more likely to be of greatest clinical value in acute, painful conditions, or when treating frail, sensitive, compromised individuals, rather than in low-grade chronic situations.

Terminology

Barriers, bind, ease, tight, loose, etc.

In osteopathic positional release methodology (strain/counterstrain, functional technique, etc.) the terms 'bind' and 'ease' are often used to describe what is noted as unduly 'tight' or too 'loose' (Jones 1981).

In manual medicine generally, when joint and soft-tissue 'end-feel' is being evaluated, it is common practice to make sense of such findings by comparing sides – identifying assymetry, which is one of the main features of the spectrum of palpation/assessment findings, described below in the notes on TARTT.

The characterization of features described as having a soft or hard end-feel; or as being 'tight or loose'; or as demonstrating feelings of ease or bind, may be a deciding factor as to which therapeutic approaches are introduced, and in what sequence (Kaltenborn 1985).

These findings (tight–loose, ease–bind, etc.) have an intimate relationship with the concept of barriers, which need to be identified in preparation for direct treatment methods (i.e. where action is forcefully directed towards the restriction barrier, towards bind, tightness) or indirect techniques (where action involves movement away from barriers of restriction, towards ease, looseness and comfort in order to allow change to evolve).

Ward (1997) has noted, 'tightness suggests tethering, while looseness suggests joint and/or soft tissue laxity, with or without neural inhibition'.

It is worth re-emphasizing that the tighter side may be the more normal side, and also that clinically, it is possible that in some circumstances, restriction barriers may best be left unchallenged, in case they are offering a degree of protective benefit (see Fig. 1.1).

A therapeutic formula

When confronted with acute or chronic symptoms, emerging from a background of failed or failing adaptation, a suggested formula for management can be summarized:

- Reduce or remove adaptive demands without imposing excessive additional adaptive load.
- Enhance functionality so that adaptive demands can be better managed – possibly by encouraging a more resilient adaptation potential (see below).
- Treat symptoms, for example modify pain in situations where neither of the other options are possible.

PALPATORY LITERACY: INTRODUCING 'TARTT'

The application of positional release methodology requires a high degree of palpation skill – *palpatory literacy* – since the ability to 'read' the responses of tissues to positioning is critical, especially in application of functional methodology.

Skilful palpation allows for discrimination between the various states and stages of dysfunction, with some degree of accuracy.

When somatic dysfunction is palpated, a number of characteristic qualities are usually identifiable.

To remember these features, various acronyms have been suggested involving the first letters of keywords, such as sensitivity (or tenderness); tissue texture changes; asymmetry and range of motion – resulting variously in STAR, ARTT or TART. By adding a fifth element – temperature, we end up with our preferred acronym, TARTT:

T = tissue texture changes. The identification of tissue texture change is important in the diagnosis of somatic dysfunction. Palpable changes may be noted in superficial, intermediate and deep tissues. It is important for clinicians to be able to distinguish normal from abnormal (Fryer & Johnson 2005).

A = asymmetry. DiGiovanna (1991) links the criteria of asymmetry to a positional focus stating that the 'position of the vertebra or other bone is asymmetrical'. Greenman (1996) broadens the concept of asymmetry by including functional in addition to structural asymmetry.

R = restricted range of motion. Alteration in range of motion can apply to a single joint, several joints or a region of the musculoskeletal system. The abnormality may relate to either restriction or increased mobility, and includes assessment of *quality* of movement and 'end-feel'.

T = **tenderness to palpation pressure**. Undue tissue tenderness may be evident – such local areas of sensitivity have been termed 'hyperalgesic skin zones' (Lewit 1999). Pain provocation and reproduction of familiar symptoms are often used to localize somatic dysfunction.

T = **temperature change** (most probably warmer if acute; cooler if chronic).

Not all these features are always apparent on palpation of somatic dysfunction, however changes in tissue texture and range of motion are almost always apparent (Gibbons & Tehan 2009).

A TARTT shortcut: drag palpation

Czech physical medicine pioneer, Karel Lewit (1999), suggested that:

- A light stroking of the skin that produces a sensation of 'drag' (apparently the result of increased hydrosis), may offer pinpoint accuracy of location of local dysfunction. The degree of pressure required is minimal – skin touching skin is all that is necessary – a 'feather-light touch'. Try removing a watch or bracelet and then lightly run a finger across the skin that was under the strap, as well as over the adjacent skin. 'Drag' will be immediately apparent as a result of increased friction/resistance.
- Reflexogenic activity may be involved, indicating the possible presence of a 'hyperalgesic skin zone', potentially related to dysfunction, such as myofascial trigger points.
- Other features of hyperalgesic skin zones ('tender point areas') include local loss of skin elasticity – as well as resistance to smooth gliding of skin as it is moved on underlying tissues. These palpation methods can be used to refine identification of the location of tender points that may reflect underlying dysfunction.
- And of course they also contain the major elements of TARTT – altered texture, asymmetry, tenderness and reduced range of motion.

Note: TARTT palpation exercises can be found in Chapter 6, together with video demonstrations.

COMPARING SCS PALPATION WITH STANDARD METHODS

McPartland & Goodridge (1997) tested the value of osteopathic palpation procedures (modifying the acronym STAR or ARTT to TART) specifically to evaluate the accuracy of positional release palpation, using Jones's strain/counterstrain methodology.

This study addresses five questions:

1. What is the inter-examiner reliability of diagnostic tests used in strain/counterstrain technique?
2. How does this compare with the reliability of the traditional osteopathic examination ('TARTT' exam)?
3. How reliable are different aspects of the TARTT exam?
4. Do positive findings of Jones's points correlate with positive findings of spinal dysfunction?
5. Do osteopathic students find TARTT tests reliable when using SCS?

In this study examiners palpated for tender points which corresponded to those listed by Jones (1981) for the first three cervical segments (Fig. 2.3). (See also Figure 4.4, Chapter 4.)

These points were located by means of their anatomical position as described in Jones's original strain/counterstrain textbook, and were characterized as being areas of 'tight' nodular myofascial tissue.

The TART examination did not palpate for temperature, but comprised assessment for:

- Tender paraspinal muscles
- Asymmetry of joints
- Restriction in ROM
- Tissue texture abnormalities.

Of these, zygapophyseal joint tenderness and tissue texture changes were the most accurate.

In Jones's methodology, the location of the tender point is meant to define the *nature* of the dysfunction.

However, McPartland & Goodridge found that: *'Few Jones points correlated well with the cervical articulations that they presumably represent'*. Nevertheless, they did find that overall use of Jones's tender points (i.e. seeking soft-tissue tenderness) was a more accurate method of localizing dysfunction in symptomatic patients, than use of joint tenderness evaluation in the TARTT exam, and that *'students performed much better at SCS diagnosis than TARTT diagnosis'*.

Paulet & Fryer (2009) evaluated the reliability of palpation for tissue texture changes paraspinally in the TARTT examination, in individuals with reported tenderness, and found that agreement between therapists was 'fair'.

It is suggested that practitioners and therapists should have the opportunity to evaluate and palpate normal individuals and tissues, where pliable musculature, mobile joint structures and sound respiratory function is evident, so that when dysfunctional examples are assessed, these can be more readily identified.

Apart from standard functional examination, it is important for practitioners and therapists to acquire the abilities to assess by observation and touch, re-learning skills familiar to older generations of 'low-tech' healthcare providers.

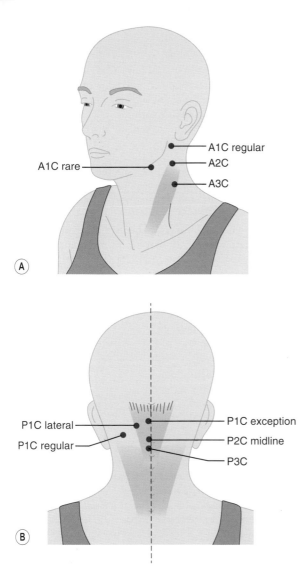

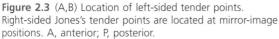

Figure 2.3 (A,B) Location of left-sided tender points. Right-sided Jones's tender points are located at mirror-image positions. A, anterior; P, posterior.

WHAT ARE THE LOCAL SIGNS AND FEATURES OF DYSFUNCTION?

Evaluation of global, whole-body patterns by observation, palpation and assessment should seek evidence of:

- What's short?
- What's tight?
- What's contracted?
- What's restricted?
- What's weak?

- What's out of balance?
- Are firing sequences abnormal?
- What has happened – overuse, misuse, trauma (abuse), disuse – to encourage or maintain dysfunction?
- What is the patient doing, or not doing, that aggravates these changes?
- What can be done to help these changes to improve or to normalize?

The question of *why* tissues become '*functionally and structurally, three-dimensionally asymmetrical*' needs some consideration, since out of the reasons for the development of somatic dysfunction emerge possible therapeutic and rehabilitation strategies.

The therapeutic objectives include the need to reduce the adaptive burden that is making demands on the structures of the body, while, at the same time, attempting to enhance functional integrity, so that the structures and tissues involved can better handle the abuses and misuses to which they are routinely subjected.

Once assessment and palpation evidence is available the application of clinical reasoning is required, based on a combination of evidence and experience, in order to determine optimal treatment approaches – in particular whether positional release methods are pertinent to the patient's needs.

Identifying general somatic dysfunction

The identification of local dysfunction – utilizing the TARTT approach – has been described because a key element of the successful use of SCS involves identification and monitoring of localized inappropriate areas of tissue tenderness – tender points.

In some cases, it may be necessary and useful to assess individual joints for their ranges of motion, and individual muscles, and groups of muscles, for flexibility, strength, stamina, shortness, etc., as well as for the presence or not of myofascial trigger points within them.

Investigation of the nature and character of general somatic dysfunction is not a feature of this book, as it is assumed that practitioners and therapists will have been trained in the skills required to identify and differentiate the multiple forms of musculoskeletal distress with which they are regularly confronted.

Observation, palpation, functional assessments and tests, as well as the use of imaging in relation to clinically relevant symptoms – provide the evidence from which to build a clinical picture.

All such assessments and evaluations are necessary in specific circumstances, however it is also useful to have – along with the Zink sequence (Box 2.2) – a number of more general screening tools which indicate current levels of functionality, and that can be repeated over time to evaluate progress, as outlined in Box 2.3.

Box 2.3 General dysfunction indicators

Three general indicators that offer rapid, clinically useful indications of function/dysfunction, are briefly outlined in this section:

- Crossed syndrome patterns – indicators of relative postural alignment (Janda 1983) together with representative functional assessments.
- Assessment of one-legged balance, eyes open and eyes closed – indicator of neurological integration between intero- and exteroceptor input, central processing efficiency and motor control (Bohannon et al. 1984).
- Evaluation of core stability – an indicator of relative efficiency of core muscles in protection of the spine (Norris 2000).

Crossed syndrome patterns

Upper crossed syndrome (Fig. 2.4)

This pattern is characterized by the following features:

- shortness and tightness of pectoralis major and minor, upper trapezius, levator scapulae, the cervical erector spinae and sub-occipital muscles, along with
- lengthening and weakening of the deep neck flexors, serratus anterior, lower and middle trapezii.

As a result, the following features develop:

1. The occiput and C1/2 become hyperextended with the head pushed forward ('chin-poke').
2. The lower cervical to fourth thoracic vertebrae becomes posturally stressed as a result.
3. The scapulae becomes rotated and abducted.
4. This alters the direction of the axis of the glenoid fossa, resulting in the humerus needing to be

stabilized by additional levator scapula and upper trapezius activity, together with additional activity from supraspinatus.

The result of these changes is greater cervical segment strain plus referred pain to the chest, shoulders and arms. Pain mimicking angina may be noted plus a decline in respiratory efficiency.

The solution, according to Janda, is to be able to identify the shortened structures and to release (stretch and relax) them, followed by re-education towards more appropriate function. Positional release alternatives are described in later chapters.

Lower crossed syndrome (Fig. 2.4)

This pattern is characterized by the following features:

- shortness and tightness of quadratus lumborum, psoas, lumbar erector spinae, hamstrings, tensor fascia lata and possibly piriformis, along with
- lengthening and weakening of the gluteal and the abdominal muscles.

The result of these changes is that the pelvis tips forward on the frontal plane, flexing the hip joints and producing lumbar lordosis and stress at L5–S1 with pain and irritation.

A further stress commonly appears in the sagittal plane leading the pelvis to be held in increased elevation, accentuated when walking, resulting in L5–S1 stress in the sagittal plane. One result of this is low back pain. The combined stresses described produce instability at the lumbodorsal junction, an unstable transition point at best.

Part of the solution for an all too common pattern such as this, is to identify the shortened structures and to

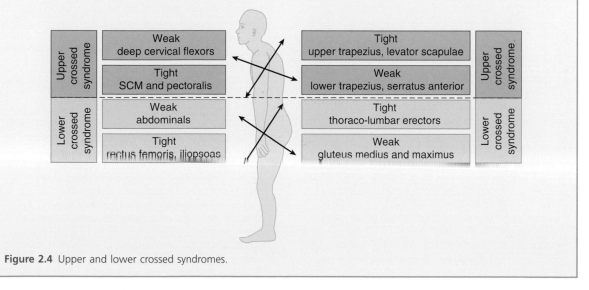

Figure 2.4 Upper and lower crossed syndromes.

Box 2.3 Continued

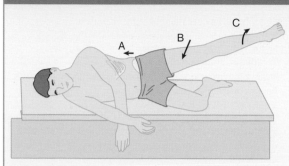

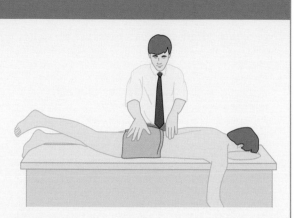

Figure 2.5 Janda's hip abduction test which, if normal, occurs without: A, 'hip hike'; B, hip flexion or C, hip external rotation.

Figure 2.6 Janda's hip extension test. The normal activation sequence is thought to be gluteus maximus, hamstrings, contralateral erector spinae, ipsilateral erector spinae (Janda 1986).

release them, followed by re-education of posture and use. Positional release approaches are described in later chapters.

Upper and lower crossed syndromes
Specific functional assessments

Hip abduction test (Janda 1983) (Fig. 2.5)

Observation assessment and/or palpation assessment may be utilized.

Observation:

- The patient lies on the side, ideally with head on a cushion, with the upper leg straight and the lower leg flexed at hip and knee, for balance.
- The practitioner, who is observing, not palpating, stands in front of the person and toward the head end of the table.

Normal is represented by pure hip abduction to 45° with 'hinging' occurring at the hip joint level.

Abnormal is represented by hinging occurring at the waist level and/or:

- hip flexion during abduction, suggesting tensor fascia lata (TFL) shortness
- the leg externally rotating during abduction, suggesting piriformis shortness
- 'hip-hiking', suggesting quadratus lumborum shortness (and gluteus medius weakness)
- posterior pelvic rotation, suggesting short antagonistic hip adductors.

Palpation:

- The practitioner stands behind the side-lying patient, with one or two finger pads of the cephalad hand on the tissues overlying quadratus lumborum (QL), approximately 2 inches (5 cm) lateral to the spinous process of L3.
- The caudad hand is placed so that the heel rests on gluteus medius and the finger pads on tensor fascia lata (TFL).

- The firing sequence of these muscles is assessed during hip abduction.
- If the QL fires first (indicated by a strong twitch or 'jump' against the palpating fingers), it is overactive and short.
- The ideal sequence is the TFL contracting first, followed by gluteus medius and finally QL (but not until about 20–25° of abduction of the leg).
- If either TFL or QL are overactive (fire out of sequence) then they will have shortened, and gluteus medius will be inhibited and weakened (Janda 1986).

Hip extension test (Fig. 2.6)

- The patient lies prone and the therapist stands to the side, at waist level, with the cephalad hand spanning the lower lumbar musculature and assessing erector spinae activity, left and right (Fig. 2.6).
- The caudal hand is placed so that its heel lies on the gluteal muscle mass, with the fingertips resting on the hamstrings on the same side.
- The person is asked to raise that leg into extension as the therapist assesses the firing sequence.
- Which muscle fires (contracts) first?
- The normal activation sequence is: (1) gluteus maximus, (2) hamstrings, followed by (3) contralateral erector spinae and then (4) ipsilateral erector spinae.
- *Note*: Not all clinicians agree that this sequence is correct; some believe the hamstrings should fire first, or that there should be a simultaneous contraction of hamstrings and gluteus maximus – but all agree that the erector spinae should not contract first.
- If the erectors on either side fire (contract) first, and take on the role of gluteus maximus as the prime movers in the task of extending the leg, they will

Box 2.3 **Continued**

become shortened and will further inhibit/weaken the gluteus maximus.

- Janda et al. (1996) observed: *'The poorest pattern occurs when the erector spinae on the ipsilateral side, or even the shoulder girdle muscles, initiate the movement and activation of gluteus maximus is weak and substantially delayed … the leg lift is achieved by pelvic forward tilt and hyperlordosis of the lumbar spine, which undoubtedly stresses this region'*.
- If on extension of the leg hinging occurs in the low back rather than at the hip, this is regarded as indicating an imbalanced response.

Assessment of balance

The extremely complex relationship between balance and the nervous system (with its interoceptive, proprioceptive and exteroceptive mechanisms) also involves a variety of somatic and visceral motor output pathways (Charney & Deutsch 1996). Maintaining body balance and equilibrium is a primary role of functionally coordinated muscles, acting in task specific patterns, and this is dependent on normal motor control (Winters & Crago 2000).

Single leg stance balance tests (Bohannon et al. 1984)

This is a reliable procedure for information regarding vulnerability and stability, as well as regarding neurological integration and efficiency (Fig. 2.7).

Method:

- The barefoot patient is instructed to raise one foot up without touching it to the support leg.
- The knee can be raised to any comfortable height.
- The patient is asked to balance for up to 30 seconds with eyes open.
- After testing standing on one leg, the other should be tested.
- When single leg standing with eyes open is successful for 30 seconds, the patient is asked to:
  - identify something on a wall opposite, and to then close the eyes while visualizing that spot
  - an attempt should be made to balance for 30 seconds.

Scoring: The time is recorded when any of the following occurs:

- The raised foot touches the ground or more than lightly touches the other leg.
- The stance foot changes (shifts) position or toes rise.
- There is hopping on the stance leg.
- The hands touch anything other than the person's own body.

By regularly (daily) practising this balance exercise, the time achieved in balance with eyes closed will increase.

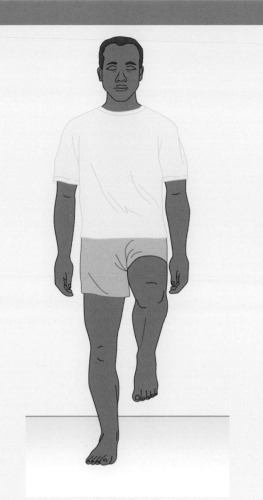

Figure 2.7 Single legged stance for balance assessment.

More challenging balance exercises can also be introduced, including use of wobble boards and balance sandals.

As relative imbalances between antagonist muscle groups are normalized ('tight–loose'), eyes closed balance as a function dependent on proprioceptive input and interpretation should improve spontaneously. Positional release methods can assist in this process.

Core stability assessment

Core stabilization assessment and exercises

Both the abdominal musculature and the trunk extensors are important in offering stability to the spine (Cholewicki & McGill 1996).

Box 2.3 **Continued**

A variety of exercises have been developed to achieve core stability involving the corset of muscles which surround, stabilize and, to an extent, move the lumbar spine, such as transversus abdominis, the abdominal oblique muscles, diaphragm, erector spinae, multifidi, etc. (Liebenson 2004).

In order to evaluate the current efficiency of stabilization the following method can be used (it can also be turned into a training exercise if core stability is deficient).

Basic 'dead-bug' exercise/test

A 'coordination' test that assists in evaluating the patient's ability to maintain the lumbar spine in a steady state during different degrees of loading has been developed by Hodges & Richardson (1999).

This 'dead-bug' exercise easily becomes a core stability exercise if repeated regularly:

- The patient adopts a supine hook-lying position (Fig. 2.8).
- One of the patient's hands can usefully be placed in the small of the back so that (s)he can be constantly aware of the pressure of the spine towards the floor – an essential aspect of the exercise.
- The patient is asked to hollow the back, bringing the umbilicus toward the spine/floor, so initiating co-contraction of transversus abdominis and multifidus, and to maintain this position as increasing degrees of load are applied by either:

  a. Gradually straightening one leg by sliding the heel along the floor. This causes the hip flexors to work eccentrically and if this overrides the stability of the pelvis it will tilt. Therefore, if a pelvic tilting/increased lumbar lordosis is observed or palpated before the leg is fully extended, this suggests *deep abdominal muscular insufficiency* involving transversus abdominis and internal obliques.

  b. Once the basic stabilization exercise of hollowing the abdomen – while maintaining pressure to the floor, is achievable without the breath being held,

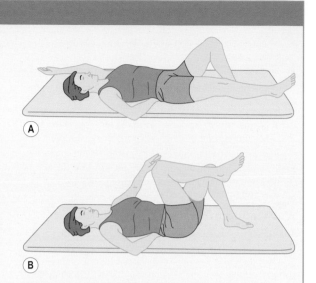

Figure 2.8 (A,B) Basic 'dead-bug' exercise to test and enhance core stability.

more advanced stabilization exercises may be introduced.

  c. These involve, in a graduated way, introducing variations on lower limb or trunk loading – for example raising one leg from the floor, then when this is easily achieved, both legs, then when this is easily achieved raising these further and 'cycling' – all the while maintaining a braced core abdominal region, with the lumbar spine pressed toward the floor (confirmed by observation) while breathing normally.

As well as abdominal tone and stability, it is necessary to encourage extensor function to be optimal and coordinated with abdominal muscle function.

All these toning and stabilizing activities are enhanced by normalizing the imbalances demonstrated in the crossed syndrome patterns (above), and positional release methodology can be a key element in those processes.

Recommended further reading:
Cook G. 2010. Movement: functional movement systems: screening, assessment, corrective strategies. Lotus Publishing, Chichester, UK.
Johnson J. 2012. Postural assessment. Human Kinetics, Champaign, IL.
Key J. 2010. Back pain – a movement problem: a clinical approach incorporating relevant research and practice. Elsevier, Edinburgh.
Myers T. 2008. Anatomy trains: myofascial meridians for manual and movement therapists, 2nd edn. Elsevier, Edinburgh.
Page P, Frank C, Lardner R. 2012. Assessment and treatment of muscle imbalance. Human Kinetics, Champaign, IL.

Myofascial trigger point assessment

In addition to these assessments, the presence of localized dysfunction, such as myofascial trigger points, within the soft tissues requires identification, for example using the TARTT approach. A question arises as to the similarities and differences between 'tender points' and 'trigger points' and this is discussed in Box 2.4.

Box 2.4 Trigger points–tender points – similarities and differences

The most basic comparison of tender and myofascial trigger points (MTP) can be:
- Trigger points are always tender.
- Tender points are not always trigger points.

In the therapeutic use of SCS, a tender point is employed as a monitor during positioning of the associated tissues – in an attempt to reduce perceived discomfort by 70% or more – in order to identify the 'position of ease'.

In that context – whether the tender point is or is not also a trigger point is irrelevant.

In the context of the treatment of myofascial pain, where MTP are thought to be major factors in pain production, the level of pain or tenderness of the point, when compressed or stretched, may be used as a means of establishing pain levels before and after treatment – whatever form that takes.

In some instances, SCS alone is used to attempt deactivation of trigger points. In Chapter 6, an integrated sequence of manual methods, including SCS, is described (INIT – integrated neuromuscular inhibition technique).

A variety of other manual – and instrument assisted – methods are also used in treatment of MTP.

Simons et al. (1999) discussed a variety of what they term *'trigger point release' procedures, ranging from direct pressure to a range of stretching possibilities, and including PRT routines (such as SCS), which they refer to as 'indirect techniques'.* They conclude that the most successful use of PRT in treating trigger points is likely to be for those points which are close to attachments, rather than the triggers found in the belly of muscles, which Simons and Travell suggest are likely to benefit from more robust treatment methods.

Positional release in general and SCS in particular, as well as further details on the trigger point phenomenon are outlined in Chapter 6.

GENERAL TREATMENT OPTIONS

PRT and a broad therapeutic approach

Ward (1997) has described methods for restoration of *'three-dimensionally patterned functional symmetry'.*

Identification of patterns of ease–bind or loose–tight, in a given body area, or the body as a whole, should emerge from sequential assessment of muscle shortness and restriction, palpation or any comprehensive evaluation of the status of the soft tissues of the body.

- Appropriate methods for release of areas identified as tight, restricted or tethered might usefully involve soft-tissue manipulation methods, such as myofascial release (MFR) – direct or indirect; muscle energy techniques (MET); neuromuscular technique (NMT); positional release technique (PRT), singly or in combination, plus other effective manual approaches.
- Identification and appropriate deactivation of myofascial trigger points contained within these soft tissue structures should be a priority (Box 2.4).
- If joints fail to respond adequately to soft-tissue mobilization, the use of articulation/mobilization or high-velocity thrust methods may be incorporated, as appropriate to the status (age, structural integrity, inflammatory status, pain levels, etc.) of the individual.
- It is suggested, however, that in sensitive or acute situations, positional release methods offer a useful first-line of treatment with little or no risk of exacerbating the condition.
- Re-education and rehabilitation (including homework) of posture, breathing and patterns of use, in order to restore functional integrity and prevent recurrence, as far as is possible.
- Exercise (homework) has to be focussed, time-efficient and within the patient's easy comprehension and capabilities, if compliance is to be achieved.

A study that illustrates the potential clinical benefit of use of positional release methods was conducted by Barnes et al. in 2013 and this is described in Box 2.5.

What we can learn from this study

The study detailed in Box 2.5 emphasizes several important points. First, that the palpation of somatic dysfunction can be accurate and relevant clinically, and that quantification of the degree of soft-tissue change may be enhanced by use of modern technology, such as – in this case – a durometer. Second, and possibly counterintuitively, one of the least invasive approaches, an indirect counterstain method, produced the most immediate changes in stiffness in dysfunctional tissues.

Box 2.5 **The Barnes study**

One way of evaluating the potential for manual treatment methods is to measure the degree of 'tissue stiffness' – before and after treatment – to evaluate change. Any change – whether an increase or a reduction in stiffness in tissues, following treatment or activity, is termed *hysteresis*. A study to measure hysteresis (fascial stiffness modification), in response to different manual methods, was undertaken by Barnes et al. (2013).

The protocol was as follows:

1. Cervical articular somatic dysfunction (SD) was identified in 240 individuals, using carefully controlled palpation assessment methods – involving the TART(T) palpation protocol – as described earlier in this chapter.

2. Once SD had been identified, and before treatment (or sham treatment) was applied, tissue stiffness was measured using an instrument designed for that purpose – a durometer.

3. Four different techniques (balanced ligamentous tension – as described in Chapter 8; muscle energy technique – which is not discussed in this book covering indirect methods; high velocity manipulation, also not discussed; and strain/counterstrain, see Chapters 3 and 4. These four methods, as well as a sham technique, were randomly applied (once) to the participants in the study, to the most severe area of identified somatic dysfunction – after which (10 minutes after treatment) the changes in tissue 'stiffness' (i.e. hysteresis) were measured, using a durometer.

4. The durometer measurement of the myofascial structures overlying each cervical segment (pre- and post-treatment) used a single consistent piezoelectric impulse. This helped to identify four different characteristics: fixation, mobility, frequency and motoricity (described as '*the overall degree of change of a segment*'), including 'resistance' and range of motion. Put simply, the measurement identified changes on mobility and stiffness.

5. When the degree of restriction/stiffness present, before and after the single use of one of the four (or sham) methods were used, the results showed that strain/counterstrain (see Chapters 3 and 4 in particular) produced the greatest changes, compared with the other methods used, or sham treatment.

The results of this study suggest that the behaviour of soft tissues associated with restricted joints (neck in this case) can be rapidly modified (becoming 'less stiff') using *any of the four methods* tested – *with the greatest effect observed following strain/counterstrain*.

Of possible interest are some of the concluding remarks of the researchers in this study:

- '*It became apparent that in many instances, treating a single identified key dysfunction sometimes modified other underlying or adjacent somatic dysfunctions*'.
- The results 'seemed to suggest that different cervical levels responded better to specific treatments'.
- '*Classification of the dysfunctions as "acute" (ostensibly containing more fluid in the tissues) or "chronic" (ostensibly stiffer tissues) might also lead to sub analysis and better interpretation of the … changes*'.

But how could such significant changes in 'stiff' tissues result from what is effectively a 'non-treatment', where tissues are simply placed into a position of reduced tension for a brief period?

A series of research studies are discussed in Box 2.6 and Chapter 3, which offer possible explanations of mechanisms involved when indirect methods, such as counterstrain, and indirect myofascial release, are used clinically.

Both of these positional release variants – and others – are described in Chapter 4.

Precautions

Positional release methods, such as SCS should be used with care in cases involving:

- Open wounds
- Recent sutures
- Healing fractures
- Haematoma
- Hypersensitivity of the skin
- Systemic localized infection

- Where soft tissue rigidity/extreme stiffness may represent protective guarding of vulnerable structures.

THIS CHAPTER

The focus of this chapter has been to offer an overview of some of the key elements that lead to somatic dysfunction, together with options for identifying the patterns that develop locally and globally.

Therapeutic options emerge from that background – with evidence that positional release methodology should be considered in a wide range of conditions and situations, in isolation or in combination with other methods, since these methods impose a minimal adaptive load on already decompensated tissues or systems.

NEXT CHAPTER

Christopher Kevin Wong offers a detailed evaluation of the research evidence that supports the use of strain/counterstrain.

Box 2.6 **Understanding the effects of SCS**

Various explanations have been suggested that may account for the clinical effects of positional release in general, and SCS in particular, for example:

- *Neurological changes* might involve muscle, fascial and joint mechanoreceptors (such as Ruffini corpuscles, Golgi tendon organs, muscle spindles) (Jones 1995) as well as pain receptors (Howell et al. 2006). Alterations in load application, for varying durations, have been shown to modify neural function (Collins 2007; Peters et al. 2013). To what degree these features are operating during application of PRT/SCS remains to be more definitively established.

- *Proprioceptive theory* is probably the most commonly discussed explanation for the efficacy of SCS. It is suggested that when a disturbed relationship exists between muscles and their antagonists, following strain, the positioning of these tissues into an unloaded, ease position, may allow spindle re-setting and partial or total resolution of inappropriate motor impairment. See Chapter 3 for further discussion of this concept (Huijing & Baar 2008; Kreulen et al. 2003).

- *Altered fibroblast responses* – Changes in the shape and architecture of cells by means of mechanotransduction (cellular responses to different degrees and forms of load) can lead to reduced inflammation. Meltzer et al. (2010) have observed that traumatized fascia disrupts the normal functions of the body, causing myofascial pain and reducing ranges of motion. They found that resulting inflammatory responses – involving fibroblast cells – can be reversed by changes in load on the tissues, delivered either by counterstrain or myofascial release, and that such changes may take as little as 60 seconds to manifest. In 2007, Standley & Meltzer observed that: 'fibroblast proliferation and expression/secretion of pro-inflammatory and anti-inflammatory interleukins may contribute to the clinical efficacy of indirect osteopathic manipulative techniques … such as SCS'. Standley & Meltzer (2008) reported that 'it is clear

that strain direction, frequency and duration, impact important fibroblast physiological functions known to mediate pain, inflammation and range of motion'.

- *Ligamentous reflexes* – Solomonow (2009) spent many years researching the functions of ligaments. He identified their sensory potential and major ligamentomuscular reflexes that have inhibitory effects on associated muscles. He states: '*If you apply only 60–90 seconds of relaxing compression on a joint … an hour plus of relaxation of muscles may result. This may come not only from ligaments, but also from capsules and tendon*' (personal communication 2009).

  - A possible clinical application of this ligamentous feature may be seen when joint crowding is induced as part of facilitated positional release and/or strain/counterstrain protocols. Such effects would be temporary (20–30 minutes) but this would be sufficient time to allow an enhanced ability to mobilize or exercise previously restricted structures.

  - Wong (2012) summarizes current thinking regarding ligamentomuscular reflexes and SCS: ligamentous strain inhibits muscle contractions that increase strain, or stimulates muscles that reduce strain, to protect the ligament (Krogsgaard et al. 2002). For instance, anterior cruciate ligament strain inhibits quadriceps and stimulates hamstring contractions to reduce anterior tibial distraction (Dyhre-Poulsen & Krogsgaard 2000). Ligamentous reflex activation also elicits regional muscle responses that indirectly influence joints (Solomonow & Lewis 2002). Research is needed to explore whether SCS may alter the protective ligamentomuscular reflex and thus reduce dysfunction by shortening joint ligaments or synergistic muscles (Chaitow 2009).

- *Water and SCS* – Coincidentally, crowding (compression) of soft tissues would have an effect on the water content of fascia, leading to temporary (also 20–30 minutes) of reduced stiffness of fascial structures – with similar enhanced mobility during that period (Klingler & Schleip 2004).

REFERENCES

AACOM, 2011. Glossary of Osteopathic Terminology. American Association of Colleges of Osteopathic Medicine, Chevy Chase, MD. Online. Available: <http://www.aacom.org>.

Barnes, P., Laboy, F., Noto-Bell, L., et al., 2013. A comparative study of cervical hysteresis characteristics after various

osteopathic manipulative treatment (OMT) modalities. Journal of Bodywork and Movement Therapies 17, 89–94.

Bohannon, R., Larkin, P., Cook, A., et al., 1984. Decrease in timed balance test scores with aging. Physical Therapy 64, 1067–1070.

Chaitow, L., 2009. Editorial. Journal of Bodywork and Movement Therapies 13, 115–116.

Charney, D., Deutsch, A., 1996. A functional neuroanatomy of anxiety and fear: implications for the pathophysiology and treatment of anxiety disorders.

Critical Reviews in Neurobiology 10, 419–446.

Cholewicki, J., McGill, S., 1996. Mechanical stability of the in vivo lumbar spine: implications for injury and chronic low back pain. Clinical Biomechanics 11, 1–15.

Collins, C.K., 2007. Physical therapy management of complex regional pain syndrome I in a 14-year-old patient using strain counterstrain: a case report. Journal of Manual and Manipulative Therapy 15, 25–41.

Davis, M.F., Worden, K., Clawson, D., et al., 2007. Confirmatory factor analysis in osteopathic medicine: fascial and spinal motion restrictions as correlates of muscle spasticity in children with cerebral palsy. Journal of the American Osteopathic Association 107, 226–232.

DiGiovanna, E., 1991. Somatic dysfunction. In: DiGiovanna, E., Schiowitz, S. (Eds.), An Osteopathic Approach to Diagnosis and Treatment. Lippincott, Philadelphia, pp. 6–12.

Dyhre-Poulsen, P., Krogsgaard, M.R., 2000. Muscular reflexes elicited by electrical stimulation of the anterior cruciate ligament in humans. Journal of Applied Physiology 89, 2191–2195.

Fryer, G., Johnson, J., 2005. Dissection of thoracic paraspinal region – implications for osteopathic palpatory diagnosis. International Journal of Osteopathic Medicine 8, 69–74.

Gibbons, P., Tehan, P., 2009. Manipulation of the Spine, Thorax and Pelvis, with DVD: An Osteopathic Perspective, third ed. Churchill Livingstone, Oxford.

Greenman, P., 1996. Principles of Manual Medicine, second ed. Williams & Wilkins, Baltimore.

Hodges, P., Richardson, C., 1999. Altered trunk muscle recruitment in people with LBP with upper limb movement at different speeds. Archives of Physical Medicine Rehabilitation 80, 1005–1012.

Howell, J.N., Cabell, K.S., Chila, A.G., et al., 2006. Stretch reflex and Hoffmann reflex responses to osteopathic manipulative treatment in subjects with Achilles tendinitis. Journal of the American Osteopathic Association 106, 537–545.

Huijing, P.A., Baar, G., 2008. Myofascial force transmission via extramuscular pathways occurs between antagonistic muscles. Cells, Tissues, Organs 188, 400–414.

Janda, V., 1983. Muscle Function Testing. Butterworth, London.

Janda, V., 1986. Muscle weakness and inhibition in back pain syndromes. In: Grieve, G. (Ed.), Modern Manual Therapy of the Vertebral Column. Churchill Livingstone, Edinburgh.

Janda, V., Frank, C., Liebenson, C., 1996. Evaluation of muscular imbalance. In: Liebenson, C. (Ed.), Rehabilitation of the Spine: A Practitioner's Manual. Williams & Wilkins, Baltimore.

Jones, L., 1981. Strain and Counterstrain. Academy of Applied Osteopathy, Colorado Springs.

Jones, L.H., 1995. Strain-Counterstrain. Jones Strain-Counterstrain Inc., Indianapolis, IN.

Kaltenborn, F., 1985. Mobilization of the Extremity Joints. Olaf Norlis Bokhandel, Oslo, Norway.

Kappler, R.E., Jones, J.M., 2003. Thrust (high-velocity/low-amplitude) techniques. In: Ward, R.C. (Ed.), Foundations for Osteopathic Medicine, second ed. Lippincott, Williams & Wilkins, Philadelphia, pp. 852–880.

Klingler W, Schleip R. 2004. European Fascia Research Project report 2005. Paper presented at the 5th World Congress on Low Back and Pelvic Pain, Melbourne Australia, 10–16 November.

Kreulen, M., Smeulders, M., Hage, J., et al., 2003. Biomechanical effects of dissecting flexor carpi ulnaris. Journal of Bone and Joint Surgery 85, 856–859.

Krogsgaard, M.R., Dyhre-Poulsen, P., Fischer-Rasmussen, T., 2002. Cruciate ligament reflexes. Journal of Electromyography and Kinesiology 12, 177–182.

Lewit, K., 1999. Manipulative Therapy in Rehabilitation of the Locomotor System, third ed. Butterworths, London.

Liebenson, C., 2004. Spinal stabilization – an update. Part 2 – Functional assessment. Journal of Bodywork and Movement Therapies 8, 199–210.

McPartland, J., Goodridge, J., 1997. Counterstrain and traditional osteopathic examination of the cervical spine compared. Journal of Bodywork and Movement Therapies 1, 173–178.

Meltzer, K.R., Cao, T.V., Schad, J.F., et al., 2010. In vitro modeling of repetitive motion injury and myofascial release. Journal of Bodywork and Movement Therapies 14, 162–171.

Norris, C., 2000. Back Stability. Human Kinetics, Champaign, IL.

Paulet, T., Fryer, G., 2009. Inter-examiner reliability of palpation for tissue texture abnormality in the thoracic paraspinal region. International Journal of Osteopathic Medicine 12, 92–96.

Peters, T., MacDonald, R., Leach, C., 2013. Counterstrain manipulation in the treatment of restless legs syndrome: a pilot single-blind randomized controlled trial; the CARL Trial. International Musculoskeletal Medicine 34, 136–140.

Pope, R.E., 2003. The common compensatory pattern: its origin and relationship to the postural model. American Academy of Osteopathy Journal 14, 19–40.

Selye, H., 1956. The Stress of Life. McGraw Hill, New York.

Simons, D., Travell, J., Simons, L., 1999. Myofascial Pain and Dysfunction: The Trigger Point Manual, second ed. Williams & Wilkins, Baltimore.

Solomonow, M., 2009. Ligaments: a source of musculoskeletal disorders. Journal of Bodywork and Movement Therapies 13, 136–154.

Solomonow, M., Lewis, J., 2002. Reflex from the ankle ligaments of the feline. Journal of Electromyography and Kinesiology 12, 193–198.

Standley, P., Meltzer, K., 2007. Modeled repetitive motion strain and indirect osteopathic manipulative techniques in regulation of human fibroblast proliferation and interleukin secretion. Journal of the American Osteopathic Association 107, 527–536.

Standley, P., Meltzer, K., 2008. In vitro modeling of repetitive motion strain and manual medicine treatments: potential roles for pro- and anti-inflammatory cytokines. Journal of

Bodywork and Movement Therapies 12, 201–203.

Ward, R., 1997. Foundations for Osteopathic Medicine. Williams & Wilkins, Baltimore.

Winters, J., Crago, P. (Eds.), 2000. Biomechanics and Neural Control of Posture and Movement. Springer, New York.

Wolf, A.H., 1970. Osteopathic manipulative procedure in disorders of the eye. In: American Academy of Osteopathy Year Book. Colorado Springs, CO, pp. 71–75.

Wong, C.K., 2012. Strain counterstrain: current concepts and clinical evidence. Manual Therapy 17, 2–8.

Zink, G., Lawson, W., 1979. Osteopathic structural examination and functional interpretation of the soma. Osteopathic Annals 7, 433–440.

Chapter | 3 |

Strain/counterstrain research

Christopher Kevin Wong

INTRODUCTION

Strain/counterstrain has been emerging as an evidence-based osteopathic manipulative therapy since the first effects were described based on the clinical experience of Lawrence Jones, over 60 years ago (Jones 1964). The development of strain/counterstrain has been strongly influenced by the empirical clinical observations of Dr Jones (Jones 1995).

Individual treatment successes with patients have led thoughtful clinicians to develop plausible theories to explain their observed clinical phenomenon. While some may accept clinical theories at face value, inquiring clinician–scientists pose and test hypotheses to confirm or deny foundational theories.

Clinical researchers seeking to determine the physiological effects of strain/counterstrain have used a variety of research methods to increase understanding of multiple aspects of strain/counterstrain. Ultimately, more research into the effects of strain/counterstrain on symptomatic patients measuring functional ability and participation restriction outcomes – as defined by the International Classification of Functioning, Disability and Health (WHO 2001) – must be conducted to provide sound rationales for its use in health care (Fig. 3.1).

The path of discovery from inception to evidence-based clinical practice for strain/counterstrain is the same as for any medical innovation. This chapter defines evidence-based practice, describes the different levels of evidence available and reviews the available scientific literature that inform clinical decision-making related to strain/counterstrain in the context of the individual patient.

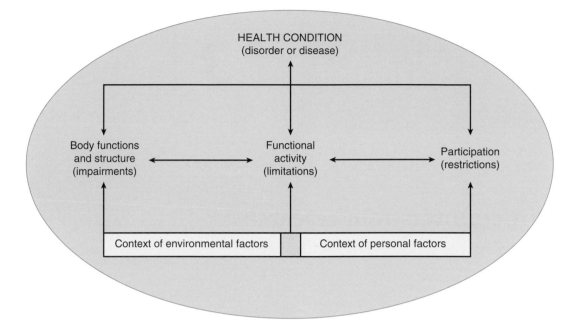

Figure 3.1 International Classification of Functioning, Disability and Health. *(Adapted from the World Health Organization.)*

EVIDENCE-BASED PRACTICE

Evidence-based medicine has been described as the 'conscientious, explicit, and judicious use of the current best evidence in making decisions about the care of individual patients' (Sackett et al. 1996). Evidence-based medicine requires the integration of each practitioner's clinical expertise with the best available research evidence in the context of the individual patient's needs and preferences. Inherent is the need for the practitioner to make a professional analysis of the facts related to each case in making judgements as to the best clinical decisions for each individual patient (Fig. 3.2).

The clinical interaction

Each clinical interaction begins with the individual patient seeking care. Their visit is typically prompted by a health problem. However, each health problem is often not as simple as the identified pathological entity. Major medical problems can lead to other system involvement beyond the primary diagnosis that becomes apparent once the medical crisis is averted. For instance:

- Myocardial infarct may lead to inactivity that affects the pulmonary and digestive system.
- Pathology of various body systems can lead to residual musculoskeletal system dysfunctions.
  - Open-heart surgery for a coronary artery bypass graft may later affect shoulder function.

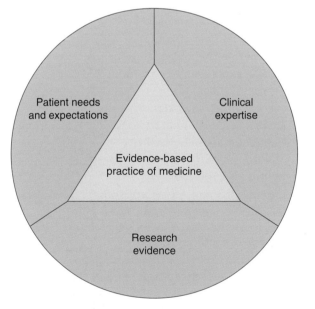

Figure 3.2 Model of evidence-based practice. *(Adapted from the Oxford Centre of Evidence-Based Medicine.)*

- A stroke can lead to joint contractures that persist even after neurological function returns.
- Autoimmune disorders can lead to delayed connective tissue and joint healing.

- Similarly, musculoskeletal problems can impact the function of other physiological systems.
  - For instance, the common problem of chronic nonspecific low back pain can lead to decreased activity, poor cardiac health and depression (Waddell 1998).

Patient needs and expectations

Beyond the precipitating health problem, the patient brings their own health and healthcare expectations related to their individual and cultural characteristics to every healthcare interaction. Patients may respond to treatment differently depending on their backgrounds, preferences and the settings in which they receive care. Pain tolerance, personal preference and individual participation goals may influence the type of care received.

Clinical expertise

Each clinical practitioner brings different levels of knowledgeable expertise, skill sets and empathy for the patient's unique sociocultural background. The practitioner's academic background, clinical practice and life experience shape their professional ability. How each practitioner uses these assets to make a clinical decision varies.

Clinical decision-making

During teaching rounds, clinical decisions may be arrived at through a hypothetical deductive process that involves the collection of clinical data to analyse that can prove or disprove clinical hypotheses and ultimately results in logical clinical decisions (Rothstein 2003). In the busy treatment room, clinical decisions may be made in a less circumspect manner based on recognition of a familiar clinical pattern (Croskerry 2009), what a practitioner has seen done before by more experienced clinicians (Tichelaar 2010), heuristic trial and error problem-solving (Hicks & Kluemper 2011) or other intuitive processes.

Sometimes left unexplored are the many subtle biases that can affect our decision-making process. Clinician personality (Dunphy 2009), individual preferences and skills (Hicks & Kluemper 2011) and social biases (Greenberger et al. 2012; Poon & Tarrant 2009; Steed 2010) may all influence our clinical decisions without conscious consideration.

These biases may especially affect care when external professional input or collaboration is absent, as unexamined experiences can reinforce the existing viewpoints. As a result, making clinical decisions based solely on one's clinical expertise is inherently tainted by bias. Although individually we can all recount clinical successes, it is impossible to separate those successes from our biases and uncontrolled variables, such as the natural healing process, over time.

Even when a treatment was successful, do we truly know why it was successful? And from a larger perspective, even when one practitioner has success using a treatment, should the treatment be taught if it cannot be shown as effective for other practitioners?

Research evidence

While not specific to any case and separate from clinical experience, evidence derived from research provides a critical element to the clinical decision-making of expert practitioners (Tichelaar 2010). The best available research evidence can be considered a source of external professional input.

Research provides additional insight regarding many elements that go into clinical decision-making for different patient scenarios. Research findings on strain/counterstrain address issues from the theoretical assumptions underlying clinical judgements, the reliability and validity of clinical examinations and the effectiveness of a treatment for a given condition considered across subjects, settings and practitioners.

The use of research evidence in clinical decision-making may ameliorate some natural biases in the patient–clinician interaction, although research findings do not prescribe a course of action for any individual patient. Integrating each individual patient's needs and preferences with a thoughtful and experienced analysis of the clinical presentation and consideration of the available research evidence to determine the best possible clinical decisions is the basis of evidence-based medicine.

LEVELS OF RESEARCH EVIDENCE

The level of research evidence in Table 3.1 depicts different levels of evidence derived from different research study designs and denotes the type of conclusions that can be drawn from the evidence. Each level of evidence has value, particularly for a relatively new treatment method such as strain/counterstrain.

- **Laboratory research** testing physiological responses provides the rationale for the development of the fundamental theories upon which strain/counterstrain has been based.
- **Methodological studies** provide insight into the validity and reliability of the methods used to assess the outcomes.
- **Case studies and expert opinions**, with or without case examples, describe a range of possible applications for a treatment and the theories upon which it is based. Included in this level are incidental findings extrapolated from other study designs.

Table 3.1 Levels of research evidence

Level of evidence	Syntheses	Single studies	Non-studies	Recommendation grades	Possible conclusions
I	SRs and meta-analyses of RCTs	RCTs	–	A	It is shown that …
II	SRs of cohort studies	Cohort studies, low quality RCTs	–	B	It is likely that …
III	SRs of case–control studies	Case–control studies	–	B	It is possible that …
IV	Case series, small or low quality cohorts	Single cases	Extrapolated findings of Level II–II evidence	C	There are signs that …
V	Clinical practice guidelines	Methodological and laboratory research	Expert opinions	D	Experts think that …

SR, systematic reviews; RCT, randomized control trials.

- **Quasi-experimental designs** such as case–control and cohort studies are preliminary tests of the theories applied to groups of subjects. While quasi-experimental studies lack the controls required to draw firm conclusions regarding cause and effect, such studies show potential effects that can generate or refine theory and application for further study (Portney & Watkins 2009).
- **Experimental studies** shed light on the cause and effect of treatments through more stringent bias control – primarily randomization, comparison groups and blinding.
- **Systematic reviews** of multiple studies, particularly when outcomes are combined and analysed through meta-analysis, demonstrate the strength of compiled evidence for the cause and effect of treatments from multiple trials in various settings conducted with different subject populations by different researchers.

While not extensive, the available evidence for strain/counterstrain represents all levels of evidence.

Quality research methodology

Beyond the study design, other basic tenets of good research apply to strain/counterstrain research. Studies should specifically define the purpose and hypotheses to be tested. Incidental findings extrapolated from the primary study are not as credible, since the study was intended and designed for another purpose and factors potentially affecting the incidental findings may not have been controlled for. Study methods should be clearly described to allow duplication of the research, including the experimental treatment, outcome assessment and data analysis. The research method should isolate the experimental treatment to avoid confounding of the results by co-interventions.

In order to provide the strongest evidence for a causal relationship between a treatment and the observed effect, the effect of the isolated treatment should be compared with a comparison treatment, involving subject groups similar in composition (Portney & Watkins 2009).

While research into some treatments can be effectively compared with placebo treatment, such as detuned ultrasound, the most stringent studies of manual therapy techniques, including strain/counterstrain, use a sham manual treatment. Sham manual treatment accounts for the potential positive effect of simple human touch on the measured outcomes. To be most clinically applicable, subjects should have characteristics and symptomatic conditions analogous to patients seen commonly by clinical practitioners.

Well-designed and thoroughly reported research can promote greater understanding of the theoretical foundations and clinical effects of strain/counterstrain. Knowledge of the quality and key findings of the available evidence, when combined with the practitioner's clinical experience and understanding of the patient's needs, contributes to sound clinical judgements.

The rest of this chapter summarizes the available strain/counterstrain research starting with the foundational level and continuing through clinical research to the top level of evidence, noting relevant research design and methods, with potential connections drawn to clinical application of strain/counterstrain techniques.

STRAIN/COUNTERSTRAIN RESEARCH

Theoretical foundations

Much of the theoretical foundation for strain/counterstrain was based on the work of Korr (1975) who described a potential mechanism of action to explain the effects of strain/counterstrain and other manual therapies. His analysis and explanation of the neurophysiological research led to the proposed theoretical link between the proprioceptors, particularly the muscle spindle and musculoskeletal dysfunction (Korr 1975).

Korr's foundational work formed the basis of the proprioceptive and nociceptive theories of strain/counterstrain (D'Ambrogio & Roth 1997). More recent research has attempted to test the theoretical underpinnings of strain/counterstrain by measuring physiological responses in laboratory research.

Neurophysiological reflexes

Research using human physiological testing has explored the effect of strain/counterstrain on neurophysiological reflexes. To explore the role of the muscle spindle and the hypothesis that sensitivity of the deep tendon monosynaptic stretch reflex contributes to range-of-motion restrictions, Howell et al. (2006) measured stretch and H-reflex latency and amplitude before and after strain/counterstrain treatment (Box 3.1).

1. Achilles tendonitis

Standardized treatment was directed specifically to the Achilles musculotendinous complex in people with Achilles tendonitis, and compared with a sham strain/counterstrain treatment of asymptomatic control subjects, using a case–control design study.

The control group experienced no changes. In the treatment group there was an 18–26% reduction in gastrocnemius and soleus stretch reflex amplitudes. This occurred without any apparent change to the H-reflex. The H-reflex is stimulated directly in the popliteal fossa, and measured

at the Achilles tendon, bypassing stretch stimulation of the muscle spindle. The results suggest that strain/counterstrain treatment affected the sensitivity of the muscle spindle, thought to be heightened by the existence of tendonitis (Howell et al. 2006).

Questions about the role of the H-reflex in the stretch reflex loop, and comparison between non-equivalent groups in this case–control study precluded a firm conclusion. Asymptomatic control subjects may have had normal reflex amplitudes at the outset, which would make treatment effects unlikely.

2. Plantar fasciitis

A similar study from the same laboratory sought to confirm the finding that strain/counterstrain decreased stretch reflex amplitude. Subjects with plantar fasciitis received strain/counterstrain to the foot, ankle and lower leg but did not experience the same reflex effects on the Achilles tendon (Wynn et al. 2006).

While the results of these two studies appear to conflict, the study by Wynn et al. (2006) did not standardize or describe the specific treatment, and the Achilles musculotendinous unit may not have been consistently targeted by the strain/counterstrain treatment.

Without a standardized strain/counterstrain treatment, specifically directed to the tissue in question, a neurophysiological reflex effect of the target tissue – in this case the Achilles tendon – would be unlikely.

The findings by Howell et al. (2006) are the strongest evidence to date for a strain/counterstrain effect on the stretch reflex but require confirmation through additional well-controlled research.

Muscle excitability and stretch reflex

Other laboratory research exploring the possibility that strain/counterstrain can affect stretch reflex amplitude, as a measure of muscle excitability, has demonstrated that a combination of non-thrust manual therapies, including strain/counterstrain, can reduce the amplitude and reduce side-to-side asymmetries (Goss et al. 2012).

The existence of co-interventions makes it impossible to draw conclusions from this research. Potential alteration of neuromuscular reflex activity or muscular excitability after strain/counterstrain, supports the notion that reducing spasm could interrupt the pain–spasm cycle. Evidence to support the notion of a circular pain–spasm cycle, however, is lacking, and the theory has been recently questioned. Laboratory research to stimulate noxious stimuli to muscle and subcutaneous tissues of conscious humans, generally decreased muscle spindle activity and did not increase muscle activity consistent with spasm (Birznieks et al. 2008). Pain is a complex entity influenced by more than local stimuli and this study did not examine whether pain, related to preexisting spasm, could be reduced by decreased muscle excitability.

> **Box 3.1 Stretch and H-reflex stimulation for measurement**
>
> Stretch reflex:
> - Elicited by rapid movement into 5 degrees of ankle dorsiflexion.
>
> H-reflex:
> - Elicited by tibial nerve stimulation in the popliteal fossa.

Circulatory effects theory of strain/counterstrain

Another line of inquiry has explored the theoretical under-pinning of the circulatory theory of strain/counterstrain (D'Ambrogio & Roth 1997).

The most often cited study observed that in a cadaveric shoulder, dye injected into the vasculature of the rotator cuff of the shoulder remained static when the shoulder was positioned in neutral, but circulated freely when posi-tioned in flexion–abduction–external rotation – the posi-tion for strain/counterstrain release of the rotator cuff (Rathbun & Macnab 1970).

This finding, however, was an incidental finding, as the study was not intended to test the circulatory theory of strain/counterstrain but rather to explore the circulation of the rotator cuff and its potential impact on healing and injury.

A different study, potentially related to circulatory effects, found that temperature measured with thermo-graphy decreased at tender points after a mixed interven-tion of three osteopathic techniques, including strain/counterstrain (Walko & Janouschek 1994). This finding also cannot be attributed to strain/counterstrain due to the existence of co-interventions, and the impact of decreased tissue temperature on healing remains unclear.

Cellular inflammation and healing

A study related to the cellular effects of injury and healing was performed on fibroblasts in tissues that had been exposed to strain, compared with control tissue (Dodd et al. 2006). Strain conditions of >10% increased inter-leukin (IL6) concentrations and cell proliferation, indicat-ing cell healing in response to injury, over the non-strain control condition. Once strain conditions increased by 30%, cell viability and metabolic response decreased pre-cipitously (Dodd et al. 2006). Whether strain/counterstrain may provide benefit to tissues through a circulatory effect has been examined at the cellular level. Meltzer & Standley (2007) sought to assess the potential effect of strain/counterstrain on inflammatory interleukins that could influence tissue healing. This laboratory study attempted to mimic a condition of chronic repetitive strain in tissue samples and to explore the effect of tissue shortening, similar to a strain/counterstrain treatment, applied to that tissue.

Cells exposed to repetitive strain demonstrated an inflammatory response measured by increased secretion of pro-inflammatory interleukins and decreased cell prolif-eration. When the strained cells were then treated with tissue shortening designed to approximate the clinical effect of strain/counterstrain, the cells secreted less pro-inflammatory interleukins including IL6 and had increased cell proliferation compared with the conditions that had

only repetitive strain and recovery conditions (Meltzer & Standley 2007).

The findings suggest that tissue shortening, characteris-tic of strain/counterstrain treatment, can reduce some inflammatory mediators when inflammation is excessive and reverse the decreased cell proliferation that occurs after repetitive strain. While the results support the hypoth-esis that strain/counterstrain can promote a healing environment for strained tissues, confirmation through additional research is needed. This kind of laboratory research is critical to test and potentially confirm the theo-retical underpinnings of strain/counterstrain and provide insight into the biophysiological processes that result.

The tender point phenomenon

The treatment of strain/counterstrain depends heavily on the local identification and assessment of the palpa-tion tenderness of defined tender points. An underlying assumption is that the tender points are quantifiably dif-ferent from other tissues. If such tender points exist, treat-ment of them is also based on the assumption that tender points can be validly and reliably assessed.

The uniqueness of tender points compared with healthy tissue has been explored. Lewis et al. (2010b) examined electrical, temperature and vibratory detection thresholds, as well as electrical, temperature and pressure pain thresh-olds. A single examiner assessed a preselected set of tender points in the lumbo-pelvic region of 15 subjects with low back pain and 15 asymptomatic controls.

Significantly lower electrical detection and pain thresh-olds were found for the symptomatic tender points of subjects with low back pain compared with corresponding asymptomatic contralateral tender points. Significantly lower tender point thermal pain thresholds were found for subjects with low back pain compared with asymptomatic control subjects and asymptomatic contralateral tender points, although not consistently at all tender points (Lewis et al. 2010b). Based on the results of this single study, tender points appear different from surrounding tissues, corresponding points on asymptomatic subjects or non-tender contralateral points.

Methodological research

Assuming that tender points exist as identifiable entities, the reliability and validity of tender point palpation must also be established. Methodological studies play an impor-tant role because valid and reliable measurement methods are necessary to test the theories upon which strain/counterstrain has been based. Perhaps the most central assumption is the validity of the palpation method gener-ally used in strain/counterstrain treatment. Most SCS prac-titioners and texts (D'Ambrogio & Roth 1997; Jones 1995) describe a tender point palpation pain assessment derived from Travell's work with trigger points in which the tenderness of the point is assessed based on the response of the patient.

A 'jump sign' or withdrawal reaction denotes significant tenderness (Simons et al. 1999). Patient response, however, can vary with individual characteristics and culture (Green 2006). When manual tender point palpation tenderness commonly identified by strain/counterstrain practitioners was compared with a subject-reported visual analogue scale of pain, the commonly used tender point palpation technique was not as reliable as the visual analogue scale for determining tender point palpation tenderness (Wong & Schauer 2004).

It was noted, however, that in clinical practice, a visual analogue scale, which would have to be repeated for each tender point treated, may be too unwieldy to be practical.

Testing tender point identification

The ability to reliably identify tender points has been tested in a study of experienced clinicians examining both symptomatic and asymptomatic subjects (McPartland & Goodridge 1997). The two testers showed moderate agreement with a Cohen's kappa value κ = 0.45 for symptomatic subjects. Agreement was low for asymptomatic subjects κ = 0.19.

While the percentage agreements for asymptomatic and symptomatic subjects were 59% and 73%, respectively, adjusting for chance agreements using the kappa statistic makes the kappa value a more realistic picture of the reliability of the tender point palpation. Substantial agreement would be indicated by kappa values >0.6 and excellent agreement indicated by values >0.8 (Portney & Watkins 2009).

While agreement was only moderate, identification of strain/counterstrain tender points was more reliable than identification of somatic dysfunction using the traditional osteopathic TART examination system (Tissue texture, Asymmetry, joint Restriction and Tenderness, see Chapter 2), which demonstrated only fair agreement (McPartland & Goodridge 1997).

Tender points in osteopathic education

The teaching of practitioners to identify different tender points should also be established. A recent multi-institutional study of five osteopathic schools identified strain/counterstrain points that were tender, a majority of the time, among osteopathic medicine students. These high yield strain/counterstrain points, as well as others deemed clinically useful, based on expert opinion, were compiled in a recommendation of strain/counterstrain points to teach in Doctor of Osteopathy schools (Snider et al. 2013).

An interesting finding of the study was the number of tender points found to be positive in the sample of asymptomatic students. A total of 40 of the 78 tender point groups studied had at least one positive tender point in over 50% of the students. The effectiveness of strain/counterstrain teaching has not been studied.

Case reports and expert opinions

Published case reports and expert opinions and recommendations provide examples of potential applications for strain/counterstrain. In a sense, reading expert opinions and case reports is like sharing the experiences of other clinicians in a larger forum.

Clinical experiences have great face validity, as they are real life experiences and capture the complexities of clinical practice in a way that a randomized control study cannot. The outcomes are individual and not average group outcomes, as reported in single or multiple group studies. Case studies, however, carry implicit bias. Authors tend to only report successful outcomes, and journals tend not to publish reports of unsuccessful cases. In addition, the conduct of most cases would not be stringently controlled.

Regardless of the outcome, without controlled comparison among multiple subjects of the isolated use of strain/counterstrain, no conclusion can be drawn with respect to cause and effect. In this regard, studies that use strain/counterstrain as one undifferentiated aspect of an experimental osteopathic manipulative treatment (OMT) provide the same information as case studies (Box 3.2).

This section summarizes the available published peer-reviewed case reports, thus eschewing editorials and clinical recommendations, texts, continuing education manuals and other non-peer-reviewed work. Selected studies, in which strain/counterstrain was applied as one aspect of a more OMT, have also been included. The combined reports provide insight into the potential applications of strain/counterstrain in various healthcare settings, for different diagnoses and presentation severities, involving multiple body segments and using a range of durations and frequencies.

Acutely ill, hospitalized patients

While most strain/counterstrain treatment is applied in outpatient settings, use of strain/counterstrain has been reported in studies with mixed interventions. Strain/counterstrain has been used in combination with other treatments in cases of visceral problems, such as pancreatitis (Radjieski et al. 1998).

In total, 15 patients with pancreatitis were randomly assigned to receive standard medical care or standard care and daily OMT including strain/counterstrain. The attending physician was blinded to group allocation. The strain/

Box 3.2 **Osteopathic manipulative treatment**

Osteopathic manipulative treatment (OMT) typically refers to the many manual techniques performed by osteopathic physicians to alleviate dysfunction within the body's structural framework, including skeletal, arthrodial, myofascial and associated vascular, lymphatic and neural structures. The most common techniques included in OMT are soft tissue, high-velocity low-amplitude thrust, muscle energy, counterstrain, myofascial release; but the range of techniques also include cranial sacral (Johnson & Kurtz 2003).

Clinicians in other professions including physical therapists and chiropractors use similar techniques. Varying nomenclature and intended effects among the professions can make comparisons between disciplines or systematic syntheses of study findings difficult (Licciardone et al. 2005).

Regardless of the profession, combining multiple techniques in a single treatment causes confounding among the co-interventions and precludes conclusions regarding the effect of any specific technique. Similarly, varying the technique or combination of techniques from subject to subject causes confounding among the subjects. Although understandable in a clinical setting to address each person's individual characteristics, varying treatment among research subjects confounds the results and prevents confirmation of the findings through independent reproduction of the study methods.

Osteopaths diagnose the specific function based on the four TART criteria: tissue texture abnormality, asymmetry, restriction of motion or tenderness (Licciardone & Kearns 2012) – as described in Chapter 2.

counterstrain group was discharged in 3.5 fewer days on average than the control group (Radjieski et al. 1998). The suggestion that strain/counterstrain can be utilized with acutely ill patients was described earlier in an opinion by Schwartz (1986) and has been explored clinically by other strain/counterstrain practitioners.

With comparatively few cases of in-patient hospital-based care reported, strain/counterstrain appears most often utilized in the outpatient setting. Patient cases with musculoskeletal diagnoses of various severities affecting both lower and upper quarters have been reported.

Complex regional pain syndrome of the foot and ankle

Strain/counterstrain has been applied in an outpatient setting to an adolescent in a case of complex regional pain syndrome of the foot and ankle (Collins 2007). Complex regional pain syndrome presents musculoskeletal deficits but has neurologic origins. In this case, the subject was

treated once or twice per week over 6 months with benefits observed in pain, range of motion, balance and gait functions. Descriptions of the foot and ankle techniques used in Collins (2007) were first published by Jones (1973).

Iliotibial band friction syndrome

Pedowitz (2005) described a case of an athletic man with lateral knee pain attributed to iliotibial band friction syndrome treated with strain/counterstrain within a comprehensive treatment plan that also included modalities, exercise, orthotics and medication, five times over a 2-week period with success.

Low back pain

Lewis & Flynn (2001) reported four cases seen in an outpatient rehabilitation department that received strain/counterstrain three times over 1 week to treat low back pain with success. While no other treatment occurred during the strain/counterstrain treatment period, total care also included joint manipulation and soft tissue mobilization, exercise and ergonomic training. The sacral points treated were the topic of earlier expert opinion by (Cislo et al. 1991) in collaboration with (Ramirez et al. 1989).

Neck and jaw pain

In the upper quarter, strain/counterstrain to the cervical region has been used for three sessions for four cases of musculoskeletal torticollis in which pain was decreased, ROM and function increased after strain/counterstrain (Baker 2013). Strain/counterstrain has also been combined with massage to the neck and upper anterior chest to reduce jaw pain and increase jaw opening (Eisensmith 2007).

Tension-type headache

Another single case report of an individual with tension-type headaches also derived benefit from passive positioning treatment similar to strain/counterstrain applied over three sessions to address common neck trigger points: upper trapezius, spinalis, SCM and suboccipital muscles (Mohamadi et al. 2012). The emphasis in this study on the use of passive positioning to treat trigger points, which reside primarily in muscle tissue, may not capture the scope of strain/counterstrain tender points that are often located on osteopathic structures but still provides examples of strain/counterstrain application.

Fibromyalgia

Management of more generalized pain was addressed in a case of myofascial pain syndrome that progressed to fibromyalgia severe enough to include an earlier hospitalization (Dardzinski et al. 2000).

In another study of people with fibromyalgia seen weekly over 23 weeks, four randomly assigned groups including mixed OMT, OMT and teaching, moist heat placebo or current medication only. The OMT treatment consisted of counterstrain and any combination of soft tissue mobilization, myofascial release, cranial-sacral therapy or muscle energy techniques. Pain and daily function outcomes favoured the strain/counterstrain groups (Gamber et al. 2002). Though the individual hands-on attention provided to the two strain/counterstrain groups are likely to have a strong biasing effect on the results, this study shows that patients with widespread musculoskeletal pain can be treated with strain/counterstrain.

Balance impairment

Beyond musculoskeletal dysfunctions, strain/counterstrain has been used for neurological dysfunction in an outpatient setting. Balance impairment in 40 elderly community dwellers with vestibular dysfunction was treated with a combination of osteopathic treatments in a non-random control trial. After four half-hour treatments including myofascial release, counterstrain and cranial-sacral techniques for subjects in the experimental group, a significant reduction in AP sway was observed (Lopez et al. 2011).

Overall, strain/counterstrain has been applied in cases of acutely ill individuals in hospital settings as well as those less medically vulnerable in outpatient settings. Patient presentation ranged from a youth to older adults with pain of likely orthopaedic origin to complex cases with possible neurological involvement, and localized to wide spread musculoskeletal complaints. And treatment in these successful cases has ranged from as little as one session to multiple over a 6-month period.

Quasi-experimental designs: case–control or cohort studies

The process of clinical research into new treatment approaches often starts with successful cases in the clinical practice of individual practitioners shared through published case reports. While theoretical principles for strain/counterstrain were presented first in this chapter, research into the foundational theories has often been spurred by such clinical observations from case reports. After a successful case report has been documented, the next step is to determine whether the observation was unique or can be repeated.

The repeatability of the findings is important to establish because the results of a case report could be unique to the individual patient, practitioner or clinical scenario. Results may be exceptional or the analysis biased.

Quasi-experimental designs, such as cohort studies can preliminarily test the theory and strengthen the findings of a single case through the reporting of repeated cases. A cohort study can provide findings for multiple cases treated in the same manner. Cohort studies can be retrospective observations or prospective measures of a cohort of subjects.

A common form is a single group assessed before and after treatment, a simple pre-treatment and post-treatment design. Some cohort studies will report multiple measures from before and/or after treatment, such as follow-up measures. Other than the foundational research into Achilles tendon reflex changes (Howell et al. 2006), the case–control design, which uses a non-randomized non-equivalent comparison group compared with the experimental cohort, has been unusual in strain/counterstrain research.

Myofascial pain and fibromyalgia

In a retrospective cohort of people with myofascial pain syndrome, including 14 of 20 that had fibromyalgia, three sessions of strain/counterstrain were effective in improving symptoms by at least 50% in 19 of the 20 subjects and 15 of the 20 after 6 months at follow-up (Dardzinski et al. 2000).

Epicondylalgia

A prospective cohort of 10 people with lateral epicondylalgia, using strain/counterstrain in a comprehensive physical therapy plan of care was also found to be effective in significantly reducing pain and increasing wrist range of motion and strength (Benjamin et al. 1999).

While providing stronger evidence than single case studies, since the number of subjects is large enough to run statistics and generate mean results, neither of these studies yield strong causative information about the effect of strain/counterstrain. This is due to the mixed subject group in the first study, the lack of control applied to the treatment in the latter study, and the lack of comparison group in both studies.

In summary, these studies highlight possible outcome effects to measure in future studies, such as pain, range of motion, strength and function.

Experimental designs: control trials

Elements of experimental design research

Control trials provide a controlled environment that allows cause and effect of strain/counterstrain to be interpreted with more confidence.

One primary element of a control trial is the use of a control group to compare with the experimental group that receives the treatment of interest. Another primary element is the random assignment of a homogenous set of subjects to the control and experimental groups.

Comparisons among the randomly assigned experimental and control groups – the classic randomized control trial – allow the effects of the different conditions to be compared with confidence and thus causation to be determined. Multiple elements of study design affect the strength of any eventual findings derived from a randomized control trial. The treatment provided to the comparison group is a critical element.

- **No-treatment** control conditions are common and demonstrates the difference between no treatment and the experimental treatment. Receiving no treatment, however, can bias subject experience positively towards the experimental treatment because the control subjects may easily perceive that they received no treatment.
- **Placebo treatment** can be used to ameliorate this effect. An inert pill, a detuned ultrasound head, or an educational video are all examples of placebo treatments designed to suggest to the subject that a treatment has been received. Placebo treatments, however, are vulnerable to bias when the experimental treatment is a hands-on manual therapy treatment, such as strain/counterstrain. The simple human act of touching may confer warmth, caring or other beneficial effects regardless of specific treatment effect.
- **Sham treatment** can be used to address this source of bias in manual therapy studies by including human touch instead or in addition to a control or placebo condition. In this way, the effect of the manual therapy treatment can be differentiated from the effect of simple human touch.

Strain/counterstrain as a sham treatment comparison

Regardless of the comparison condition, determining whether the group allocations remained blind throughout the trial by surveying the subjects, for instance, is a very stringent methodology that helps validate the study findings. Blinded sham comparison treatments are research design elements to attend to when reviewing randomized control trials.

One study specifically examined whether a simulated strain/counterstrain treatment including palpation, positioning and a 90-second holding time could be used as a sham without the subject or assessor detecting the group allocation (Brose et al. 2013). This randomized control trial stratified subjects by pain level and randomly assigned them to sham or strain/counterstrain treatment groups. The 26 subjects were not able to detect which group they had been assigned to even though pain reduction was associated with receiving real strain/counterstrain treatment. In addition, the blinded assessor was not able to detect the group allocation based on interactions with the subjects (Brose et al. 2013). These results suggest that strain/counterstrain can be effectively simulated and used as a sham treatment in manual therapy research.

Table 3.2 Methodological study quality tool	
Methodological study criteria	**Yes–Unclear–No**
Groups were randomly assigned	
Treatment group allocation was concealed	
Subject was blinded to treatment allocation	
Care provider was blinded to treatment allocation	
Outcome assessor blinded to treatment allocation	
The recruitment and drop-out rates were reported	
Data from all subjects that began the study were analysed	
Groups were similar at baseline	
Treatments clearly described avoiding co-interventions/ confounders	
Compliance with the treatment conditions acceptable in all groups	
The outcome assessment timing similar in all groups	
All planned outcomes were reported	
Number of criteria met (yes)	

Methodological study quality criteria

Other aspects of research design weigh heavily on the quality of the study design and the eventual interpretation of the results as well. Study methodological quality can be assessed in a critical appraisal of the research using standard criteria (Table 3.2) often addressed in the publication process of many journals. Related to random group assignment is whether allocation to the experimental or control group remains concealed to the subjects and assessors. While possible in a study using placebo pills, it seems impossible to keep the care provider blinded from a manual therapy treatment study.

1. Complete subject data

Completeness of the data is also important in not biasing study findings: keeping track of the recruitment rate for subjects to enter a study and the number of subjects that do not complete the study is important. Subjects may not complete a study when they perceive little improvement, thus analysis without this group that was intended to receive treatment may bias the results. The subjects that are recruited to the different groups should be similar in characteristics in order to be compared.

2. Complete description of independent treatments

All treatment conditions whether sham or strain/counterstrain must be reported with enough specificity to be reproduced. To understand clearly what the effect of one treatment was, the study treatment should be independent from other co-interventions. This separation of one treatment from another is not common in clinical practice and occurs in the research treatment protocols within the literature as well. However, any finding that results from such a mixed intervention cannot be applied to any specific treatment. The treatment protocol should be consistently adhered to and the outcome consistently assessed.

3. Complete description of all outcomes

Missed treatment sessions, lack of information about home exercise adherence and variability of the follow-up time, are all research design elements that can bedevil the clinical researcher because subject behaviour falls outside the control of the researcher. Reporting all planned outcomes, however, is the researcher's responsibility and the selective reporting of some results while not reporting others denies the consumer of research full understanding of the findings.

A summary of methodological study criteria can be documented with various standardized rating tools like that used by the Cochrane Back Review Group (Furlan et al. 2009) to consistently record important elements of research methods (Table 3.2).

Overall, randomized control trials test specific hypotheses related to the effect of an experimental treatment on defined measureable subject outcomes, while controlling as many other aspects as possible. The controlled study environment allows conclusions to be drawn about the causative factors leading to the measured effects.

Because average outcomes for homogenous subject groups are typically reported for randomized control trial designs, however, the findings may not apply to an individual clinical case with unique characteristics. Outcomes resulting from experimental studies investigating strain/counterstrain include pain, tissue texture, range of motion, strength and function measures.

Pain

Musculoskeletal pain is one of the most frequent complaints of patients seeking care by their physicians (Jordan et al. 2010). The effect of strain/counterstrain on painful musculoskeletal conditions has been relatively rarely reported.

1. Neck pain and upper trapezius trigger points

One example is a randomized control trial of people with nonspecific neck pain and upper trapezius trigger points with blinded assessors (Nagrale et al. 2010). Subjects were randomly assigned to a control group that received a muscle energy technique described as contract–relax stretching or integrated neuromuscular inhibition technique treatment. The integrated neuromuscular inhibition technique included the same muscle energy technique applied after strain/counterstrain was applied for 20–30 seconds with three to five repetitions to reduce the discomfort resulting from ischaemic compression. The 60 subjects received 12 treatments over 4 weeks. Pain and neck disability index scores were all significantly improved with large effect sizes compared with the muscle energy technique treatment alone (Nagrale et al. 2010).

2. Upper trapezius pain and spasm

The finding of reduced neck pain after integrated neuromuscular inhibition technique stands in contrast to the findings of another randomized control trial. Perreault et al. (2009) studied 20 subjects with self-reported upper trapezius pain and spasm that were allocated to receive a single strain/counterstrain or sham touch treatment.

The subjects receiving strain/counterstrain had significant reduction in resting pain with large effect size immediately post-treatment. However, this change was not different from the sham procedure, which also had a large effect size pain reduction 24 hours after treatment (Perreault et al. 2009). Although the sham procedure was certainly different from the strain/counterstrain position for the upper trapezius, positioning the neck in slight rotation could affect other cervical tender points that can affect pain in the neck region.

Both studies included people with neck pain, but inclusion standards for the Nagrale et al. study (2010) were more stringent. Baseline pain in the Nagrale et al. study (2010) was rated on a visual analogue scale of more than 8 out of 10, while the baseline pain in Perreault et al. (2009) was 1 out of 10. The low pain rating on the visual analogue scale suggests that an essentially asymptomatic population may have little room for improvement (Perreault et al. 2009).

3. Neck pain

In extrapolated findings from a pilot randomized control trial study with 26 subjects investigating the feasibility of simulated strain/counterstrain position as a sham for use in future research, cervical pain was reduced after strain/counterstrain treatment compared with the sham condition. The incidental nature of the findings and the incomplete description of the numeric pain rating assessment used made firm conclusion impossible in this study (Brose et al. 2013).

Low back pain

One other study included people with low back pain rated from between 3 and 4 out of 10 on a visual analogue scale for both experimental and control groups. Treatment four times over 2 weeks was provided with the control group performing exercise that included abdominal bracing, knee to chest and trunk roll stretching, and the experimental group receiving strain/counterstrain combined with the exercises. Strain/counterstrain did not have a significant impact on pain level compared with exercise alone at four time points from 0 to 28 weeks (Lewis et al. 2010a).

Overall, there is limited evidence documenting reduction in general or regional pain for subjects with painful conditions after isolated strain/counterstrain treatment. The improvement in global rating of change reported by Collins (2014) in a randomized control trial of people with chronic ankle instability could be construed as a reduction in pain but was not defined as such. Reduction in tender point palpation pain has been reported more frequently and will be discussed in the systematic review section, as there were sufficient studies to perform a meta-analysis (Wong et al. 2014).

Tissue texture

Tender points in strain/counterstrain treatment are identified by palpation with the recognition that the tender point has a different tissue texture than surrounding tissue. Tissue texture can be quantified with a durometer that can measure the hysteresis, which takes into account the force applied, the responding tissue resistance and the tissue response time.

A randomized control trial with blinded subjects and assessor, by Baker et al. (2013), compared the effects of a sham and four osteopathic manipulative therapies. Strain/counterstrain appeared to significantly increase hysteresis, more than other treatments, based on a comparison of median values. Unclear recruitment inclusion criteria, inconsistent randomization methods, unspecified conditions for each treatment group and incomplete statistical analyses weaken the results of this study (Baker et al. 2013).

Range of motion

Range of motion has been less frequently measured as an outcome of strain/counterstrain than pain and tenderness.

1. Hamstring flexibility

The first study to examine the effect of strain/counterstrain on range of motion was a randomized control trial using a crossover design to study the effect on hamstring muscle flexibility measured in active knee extension from the supine 90-degree hip position. No significant difference was found between the experimental group and the control group, which received a sham manual positioning treatment (Birmingham et al. 2004).

While the result of this study was that strain/counterstrain had no effect on hamstring flexibility, this study of 33 asymptomatic individuals had research design flaws that could have affected the outcome.

- First, the asymptomatic individuals were included if they lacked at least 10 degrees of motion; a small limitation that may not have provided the potential for larger improvements in individuals who present with musculoskeletal dysfunction.
- Second, the crossover design, used by some researchers to increase the analysed sample size, exposes subjects of both groups to the same treatments. When study treatments can be reasonably expected to produce a lasting change, the results of crossover study designs can be confounded by co-intervention of the other treatment conditions. Even though this study employed a week long wash-out period between the two treatments, evidence from case reports and cohorts discussed previously suggest that beneficial effects of strain/counterstrain could last for 6 months (Dardzinski et al. 2000).
- Third, the strain/counterstrain treatment selected addressed only the lateral hamstring muscles, thus subjects with impaired motion related to the untreated medial hamstrings could be less affected.

2. Hip flexor flexibility

The effect of strain/counterstrain on lower extremity muscle flexibility was also examined in an unpublished dissertation that used a randomized control trial design with symptomatic individuals with low back pain and/or lower extremity dysfunction. The control group in this study received a manual hip flexor muscle stretch, while the experimental group received strain/counterstrain.

The strain/counterstrain group gained significantly more hip flexor flexibility than the control group, with an average difference >10 degrees (Dempsey 2001). The use of subjects with heterogeneous presentations combined with the fact that this research was never published, relegates the findings to the level of expert opinion, despite the more stringent research design.

3. Neck mobility in non-neurological neck pain

Klein et al. (2013) reported the results of a study of 61 subjects with non-neurological neck pain and a cervical joint block restricting normal joint movement of at least one cervical level. Subjects were randomly assigned to a single individual strain/counterstrain treatment, that was not described, or sham treatment before other osteopathic treatment was performed.

Cervical range of motion measured with a cervical rotation goniometer found the strain/counterstrain group increased rotation range of motion by 2%, while the manual sham group increased by an insignificant 0.6%. After the individualized osteopathic treatment, both groups had gained around 5% range of motion and there was no significant difference for the experimental group (Klein et al. 2013).

In this study, subjects were included when identified as having reduced cervical range of motion due to joint restriction. Without clear description of the treatment in Klein et al. (2013), it remains unknown whether the strain/counterstrain treatment was directed towards a joint restriction or muscle tightness. The study described earlier in the Pain section by Nagrale et al. (2010) directed treatment to muscle and produced a large effect size increase in upper trapezius flexibility assessed with lateral cervical flexion range of motion.

Because strain/counterstrain treatment can be theoretically directed to muscle, such as the upper trapezius or joint restrictions at specific cervical levels using posterior cervical release positions, without clear description of the treatment used in Klein et al. (2013) it is difficult to analyse the meaning of the results and impossible to independently reproduce the treatment or study methods.

4. Masseter trigger points and active mouth opening

Two strain/counterstrain studies produced by research collaborations with multiple shared authors have investigated range of motion changes, as measured by active mouth opening in people with masseter muscle trigger points.

The first of these studies used 90 subjects randomly divided into three treatment groups that received strain/counterstrain, repeated contract–relax masseter muscle stretching or no treatment (Blanco et al. 2006). No significant effect of strain/counterstrain on active mouth opening was found compared with no treatment. Repeated contract–relax stretching produced a significant and large effect size change in mouth opening compared with the other groups when measured immediately after the single treatment (Blanco et al. 2006).

The second study used 71 subjects using a soft-tissue mobilization technique consisting of masseter muscle longitudinal stroking instead of the contract–relax stretching. The results showed strain/counterstrain and the stroking soft-tissue mobilization technique both produced significant and large effect size changes in active mouth opening compared with control (Ibáñez-García et al. 2009).

The second study utilized three sessions scheduled once per week with outcome assessed 1 week after the last session. The repeated strain/counterstrain treatments in

this second study produced a 4 mm increase in active mouth opening range of motion, which when compared to the single session result of the first study (2 mm), may be considered more effective. This observation extrapolated from the findings of two studies is not a direct comparison. No experimental research into strain/counterstrain treatment dosing has been reported.

Differentiation of joint and muscle mobility effects in strain/counterstrain research

Range of motion outcome measures do not typically differentiate between joint mobility and muscle flexibility, although these are not identical entities. The Birmingham et al. (2004) study did ascertain that full knee joint extension was available before assessing hamstring flexibility with knee extension from a hip position of flexion. The two-joint hamstring muscle was clearly accommodated for and separate from hip joint range of motion.

Ascertaining the available joint motion in the absence of muscle tightness was not possible in the studies of active jaw opening. Although Blanco et al. (2006) and Ibáñez-García et al. (2009) directed treatment to muscle tissue, as specified by the inclusion criteria of masseter muscle trigger point, the strain/counterstrain positioning for the masseter involves lateral glide of the mandible at the temporomandibular joint.

It is possible that strain/counterstrain in this instance may have produced increased range of motion through joint alignment and mobility, since joint mobilization with lateral glides has also been reported to increase range of motion (Mulligan 2010).

Strength

As has range of motion, strength has been infrequently reported as an outcome measure after strain/counterstrain treatment.

1. Hip strength

The first study employing an experimental design with strain/counterstrain to measure strength effects – assessed as the maximal voluntary isometric contraction generated against a handheld dynamometer – included 49 subjects randomly assigned to an exercise-only control group, a strain/counterstrain group and a strain/counterstrain plus exercise group.

Subjects received strain/counterstrain for painful hip adductor and abductor tender points with all subject outcomes measured 2–4 weeks after treatment (Wong & Schauer-Alvarez 2004).

While the exercise-only group gained strength by the second session, the groups receiving strain/counterstrain with or without exercise had significant within group strength increases after the first session. The strength increases in the strain/counterstrain groups were significantly greater than the exercise group throughout the study. Total strength gains at follow-up ranged from 22% to 40% for the exercise group and 50 to 73% in the groups receiving strain/counterstrain (Wong & Schauer-Alvarez 2004).

Lack of a sham manual treatment and imprecisely standardized muscle testing and lack of assessor blinding limited the strength of the findings.

2. Arm muscle strength

A smaller study of 12 people with forearms that were tender to palpation at the supinator and pronator points, had more modest findings. This randomized control trial by the same author compared strain/counterstrain with a sham manual treatment condition in a subject and assessor blinded environment with a standard strength testing protocol that had been shown to be both reliable and valid in previous work (Wong & Moskowitz 2010).

After three sessions of strain/counterstrain for the pronator and supinator muscles over 3 weeks, increased within-group strength was apparent with significant between group pronator strength increase after strain/counterstrain (Wong et al. 2011).

Inconsistent results for supinator muscle strength, allocation of individual forearms to different groups, and analysis with one-tailed *t*-tests weakened the results of this study. Furthermore, neither of these studies examined the effects of strain/counterstrain on symptomatic individuals who may respond differently than those with symptomatic conditions.

3. Ankle strength

Another study to assess strength after strain/counterstrain treatment was a randomized control trial of a strain/counterstrain approach to treatment for people with chronic ankle instability and a history of ankle sprain (Collins 2014). The 27 study subjects were randomly assigned to strain/counterstrain or sham treatment groups for four treatment sessions over 4 weeks. Specific strain/counterstrain treatments were not detailed.

No significant strength gains were noted, despite significant improvement on functional balance testing (Collins 2014). Because treatment varied depending on individual presentation, it is unknown whether specific strain/counterstrain treatment was consistently directed to the ankle invertor and evertor muscles that were strength tested.

4. Wrist strength

A study that applied strain/counterstrain to the forearm wrist muscles found wrist extension strength increased significantly by 40% in patients with epicondylalgia (Benjamin et al. 1999). The effects of strain/counterstrain in this study, however, were confounded by other treatments including modalities, exercise and massage. Thus, strain/counterstrain may well have an effect on strength when treatment is directed specifically to the muscle to be assessed but independent confirmation with carefully designed studies is lacking.

Assessing strength effects in strain/counterstrain research

The conclusion as to whether strain/counterstrain could affect inversion and eversion muscle function after the generalized strain/counterstrain treatment reported by Collins (2014) was not possible because treatment may not have been directed to the particular muscles tested.

This was also the case in Wynn et al. (2006), which noted no change in Achilles tendon reflex amplitude after general and undefined strain/counterstrain treatment around the foot and ankle.

Specific effects on muscle contractions due to strain/counterstrain would appear to require isolated treatment directed to specific muscles. In research, the treatment and assessment of the treated muscles must be described in sufficient detail to be reproduced in order to draw conclusions about the observed effect.

Functional outcomes

If pain is the most frequent patient complaint, functional outcomes have the greatest impact on functional disability and participation limitations (WHO 2001).

1. Balance and ankle instability

Collins (2014) revealed an increase in functional balance performance in subjects with ankle instability after strain/counterstrain, although improvement in physical performance ability was not matched by subjective ability level measured by the self-reported Foot Ankle Ability Measure.

Functional balance performance was measured with the Star Excursion Balance Test, which involves balance on the affected leg, while reaching the other foot as far as possible in eight directions around a circle. Significant gains were made in seven of eight directions after strain/counterstrain compared with the sham treatment. Although subjects judged their global rate of change to be greater after strain/counterstrain, no change was noted in either the Activity of Daily Living or Sport subsections of the Foot Ankle Ability Measure (Collins 2014).

2. Global ratings

A similar result was found in a randomized control trial of 89 people with low back pain. Subjects received exercise alone or strain/counterstrain plus exercise. A significant difference in the global rating of change – patient-rated judgements about the overall improvement or worsening of their condition – favoured the strain/counterstrain group. However, no functional benefit was reported on the Oswestry Disability Index (Lewis et al. 2010a).

The apparent conflict between global ratings of change and self-reports of functional limitations or abilities may be explained by potential subject bias. Since neither study (Collins 2014; Lewis et al. 2010a) reported subject or assessor blinding, the possibility exists that subjects were biased in favour of the strain/counterstrain treatment on the global ratings of change. Global ratings of change have been shown to inadequately correlate with measures of functional change (Schmitt & Abbott 2015).

3. Neck disability scores

One study of patients with nonspecific neck pain and upper trapezius trigger points responding to integrated neuromuscular inhibition technique, demonstrated significantly improved neck disability index scores indicating less discomfort in daily activities commonly associated with neck pain (Nagrale et al. 2010).

In summary, investigations assessing functional activity and participation restriction outcomes (WHO 2001) of symptomatic patients have been infrequently reported. Treatment primarily using strain/counterstrain has more often been found to improve specific impairments in the available research.

Controlled studies investigating specific strain/counterstrain treatments for conceptually related impairment level outcomes are still needed to gain greater understanding of how strain/counterstrain affects body structures and functions. Clinical improvements in general functioning and participation gains for patients may require a more comprehensive approach than isolated strain/counterstrain treatment.

Systematic reviews and meta-analyses

Systematic reviews are a compilation of studies. Analysing studies together reduces the effect of the unique or exceptional finding of a single study by combining the results of multiple studies, not unlike collecting data from a subject cohort instead of a single case. When multiple study results present similar data with sufficient detail, the findings can be compiled and data aggregated in a meta-analysis.

The quality of the conclusions drawn from a systematic review depends on the quality of the studies reviewed. Thus, a review of cohort studies never rises to the highest level of evidence (Table 3.1).

One systematic review with meta-analysis examined the narrow question of whether strain/counterstrain affected tender point palpation tenderness (Wong et al. 2014). This review covering the 10 years from 2002 to 2012 included only experimental research examining the effect of isolated strain/counterstrain treatment on tender point palpation pain measured with a visual analogue scale.

The five studies that met the criteria demonstrated a significant pooled tender point palpation pain reduction with small (0.14) to large (1.15) effect sizes (Ibáñez-García et al. 2009; Lewis et al. 2010a; Meseguer et al. 2006; Perreault et al. 2009; Wong & Schauer 2004).

The meta-analysis for the 283 combined subjects included in the five studies demonstrated a pooled effect of an approximately 1/2 cm pain reduction on a 10 cm visual analogue scale.

The meta-analysis included asymptomatic (Ibáñez-García et al. 2009; Perreault et al. 2009; Wong & Schauer 2004) and symptomatic subjects (Lewis et al. 2010a; Meseguer et al. 2006) with tender points at the jaw (Ibáñez-García et al. 2009), upper trapezius (Meseguer et al. 2006; Perreault et al. 2009), lower back (Lewis et al. 2010a) and hips (Wong & Schauer 2004).

Heterogeneity among the studies related to the body regions examined, the mixture of asymptomatic and symptomatic subjects, and the small number of overall subjects led to a downgrading of the combined randomized control trial evidence to low quality, following the recommendations of the Cochrane Collaboration for ratings for systematic reviews of randomized control trials (Higgins & Green 2011).

The small pooled findings for tender point palpation tenderness reduction with strain/counterstrain compared to control conditions (Wong et al. 2014) when considered with the limitations of only moderate reliability for palpating tender points in the first place (McPartland & Goodridge 1997), may lead researchers to employ more objective outcome measures than palpation pain in future strain/counterstrain research.

STRENGTH OF RESEARCH RECOMMENDATIONS FOR STRAIN/COUNTERSTRAIN

Strain/counterstrain research is in a nascent stage. While support is not definitive for strain/counterstrain as the cause of the observed effects for any of the applications for which it has been recommended, this is not unusual for manual therapy in general. The evidence suggests that strain/counterstrain may well be the cause of changes in measureable outcomes, including pain, range of motion, strength and functional outcomes.

The small number of subjects included in research involving symptomatic conditions, flaws in research methodology, and conflicting results make firm conclusions impossible. The onus remains on manual therapy clinician researchers to design and conduct high quality research that will enhance our understanding of strain/counterstrain and outline evidence-based applications in health care.

Recommendation grades for research evidence

The Oxford Centre for Evidence-Based Medicine (OCEBM 2009) suggests recommendation grades for the available evidence supporting healthcare treatments.

- An A grade is given when the evidence is drawn consistently from Level I randomized control trial studies.
- A B grade is warranted when the evidence is consistently drawn from Level II–III studies, which include lower quality randomized control trials, as well as cohort and case–control studies.
- A C grade is given to Level IV evidence, such as case studies and extrapolated findings from Level II–III studies.
- A D grade is given to expert opinion, foundational laboratory research, theories developed from bench research, and other Level V evidence; or when the available studies are inconsistent, inconclusive, or have troublesome design flaws.

Any recommendation can be downgraded (–) due to limited available evidence or weaknesses within the combined evidence.

Design flaws include basic tenets of good experimental research such as employing independent interventions by eliminating co-interventions and clearly defining and describing the interventions so that other clinicians and researchers can reproduce the intervention.

A number of strain/counterstrain studies have not described the treatment protocols with enough specificity to reproduce the study or even the treatment for individual clinical cases. Such undifferentiated treatment descriptions limit all study findings. Limitations extend to the analytical interpretations of what occurred during treatment, such as whether related points may have been treated during purportedly inert sham treatments.

Many studies have included strain/counterstrain with other co-interventions making the effect of strain/counterstrain unclear. While such an approach may support the particular protocol used for the clinical research scenario, a clinician attempting to use these findings for practical purposes would not be able to differentiate which treatments were beneficial or necessary.

Overall quality of strain/counterstrain research

The overall quality of research into strain/counterstrain is low with few randomized control trials included. While the number of randomized control trials has steadily increased since 2004 when the first were published, a number of methodological quality criteria have not been consistently met.

For example, the concealment of group allocation and the effectiveness of participant and evaluator blinding were not routinely reported (Table 3.2). Another common source of potential bias has been the lack of stringently defined inclusion criteria for self-referred or recruited subjects with tender points and the lack of recruitment rate reporting.

Careful reporting of the inclusion of symptomatic participants with diagnosed pathology would mitigate these problems. It has been very encouraging, however, that sham treatments were commonly used in strain/counterstrain research. Without sham treatment conditions in manual therapy the effect of manual therapy compared to the power of simple touch cannot be differentiated.

The paucity of experimental studies and the limited number of outcomes that have been assessed, as well as limiting study design elements, limit the possible conclusions that can be drawn.

- A B recommendation can be supported by the available evidence only for use of strain/counterstrain for the relief of tender point palpation tenderness.
- While there is evidence to suggest that strain/counterstrain can increase range of motion or strength in specific target muscles and improve some functional measures, the available evidence only warrants a grade of C–.
- The many alternative applications for strain/counterstrain reported in the available case studies and suggested in continuing education courses can only receive a D grade recommendation.

The grade recommendations derived from the limited available evidence for strain/counterstrain serve as a cautionary word for clinical practitioners but also an opportunity for researchers. Since the first experimental study into the effects of strain/counterstrain only appeared in the literature 10 years ago, significant progress has been made with respect to both the clinical findings and the quality of the research methods used. It can be expected that more progress and significant discoveries related to strain/counterstrain will be made in future decades.

PRIORITIES FOR FUTURE STUDY

Evidence-based medicine is based on using clinical experience, knowledge of the available evidence and individual judgement of the patient's individual needs, to make the best clinical decisions in the care of our patients.

Strain/counterstrain is the fourth most often used osteopathic manipulative technique, though it is only used very often by 15% of osteopaths (Johnson & Kurtz 2003). Use of strain/counterstrain may be hampered by lack of supporting evidence. Recent evidence using a durometer to objectively assess tissue texture response has found that strain/counterstrain affected tissue hysteresis more than other common osteopathic techniques while providing a new research assessment method (Barnes 2013). Future research into strain/counterstrain should continue to explore the theoretical foundations of the fundamental mechanisms of strain/counterstrain. In addition to the mechanisms discussed in this chapter, future exploration of the effect of strain/counterstrain on the ligamentomuscular reflex that coordinates the synergistic functions of joint ligaments and related muscle contractions may yield relevant knowledge (Chaitow 2009).

Future strain/counterstrain research focussed on people with symptomatic pathological conditions should use objective outcome measures that can include pain and impairment level outcomes but also functional ability and participation restriction level outcomes (WHO 2001).

THIS CHAPTER

This chapter has provided an evaluation of the current understanding of the mechanisms involved in positional release approaches, particularly strain/counterstrain (SCS).

NEXT CHAPTER

The next chapter goes more deeply into the methodology of SCS/counterstrain – together with numerous exercises and clinical examples of its application in treatment of soft-tissue and joint dysfunction.

REFERENCES

Baker, R.T., Nasypany, A., Seegmiller, J.G., et al., 2013. Treatment of acute torticollis using positional release therapy: Part 2. International Journal of Athletic Therapy & Training 18, 38–43.

Barnes, P.L., Laboy, F. III, Noto-Bell, L., et al., 2013. A comparative study of cervical hysteresis characteristics after various osteopathic manipulative treatment (OMT) modalities. Journal of Bodywork Movement Therapies 17, 89–94.

Benjamin, S.J., Williams, D.A., Kalbfleisch, J.H., et al., 1999. Normalized forces and active range of motion in unilateral radial epicondylalgia. Journal of Orthopedic and Sports Physical Therapy 29, 668–676.

Birmingham, T.B., Kramer, J., Lumsden, J., et al., 2004. Effect of a positional release therapy technique on hamstring flexibility. Physiotherapy Canada 56, 165–170.

Birznieks, I., Burton, A.R., Macefield, V.G., 2008. The effects of experimental muscle and skin pain on the static stretch sensitivity of human muscle spindles in relaxed leg muscles. Journal of Physiology 586, 2713–2723.

Blanco, C.R., de las Penas, C., Xumet, J.E., et al., 2006. Changes in active mouth opening following a single treatment of latent myofascial trigger points in the masseter muscle involving post-isometric relaxation or strain-counterstrain. Journal of Bodywork and Movement Therapies 10, 197–205.

Brose, S.W., Jennings, D.C., Kwok, J., et al., 2013. Sham manual medicine protocol for cervical strain-counterstrain research. PM&R 5, 400–407.

Chaitow, L., 2009. Ligaments and positional release techniques? Journal of Bodywork and Movement Therapies 13, 115–116.

Cislo, S., Ramirez, M.A., Schwartz, H.R., 1991. Low back pain: treatment of forward and backward sacral torsions using counterstrain techniques. Journal of the American Osteopathic Association 91, 255–259.

Collins, C.K., 2007. Physical therapy management of complex regional pain syndrome in a 14-year-old patient using strain counterstrain: a case report. Journal of Manual and Manipulative Therapy 15, 25–41.

Collins, C.K., Masaracchio, M., Cleland, J.A., 2014. The effectiveness of strain counterstrain in the treatment of patients with chronic ankle instability: a randomized clinical trial. Journal of Manual and Manipulative Therapy 22, 119–128.

Croskerry, P., 2009. Clinical cognition and diagnostic error: applications of a dual process model of reasoning. Advances in Health Science Education 14, 27–35.

D'Ambrogio, K.J., Roth, G.B., 1997. Positional Release Therapy: Assessment and Treatment of Musculoskeletal Dysfunction, Mosby, St Louis.

Dardzinski, J.A., Ostrov, B.E., Hamann, L.S., 2000. Myofascial pain unresponsive to standard treatment: successful use of a strain and counterstrain technique with physical therapy. Journal of Clinical Rheumatology 6, 169–174.

Dempsey, A.V., 2001. The effect of strain/counterstrain on the flexibility of restricted hip flexors. Proquest Dissertations and Theses, Ann Arbor, MI, UMI 1401893.

Dodd, J.G., Good, M.M., Nguyen, T.L., et al., 2006. In vitro biophysical strain model for understanding mechanisms of osteopathic manipulative treatment. Journal of the American Osteopathic Association 106, 157–166.

Dunphy, B.C., Cantwell, R., Bourke, S., et al., 2009. Cognitive elements in clinical decision-making: toward a cognitive model for medical education and understanding clinical reasoning. Advances in Health Science Education 15, 229–250.

Eisensmith, L.P., 2007. Massage therapy decreases frequency and intensity of symptoms related to temporomandibular joint syndrome in one case study. Journal of

Bodywork Movement Therapies 11, 223–230.

Furlan, A.D., Pennick, V., Bombardier, C., et al., 2009. Updated method guidelines for systematic reviews in the Cochrane back review group. Spine 34, 1929–1941.

Gamber, R.G., Shores, J.H., Russo, D.P., et al., 2002. Osteopathic manipulative treatment in conjunction with medication relieves pain associated with fibromyalgia syndrome: results of a randomized clinical pilot project. Journal of the American Osteopathic Association 102, 321–325.

Goss, D.A., Thomas, J.S., Walkowski, S., et al., 2012. Non-thrust manual therapy reduces erector spinae short-latency stretch reflex asymmetries in patients with chronic low back pain. Journal of Electromyography and Kinesiology 22, 663–669.

Green, C.R., 2006. Assessing and managing pain. In: Satcher, D., Pamies, R.J. (Eds.), Multicultural Medicine and Health Disparities, McGraw Hill, New York.

Greenberger, H.B., Beissner, K., Jewell, D.V., 2012. Patient age is related to the types of physical therapy interventions provided for chronic low back pain: an observational study. Journal of Orthopaedic and Sports Physical Therapy 42, 902–911.

Hicks, E.P., Kluemper, G.T., 2011. Heuristic reasoning and cognitive biases: are they hindrances to judgments and decision making in orthodontics? American Journal of Orthodontics and Dentofacial Orthopedics 139, 297–304.

Higgins, J.P.T., Green, S. (Eds.), 2011. Cochrane Handbook for Systematic Reviews of Interventions, version 5.1.0 [updated March 2011], The Cochrane Collaboration. Online. Available: <http://www.cochrane-handbook.org> (Accessed 1 September 2012).

Howell, J.N., Cabell, K.S., Chila, A.G., et al., 2006. Stretch reflex and Hoffman reflex responses to osteopathic manipulative treatment in subjects with Achilles tendonitis. Journal of the American Osteopathic Association 106, 537–545.

Ibáñez-García, J., Alburquerque-Sendín, F., Rodríguez-Blanco, C., et al., 2009. Changes in masseter muscle trigger points following strain-counterstrain or neuro-muscular technique. Journal of Bodywork and Movement Therapies 13, 2–10.

Johnson, S.M., Kurtz, M.E., 2003. Osteopathic manipulative treatment techniques preferred by contemporary osteopathic physicians. Journal of the American Osteopathic Association 103, 219–224.

Jones, L.H., 1964. Spontaneous release by positioning. Doctor of Osteopathy 4, 109–116.

Jones, L.H., 1973. Foot treatment without hand trauma. Journal of the American Osteopathic Association 72, 481–489.

Jones, L.H., 1995. Strain-counterstrain. Jones Strain-Counterstrain Inc., Indianapolis, IN.

Jordan, K.P., Kadam, U.T., Hayward, R., et al., 2010. Annual consultation prevalence of regional musculoskeletal problems in primary care: an observational study. BMC Musculoskeletal Disorders 11, 144.

Klein, R., Barels, A., Schneider, A., et al., 2013. Strain-counterstrain to treat restrictions of the mobility of the cervical spine in patients with neck pain – a sham-controlled randomized trial. Complementary Therapies in Medicine 21, 1–7.

Korr, I.M., 1975. Proprioceptors and somatic dysfunction. Journal of American Osteopathic Association 74, 638–650.

Lewis, C., Flynn, T., 2001. The use of strain counterstrain in the treatment of patients with low back pain. Journal of Manual and Manipulative Therapy 9, 92–98.

Lewis, C., Khan, A., Souvlis, T., et al., 2010a. A randomised controlled study examining the short-term effects of strain-counterstrain treatment on quantitative sensory measures at digitally tender points in the low back. Manual Therapy 15, 536–541.

Lewis, C., Souvlis, T., Sterling, M., 2010b. Sensory characteristics of tender points in the lower back. Manual Therapy 15, 451–456.

Licciardone, J.C., Brimhall, A.K., King, L.N., 2005. Osteopathic manipulative treatment for low back pain: a systematic review and meta-analysis of randomized controlled trials. BMC Musculoskeletal Disorders 6, 43.

Licciardone, J.C., Kearns, C.M., 2012. Somatic dysfunction and its association with chronic low back pain, back-specific functioning, and general health: results from the OSTEOPATHIC trial. Journal of the American Osteopathic Association 112, 420–428.

Lopez, D., King, H., Knebl, J.A., et al., 2011. Effects of comprehensive osteopathic manipulative treatment on balance in elderly patients: a pilot study. Journal of the American Osteopathic Association 11, 382–388.

McPartland, J.M., Goodridge, J.P., 1997. Counterstrain and traditional osteopathic examination of the cervical spine compared. Journal of Bodywork and Movement Therapies 1, 173–178.

Meltzer, K.R., Standley, P.R., 2007. Modeled repetitive motion strain and indirect osteopathic manipulative techniques on regulation of human fibroblast proliferation and interleukin secretion. Journal of the American Osteopathic Association 107, 527–536.

Meseguer, A., Fernandez-de-las-Penas, C., Navarro-Poza, J.L., et al., 2006. Immediate effects of the strain-counterstrain technique in local pain evoked by tender points in the upper trapezius muscle. Clinical Chiropractic 9, 112–118.

Mohamadi, M., Ghanbari, A., Jaberi, A.R., 2012. Tension-type-headache treated by positional release therapy: a case report. Manual Therapy 17, 456–458.

Mulligan, B.R., 2010. Manual Therapy: 'NAGS', 'SNAGS', and 'MWMS' etc, sixth ed. Plane View Services Ltd., Wellington, NZ.

Nagrale, A.V., Glynn, P., Joshi, A., et al., 2010. The efficacy of an integrated neuromuscular inhibition technique on upper trapezius trigger points in subjects with non-specific neck pain: a randomized controlled trial. Journal of Manual and Manipulative Therapy 18, 37–43.

OCEBM Levels of Evidence Working Group, 2001. Levels of Evidence [updated March 2009]. Oxford

Centre for Evidence-Based Medicine. Online. Available: <http://www.cebm.net/index.aspx?o=1025> (Accessed 1 January 2014).

Pedowitz, R.N., 2005. Use of osteopathic manipulative treatment for iliotibial band friction syndrome. Journal of the American Osteopathic Association 105, 563–567.

Perreault, A., Kelln, B., Hertel, J., et al., 2009. Short-term effects of strain counterstrain in reducing pain in upper trapezius tender points. Athletic Training and Sports Health Care 1, 214–221.

Poon, M.Y., Tarrant, M., 2009. Obesity: attitudes of undergraduate student nurses and registered nurses. Journal of Clinical Nursing 18, 2355–2365.

Portney, L.G., Watkins, M.P., 2009. Foundations of Clinical Research: Applications to Research, third ed. Pearson Prentice Hall, Upper Saddle River, NJ.

Radjieski, J.M., Lumley, M.A., Cantieri, M.S., 1998. Effect of osteopathic manipulative treatment on length of stay for pancreatitis: a randomized pilot study. Journal of the American Osteopathic Association 98, 264–272.

Ramirez, M.A., Haman, J.L., Worth, L., 1989. Low back pain: diagnosis by six newly discovered sacral tender points and treatment with counterstrain. Journal of the American Osteopathic Association 89, 905–913.

Rathbun, J., Macnab, I., 1970. Microvascular pattern at the rotator cuff. Journal of Bone and Joint Surgery [Am] 52, 540–553.

Rothstein, J.M., Echternach, J.L., Riddle, D.L., 2003. The hypothesis-oriented algorithm for clinicians II (HOAC II): a guide for patient management. Physical Therapy 83, 455–470.

Sackett, D.L., Rosenberg, W.M., Gray, J.A., et al., 1996. Evidence based medicine: what it is and what it isn't. British Medical Journal 312, 71–72.

Schmitt, J., Abbott, J.H., 2015. Global ratings of change do not accurately reflect functional change over time in clinical practice. Journal of Orthopedic Sports Physical Therapy 45 (2), 106–111.

Schwartz, H.R., 1986. The use of counterstrain in an acutely ill in-hospital population. Journal of the American Osteopathic Association 86, 433–442.

Simons, D.G., Travell, J.G., Simons, L.S., 1999. Myofascial Pain and Dysfunction: The Trigger Point Manual, vol. 1. Williams & Wilkins, Baltimore, p. 70.

Snider, K.T., Glover, J.C., Rennie, P.R., et al., 2013. Frequency of counterstrain tender points in osteopathic medical students. Journal of the American Osteopathic Association 113, 690–702.

Steed, R., 2010. Attitudes and beliefs of occupational therapists participating in a cultural competency workshop. Occupational Therapy International 17, 142–151.

Tichelaar, J., Rachir, M., Avis, H.J., et al., 2010. Do medical students copy the drug treatment choices of their teachers or do they think for themselves? European Journal of Clinical Pharmacology 66, 407–412.

Waddell, G., 1998. The Back Pain Revolution. Churchill Livingstone, Edinburgh.

Walko, E.J., Janouschek, C., 1994. Effects of osteopathic manipulative treatment in patients with cervicothoracic pain: pilot study in thermography. Journal of the American Osteopathic Association 94, 135–141.

Wong, C.K., Abraham, T., Karimi, P., et al., 2014. Strain counterstrain technique to decrease tender point palpation pain compared to a control condition: a systematic review with meta-analysis. Journal of Bodywork Movement Therapies 18, 165–173.

Wong, C.K., Moskowitz, N., 2010. New assessment of forearm strength: reliability and validity. American Journal of Occupational Therapy 64, 809–813.

Wong, C.K., Moskowitz, N., Fabillar, R., 2011. Effect of strain counterstrain on forearm strength compared to placebo positioning. International Journal of Osteopathic Medicine 14, 86–95.

Wong, C.K., Schauer, C.S., 2004. Reliability, validity, and effectiveness of strain counterstrain techniques. Journal of Manual and Manipulative Therapy 12, 107–112.

Wong, C.K., Schauer-Alvarez, C.S., 2004. The effect of strain counterstrain on pain and strength. Journal of Manual and Manipulative Therapy 12, 215–224.

World Health Organization (WHO), 2001. International Classification of Functioning, Disability and Health (ICF). Online. Available: <http://www.who.int/classifications/icf/en/index.html> (Accessed 1 January 2014).

Wynn, M.W., Burns, J.M., Eland, D.C., et al., 2006. Effect of counterstrain on stretch reflexes, Hoffman reflexes and clinical outcomes in subjects with plantar fasciitis. Journal of the American Osteopathic Association 106, 547–556.

Chapter 4

Counterstrain models of positional release

The best known and most widely used positional release variation is the method developed from the clinical research of Laurence Jones – Strain Counterstrain (SCS). This pioneering work of developing SCS evolved into a method of treatment of joint and soft-tissue dysfunction of supreme gentleness (Jones 1981).

Modifications by the author and others, particularly the late George Goodheart DC, of Jones's original counterstrain methods are described in detail in this chapter, as well as a further variant, known as *positional release therapy* (D'Ambrogio & Roth 1997) (see Scanning and mapping, later in this chapter).

Evidence of efficacy of the use of SCS has been comprehensively detailed and discussed in the previous chapter and will not be amplified further in this chapter. Chapter 9, Visceral positional release: the counterstrain model, outlines counterstrain in a non-musculoskeletal setting.

HOW DOES SCS WORK?

It is important to state at the outset that the various theories as to how positional release in general, and counterstrain (SCS) in particular, achieves its effects, remain largely hypothetical. What supporting evidence there is for the theoretical models is outlined in this chapter.

Much basic scientific research remains to be conducted to validate the hypotheses discussed below, and the reader is advised to adopt a robustly critical frame of mind, while attempting to evaluate the mechanisms described, that *might* be operating.

Some of the hypotheses made are based on animal models (see Chapter 12). Some also emerge from a combination of assumption and deduction, based on clinical evidence, and an understanding of basic physiology and experience.

Very little concrete certainty exists, apart from the reality that positional release methods are safe and effective (see Chapter 3). How they achieve their benefits remains for future research.

THEORETICAL MODELS

Jones's (1981) concept as to how SCS works is based on the predictable physiological responses of muscles in particular situations, most notably in relation to acute or chronic strains. He describes how, in a balanced state, the proprioceptive functions of the various muscles supporting a joint will be feeding a flow of information, derived from the neural receptors in those muscles and their tendons, to the higher centres.

For example, the Golgi tendon organs will be reporting on tone, while the various receptors in the spindles will be firing a constant stream of information (slowly or rapidly depending upon the demands being placed on the tissues) regarding their resting length and any changes that might be occurring in that length.

In a dysfunctional state (see Neurological concepts, below) inappropriately excessive degrees of tone may be sustained, leading to chronic imbalances between agonists, antagonists and associated muscles. In some instances, excessive tone might relate to some degree of segmental or local (e.g. trigger point) facilitation.

D'Ambrogio & Roth (1997) state that:

> *Positional release therapy appears to have a damping influence on the general level of excitability within the facilitated segment. Weiselfish (1993) has found that this characteristic of PRT is unique in its effectiveness, and has utilized this feature to successfully treat severe neurologic patients, even though the source of the primary dysfunction arose from the supraspinal level.*

It is the dampening, calming, influence on the neurological features (including pain receptors) of hyperreactive and stressed tissues that seems to characterize many of the results observed following appropriate use of PRT.

Circulatory and fascial influences are also considered possible mechanisms for PRT's benefits, as outlined below.

NEUROLOGICAL CONCEPTS

The proprioceptive hypothesis

(Korr 1947, 1975; Mathews 1981)

Jones first observed the phenomenon of spontaneous release when he 'accidentally' placed a patient who was in considerable pain, and some degree of compensatory distortion, into a position of comfort ('ease') on a treatment table (Jones 1964).

Despite no other treatment being given, after just 20 minutes resting in a position of relative ease, the patient was able to stand upright and was free of pain. The pain-free position of ease into which Jones had helped the patient was one which exaggerated the degree of distortion in which his body was being held.

Jones had taken the patient into the direction of 'ease' (as opposed to 'bind'), since any attempt to correct or straighten the body would have been met by both resistance and pain. In contrast, moving the body further into distortion was acceptable and easy, and seemed to allow the physiological processes involved in resolution of spasm, etc. to operate. This position of ease is the key element in what later came to be known as strain/counterstrain.

Example

The events that take place at the moment of strain may provide the key to understanding the mechanisms of neurologically induced positional release.

Take, for example, an all too common instance of someone bending forwards from the waist. At that moment, the flexor muscles would be short of their resting length, and the neural reporting structures (muscle spindles) in the flexor muscles would be firing slowly, indicating little or no activity and no change of length taking place.

At the same time, the antagonist group of muscles – the spinal erector group in this example – would be stretched or stretching, and firing rapidly.

Any stretch affecting a muscle (and therefore its spindles) will increase the rate of reporting, which will reflexively induce further contraction (myotatic stretch reflex), as well as an increase in tone in that muscle, along with an instant inhibition (reciprocal) of the functional antagonists, so further reducing the already limited degree of reporting from the antagonists' spindle cells.

This feedback link with the central nervous system is the primary muscle spindle afferent response, and it is thought to be modulated by an additional muscle spindle function that involves the gamma-efferent system, which is controlled from higher (brain) centres. In simple terms, the gamma-efferent system influences the primary afferent

system: for example, when a muscle is in a quiescent state, when it is relaxed and short with little information coming from the primary receptors, the gamma-efferent system might fine-tune and increase ('turn up') the sensitivity of the primary afferents to ensure a continued information flow (Mathews 1981).

It is important to acknowledge that these neurological concepts are largely based on animal studies, and that definitive basic science studies to validate them have not yet been performed in humans.

Crisis

Now imagine a sudden 'alarm' situation arising (a person loses his footing while stooping, or the load being lifted shifts), which creates immediate demands for stabilization on both sets of muscles (the short, relatively 'quiet' flexors and the stretched, relatively actively firing extensors), even though they are in quite different states of preparedness for action.

- The flexors would be 'unloaded', relaxed and providing minimal feedback to the control centres, while the spinal extensors would be at stretch, providing a rapid outflow of spindle-derived information, some of which ensures that the relaxed flexor muscles remain relaxed, due to inhibitory activity.
- The central nervous system would at this time be receiving minimal information as to the status of the relaxed flexors and, at the moment when the demand for stabilization occurs, these shortened/relaxed flexors would be obliged to stretch quickly to a length that will balance the already stretched extensors.
- Meanwhile these stretched extensors will most probably be contracting rapidly, also to achieve stabilization.
- As this happens, the annulospiral receptors in the short (flexor) muscles will respond to the sudden stretch demand by contracting even more – the stretch reflex (Fig. 4.1).
- The neural reporting stations in these shortened muscles would be firing impulses as if the muscles were being stretched, even though the muscle remains well short of its normal resting length.
- Simultaneously, the extensor muscles, which had been at stretch and which, in the alarm situation, were obliged to rapidly shorten, would remain longer than their normal resting length as they attempt to stabilize the situation (Korr 1976).

Korr has described what he believes happens in the abdominal muscles (flexors) in such a situation. He says

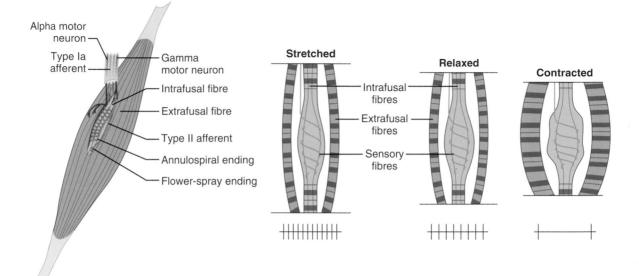

Figure 4.1 Annulospiral receptors. The sensitivity of the stretch receptors is adjusted by the innervating gamma motor neurons, and the intrafusal fibres detect stretch. When the muscle contracts gamma motor neurons fire, increasing tension on the intrafusal fibres so that muscle spindles maintain sensitivity to changes in the muscle length.

that because of their relaxed status, short of their resting length, there occurs in these muscles a silencing of the spindles; however, due to the demand for information from the higher centres, *gamma gain is increased reflexively* and, as the muscle contracts rapidly to stabilize the alarm demands, the central nervous system will receive information that the muscle, which is actually short of its neutral resting length, is being stretched.

In effect, the muscles would have adopted a restricted position as a result of inappropriate proprioceptive reporting. As DiGiovanna explains (Jones 1964):

> *With trauma or muscle effort against a sudden change in resistance, or with muscle strain incurred by resisting the effects of gravity for a period of time, one muscle at a joint is strained and its antagonist is hyper-shortened. When the shortened muscle is suddenly stretched the annulospiral receptors in that muscle are stimulated causing a reflex contraction of the already shortened muscle. The proprioceptors in the short muscle now fire impulses as if the shortened muscle were being stretched. Since this inappropriate proprioceptor response can be maintained indefinitely a somatic dysfunction has been created.*

In effect, the two opposing sets of muscles will have adopted a stabilizing posture to protect the threatened structures, and in doing so would have become locked into positions of imbalance in relation to their normal

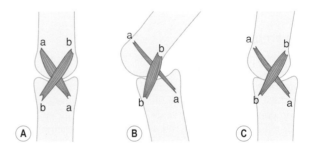

Figure 4.2 (A) Normal unstrained joint in normal position with muscles 'a' and 'b' in a non-stressed state. (B) Normal joint in an extreme position in which stress occurs which will result in strain, as illustrated in (C). (C) Joint in a strained state in which muscle 'a', which had been excessively stretched, is splinted/contracted and resists movement, and muscle 'b', short at the time of the stress, is slightly stretched and is neither splinted nor contracted. Any attempt at returning to the situation as illustrated in (A) would meet with resistance, while a return to the position of stress, (B), would be easily and painlessly achieved and could allow for a spontaneous positional release of the hypertonicity and splinting in muscle 'a'.

function. One would be shorter and one longer than its normal resting length (Fig. 4.2).

At this time, any attempt to extend the area/joint(s) would be strongly resisted by the tonically shortened flexor group. The individual would be locked into a forward-bending distortion (in this example).

The joint(s) involved would not have been taken beyond their normal physiological range, and yet the normal range would be unavailable, due to the shortened status of the flexor group (in this particular example). Going further into flexion, however, would present no problems or pain.

Walther (1988) summarizes the situation as follows:

> *When proprioceptors send conflicting information there may be simultaneous contraction of the antagonists … without antagonist muscle inhibition, joint and other strain results [and in this manner] a reflex pattern develops which causes muscle or other tissue to maintain this continuing strain. It [strain dysfunction] often relates to the inappropriate signaling from muscle proprioceptors that have been strained from rapid change that does not allow proper adaptation.*

This situation would be unlikely to resolve itself spontaneously and is the 'strain' position in Jones's SCS method.

We can recognize it in an acute setting in torticollis, as well as in acute lumbago. It is also recognizable as a feature of many types of chronic somatic dysfunction in which joints remain restricted due to muscular imbalances of this type, occurring as part of an adaptive process (as discussed in Chapter 2).

This is a time of intense neurological and proprioceptive confusion, and is the moment of 'strain'. SCS offers a means of quieting the neurological confusion and the excessive, or unbalanced, tone.

The nociceptive hypothesis

(Bailey & Dick 1992; Van Buskirk 1990)

In order to appreciate a second possible neurological influence involved in strain, we need a different example.

Let us consider someone involved in a simple whiplash-like neck stress as a car came to an unexpected halt:

- The neck would be thrown backwards into hyperextension, provoking all of the factors described above involving the flexor group of muscles in the forward-bending strain.
- The extensor group would be rapidly shortened and the various proprioceptive changes leading to strain and reflexive shortening would operate.
- At the time of the sudden braking of the car, there would occur hyperextension of the flexors of the neck, scalenes, etc. which would be violently stretched, inducing actual tissue damage.

- Nociceptive responses would occur (which are more powerful than proprioceptive influences) and these multisegmental reflexes would produce a flexor withdrawal, dramatically increasing tone in the flexor group.
- The neck would now display hypertonicity of both the extensors and the flexors; pain, guarding and stiffness would be apparent and the role of the clinician would be to remove these restricting influences layer by layer.
- Where pain is a factor in strain, this needs to be considered as producing an overriding influence over whatever other more 'normal' reflexes are operating.

In the simple example of neck strain described above, it is obvious that, in real life, matters are likely to be even more complicated, since a true whiplash would introduce both rapid hyperextension and hyperflexion as well as a multitude of layers of dysfunction.

More complex than described

The proprioceptive and nociceptive reflexes that might be involved in the production of strain are also likely to involve other factors, including chemically mediated changes.

D'Ambrogio & Roth (1997) elucidate:

> *Free nerve endings are distributed throughout all of the connective tissues of the body with the exception of the stroma of the brain. These receptors are stimulated by neuropeptides produced by noxious influences, including trauma … Impulses generated in these neurons spread centrally and also peripherally along the numerous branches of each neuron. At the terminus of the axons, peptide neurotransmitters such as substance P are released. The response of the musculoskeletal system to these painful stimuli may thus play a central role in the development (and maintenance) of somatic dysfunction.*

As Bailey & Dick (1992) explain:

> *Probably few dysfunctional states result from a purely proprioceptive or nociceptive response. Additional factors such as autonomic responses, other reflexive activities, joint receptor responses, [biochemical features] or emotional states must also be accounted for.*

It is at the level of our basic neurological awareness that understanding of the complexity of these problems commences.

PRT as a safe solution

(DiGiovanna 1991; Jones 1964, 1966)

Fortunately, the methodology of positional release does not demand a complete understanding of what is going on neurologically, since that which Jones and his followers, and those clinicians who have evolved the art of SCS to newer levels of simplicity have shown, is that by means of a slow, *painless* return to the position of strain, aberrant neurological activity currently locked into place in the strained tissues can frequently resolve itself, irrespective of the mechanisms involved.

The reaction of the body to this confusing and stressed situation apparently varies with the time available to it.

Should a deliberate and controlled response be possible, allowing the stretched muscles to slowly return to normal, then resolution of the potential problem might take place with no dysfunction arising. This can happen only if a controlled and not a panicky return towards the neutral position is achieved.

All too often, however, the situation is one of an almost-panic response, as the body makes a rapid attempt to restore stability to the region and finds the neural reporting information incoherent (one moment the abdominal muscles are saying, 'all is well, we are relaxed and short', and the next they are firing rapidly and lengthening, while there is a sudden change imposed on already stretched spinal extensors, which are trying to shorten at the same time in order to produce balance).

Restriction

The result is likely to involve the shortened muscles being 'fixed' in a position short of their normal resting length, from which they cannot easily be lengthened without pain (Fig. 4.3C).

The person bending, as described in our earlier example, would be locked in flexion, with an acute low back pain. The resulting spasm in tissues 'fixed' by this or other similar neurologically induced 'strains' causes the fixation of associated joint(s), and prevents any attempt to return to neutral. Any attempt to force the distorted spine (in this example) towards its anatomically correct position, would be strongly resisted by the shortened fibres.

It would, however, not be difficult, or indeed painful, to take the tissues/joint(s) further towards the position in which the strain occurred, effectively shortening the spasmed fibres even further, so reducing tension on affected tissues, and calming excessive proprioceptive reporting.

It is suggested that when held at 'ease', that enhanced vascular and interstitial circulatory function in previously tense and probably ischaemic tissues would moderate the activity of inflammation-enhancing chemical mediators. This model has been validated – for example in treatment of low back pain by Lewis & Flynn (2001).

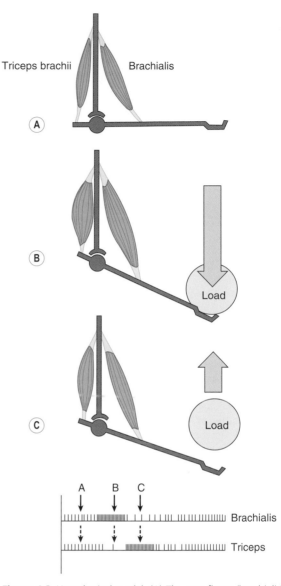

Figure 4.3 Hypothetical model. (A) The arm flexor (brachialis) and extensor (triceps brachii) muscles in an easy, normal position, as shown by the rate of firing indicated on the scale for each muscle. (B) A sudden force is applied which results in the flexors being stretched while the extensors protect the joint by rapidly shortening. The firing rate relating to hyperextension and hypershortening is indicated on the scale. (C) Flexor stretch receptors have been excited by this sudden demand and these continue to fire as though stretch were continuing even though a relatively normal position has been achieved. The rate of firing of both flexors and extensors continues to be maintained at an inappropriately high rate. This is the situation in a strained joint. DiGiovanna (1991) explains: 'The joint is restricted within its physiological range of motion (and is prevented) from achieving its full range of motion. It is therefore an active process rather than a static injury usually associated with a strain'.

Moving towards 'ease'

Jones found that by taking the joint/area close to the position in which the original strain took place an interesting phenomenon was observed, in which the proprioceptive functions were given an opportunity to reset themselves, to become coherent again, during which time pain in the area lessened.

This is the 'counterstrain' element of the system.

If the position of ease were held for a period (Jones suggests 90 seconds; see discussion of 'Timing' in Box 4.4), the spasm in hypertonic, shortened tissues commonly resolves, following which it is usually possible to return the joint/area to a more normal resting position, as long as this action is performed extremely slowly.

The muscles that had been overstretched might remain sensitive for some days, but for all practical considerations, the joint would be normal again.

Jones had found that by carefully positioning the joint, whether this be a small extremity joint or a spinal segment, into a position of neutral or 'ease' (which is frequently an exaggeration of the distorted position in which the body is holding the area, or is a close replica of the position in which the original strain took place), a resolution of spasm/hypertonia takes place.

Since the position of ease achieved during Jones's therapeutic methods is the same as that of the original strain, the shortened muscles are repositioned in such a manner as to allow the dysfunctioning proprioceptors to modulate their activity.

Korr's explanation for the physiological normalization of tissues brought about through positional release (Korr 1976) is that:

> *The shortened spindle nevertheless continues to fire, despite the slackening of the main muscle, and the CNS is gradually able to turn down the gamma discharge and, in turn enables the muscles to return to 'easy neutral', at its resting length. In effect, the [practitioner] has led the patient through a repetition of the dysfunctioning process with, however, two essential differences. First it is done in slow motion, with gentle muscular forces, and second there have been no surprises for the CNS; the spindle has continued to report throughout.*

Travell & Simons (1992) noted that in stressed soft tissues, there are likely to be localized areas of relative ischaemia – lack of oxygenated blood – and that this can be a key factor in production of pain and altered tissue status contributing to the evolution of myofascial trigger points.

Studies on cadavers have shown that when a radiopaque dye is injected into muscles, this is more likely to spread into the vessels of the muscle when a 'counterstrain' position of ease is adopted than when the muscle is in a neutral position (Rathbun & Macnab 1970). This was demonstrated by injecting a suspension into the arm of a fresh cadaver while the arm was maintained at the side. No filling of blood vessels occurred. When the other arm, following injection of a radiopaque suspension, was placed in a position of flexion, abduction and external rotation (position of 'ease' for the supraspinatus muscle), there was almost complete filling of the blood vessels by the dye, as a result.

Jacobson et al. (1989) suggested that, 'unopposed arterial filling may be the same mechanism that occurs in living tissue during the 90-second counterstrain treatment'.

More recently, studies at the University of Ulm, Germany, by Schleip and Klingler have expanded awareness of the effects of aspects of soft tissue treatment on the fluid content of tissues. For example, when tissues are compressed or crowded, as occurs in counterstrain, as well as during application of facilitated positional release (FPR) methods, water is extruded from fascial structures in a sponge-like manner. This makes the tissues more pliable for a period of up to 30 minutes (Klingler et al. 2004). As water levels drop, temporary relaxation and an increased range of movement is possible – until water is absorbed back into the tissue, after 20–30 minutes, at which time it stiffens again (Schleip et al. 2012). The 20–30 minutes of greater mobility allows tissues to move more freely and for proprioceptive functions to normalize, offering the individual an experience of reduced discomfort and greater motor control.

Wong et al. (2014) explained yet another fluid related effect of counterstrain. They noted that Standley & Meltzer (2007) demonstrated that counterstrain methods lead to a decrease in interleukin (IL-6) levels, and that these are important for mediating inflammatory healing after acute injury. This effect may explain why Achilles tendonitis patients report reduced swelling after SCS (Howell et al. 2006).

CIRCULATORY AND FLUID CONCEPTS AND PRT

There exist other mechanisms that suggest ways in which positional release methods might usefully modify distressed tissues – involving circulatory changes.

CONNECTIVE TISSUE AND COUNTERSTRAIN CONCEPTS

In summary (see also Chapter 7 for a fuller exploration of the proposed connections between positional release approaches and connective tissues), a number of fascial features and functions appear to be associated with mechanisms involved in different PRT effects.

1. *Mechanotransduction* involves a variety of cellular effects in response to mechanical load applications. Of particular interest are the effects of altered degrees and types of strain and load on fibroblasts – cells that are plentifully present in fascial structures (Dodd et al. 2006; Standley & Meltzer 2008; Meltzer et al. 2010).

2. *Ligamentous reflexes* may be a feature of the effects – albeit temporary – of facilitated positional release (FPR, see Chapter 5) and aspects of counterstrain according to Solomonow (2009) – Wong et al. (2014) has summarized current thinking regarding ligamentomuscular reflexes and SCS:

Ligamentous strain inhibits muscle contractions that increase strain, or stimulates muscles that reduce strain, to protect the ligament (Krogsgaard et al. 2002). For instance, anterior cruciate ligament strain inhibits quadriceps and stimulates hamstring contractions to reduce anterior tibial distraction (Dyhre-Poulsen & Krogsgaard 2000). Ligamentous reflex activation also elicits regional muscle responses that indirectly influence joints (Solomonow & Lewis 2002). Research is needed to explore whether SCS may alter the protective ligamentomuscular reflex and thus reduce dysfunction by shortening joint ligaments or synergistic muscles (Chaitow 2009).

CONVENTIONAL SCS AND THE MODIFIED APPROACH

The counterstrain model advocated in this book is not the same as that originally taught by Jones (1981), but is a variation largely based on refinements suggested by Goodheart. This chapter therefore focusses on modifications of Jones's original SCS model and how to use it. In order to do so, the phenomenon of the 'tender point' needs to be thoroughly grasped.

The elements that need to be kept in mind as SCS methods are summarized in Boxes 4.1 and 4.2.

The usual method for studying Jones's SCS methodology involves learning the described locations, and practising the location, of tender points, followed by practising the positioning of the body/associated area in a prescribed manner, in order to reduce discomfort in the palpated tender point.

Locating tender points depends upon palpation skills which can be learned, and which practice can refine into

---

Box 4.1 Ideal settings for application of SCS/PRT

See also Box 4.7 for contraindications and Box 4.8 for indications

- For reduction of stiffness (hypertonia) in pre- and postoperative patients
- In cases involving muscle spasm – where more direct methods would not be tolerated
- Where contraction is a feature – reducing tone before stretching tissues after use of muscle energy or other techniques
- In cases of acute and multiple strain – whiplash, for example
- As part of any treatment of chronic soft-tissue dysfunction
- As part of a sequence (INIT) of treating trigger points – after NMT and before MET
- In treatment of sensitive, frail, delicate individuals or sites
- In treatment of joint dysfunction where hypertonia is the prime restricting factor.

Box 4.2 SCS application guidelines

The four keys which allow anyone to apply counterstrain efficiently are:

1. An ability to localize by palpation soft-tissue changes related to particular strain dysfunctions, acute or chronic.
2. An ability to sense tissue change as it moves into a state of ease, comfort, relaxation and reduced resistance.
3. The ability to guide the patient as a whole, or the affected body part, towards a state of ease with minimal force.
4. The ability to apply minimal palpation force as the changes in the tissues are evaluated.

Application guidelines:

1. Locate and palpate an appropriate tender point
2. Use minimal force
3. Use minimal monitoring pressure
4. Achieve maximum ease/comfort
5. Produce no additional pain anywhere else.

---

a practical ability that allows for the very rapid location of areas of localized soft-tissue dysfunction.

Some researchers in positional release and SCS who discuss tender point characteristics speak of *sudomotor changes* as a primary feature, usually associated with increased or decreased temperature as compared with surrounding tissues (Lewit 1999). Phenomena, such as blanching, erythema and sweating of the skin overlying tense, tender and often oedematous tender points, are all used as a means of their identification (Chaitow 2003; Jones 1964, 1981; Schwartz 1986).

- The simplest method of palpation ('drag palpation') involves the light passage across the skin involving one digit, which seeks a sense of 'drag' in which the elevated sympathetic, sudomotor activity becomes apparent, as the finger or thumb feels a momentarily retarded passage over the skin, due to increased hydrosis (as described in Chapter 2 under the heading 'A TARTT shortcut: drag palpation').
- Pressure applied into the tissues below such localized skin changes (described as 'hyperalgesic skin zones' by Lewit 1999), usually evinces an increased degree of sensitivity or pain.
- Whether this or some other form of soft-tissue palpation is used, the tender points, which Jones has catalogued, need to be identified. They frequently differ from active myofascial trigger points inasmuch as Jones's tender points may refer pain elsewhere when compressed, whereas active trigger points always refer pain elsewhere.
- They commonly lie in those tissues that were shortened at the time of strain, or have been shortened in response to chronic strain, and are seldom in areas where the patient was previously aware of pain.

SCS guidelines

The general guidelines that Jones gives for relief of the dysfunction with which such tender points are related (pain, restriction, etc.) involves directing the movement of these tissues towards ease, which commonly involves using the protocols listed in Box 4.3.

Once in a 'position of ease', the optimal amount of time this position should be maintained has been subject to different opinions. The key suggestions are listed in Box 4.4. Using these guidelines, it is possible to begin to practice the use of SCS on a model, fellow student, a willing volunteer or even oneself.

Further clinical guidelines

A consensus has emerged, out of the clinical experience of thousands of practitioners, over the past 40 years, of a number of simple yet effective ways of selecting which of many areas of discomfort and 'tenderness' should receive primary attention (McPartland & Klofat 1995). The advice is summarized in Box 4.5.

Box 4.3 Counterstrain positioning guidelines

- For tender points on the anterior surface of the body, flexion, side-bending and rotation is most commonly towards the side of the palpated point, followed by fine-tuning to reduce sensitivity by at least 70%.
- For tender points on the posterior surface of the body, extension, side-bending and rotation is most commonly away from the side of the palpated point, followed by fine-tuning to reduce sensitivity by at least 70%.
- The closer the tender point is to the midline, the less side-bending and rotation is usually required, and the further from the midline, the more side-bending and rotation may be required, in order to effect ease and comfort in the tender point (without any additional pain or discomfort being produced anywhere else).
- The direction towards which side-bending is introduced when attempting to find ease, is most frequently away from the side of the palpated pain point, especially in relation to tender points found on the posterior aspect of the body.
- Despite the previous comment, there are instances in which ease will be noted when side-bending towards the direction of the painful point. These guidelines therefore offer a 'suggestion' as to the likeliest directions of ease and are not 'rules'. Individual tissue characteristics will ultimately determine the ideal directions that will achieve comfort/ease for the point being monitored.

Where to look for tender points

- Use of Jones's 'maps' (or D'Ambrogio & Roth 1997) offer one way of deciding where to palpate for a tender point. This model is formulaic, and does not take account of the unique characteristics of individuals or their dysfunctional patterns – which is why the Goodheart model is advocated (see below).
- As briefly explained in Chapter 1, Goodheart (1985) suggested a patient-specific formula for identifying the location of areas of tenderness that can be used in the counterstrain procedure.
  - If the patient displays obvious distortion, or a marked imbalance in terms of 'loose–tight' tissues, the tender points that are most likely to be useful as monitors during counterstrain application will be found in the tight (i.e. shortened) tissues, and the ease position is likely to be an exaggeration of the presenting distortion (see Chapter 1 for an elaboration of this concept). The tissues that are short are shortened and crowded (painlessly) even more, during the positioning and 'fine-tuning' process, while the tender point is monitored for a decrease in sensitivity.

Box 4.4 Timing and SCS

- Jones (1981) suggests a 90-second hold of the position of ease.
- Goodheart (in Walther 1988) suggests that if a facilitating crowding or neuromuscular manipulation of the spindle is utilized (see Fig. 1.9), a 20–30-second holding of the position of ease is usually adequate.
- Morrison (induration technique, described later in this chapter) suggests a 20-second hold in the position of ease.
- Weiselfish (1993) recommends not less than 3 minutes for neurological conditions to benefit.
- Schiowitz (1990) reduces the holding time to just 5 seconds when employing facilitated positional release (see Chapter 5).
- D'Ambrogio & Roth (1997) suggest that between 1 and 20 minutes may be needed to achieve fascial release.
- Others (e.g. Chaitow 1996) suggest that the times recommended above are approximate at best, since tissues respond idiosyncratically, depending on multiple factors which differ from individual to individual.
- As the tissues release, palpation should reveal these changes, at which time, a slow return to neutral is called for. However, the basic idea of a 90-second hold as a minimum for using Jones's methodology is endorsed, when first learning these methods.

   Additional notes on timing, and ways of modifying this, will be found later in this chapter.

Box 4.5 Which points to treat first?

- Choose the most painful, the most medial and the most proximal tender points for primary attention, within the area of the body that demonstrates the greatest aggregation of tender points.
- If a chain, or line, of tender points is identified, treat the most central of these.
- No more than five tender points should receive attention at any one treatment session, even if a relatively robust individual is involved.
- The more dysfunctional, ill, adaptively exhausted (see Zink & Lawson's evaluation in Chapter 2), pain-ridden and/or fatigued the patient, the fewer the number of tender points that should be treated at any one session (between one and three in such cases).

- If the patient demonstrates a movement that is painful, or that is restricted, then Goodheart's guidelines suggest the tender points most useful for monitoring will be located in the muscles that would perform the opposite movement to that which is painful or restricted, i.e. the practitioner should seek tender points in the antagonists to muscles active when pain or restriction is reported or observed.
  - As an example, if turning the head to the right is either painful or restricted, the muscles that produce that action would be those on the right of the neck, as well as the left sternocleidomastoid muscle.
  - Restriction in rotation to the right might therefore be expected to relate to shortening (or dysfunction) involving the muscles *on the left side of the neck*, and/or right sternomastoid.
  - According to Goodheart's guidelines ('seek tender points in antagonist muscle to those active when pain or restriction is noted'), it is in these shortened structures that a tender point can be found, and used as a monitor during SCS positioning.
  - Palpation for suitable tender points should be carried out in the muscles that would turn the head to the left, i.e. those on the left side of the neck, as well as in right side sternomastoid (as this helps to turn the head to the left).
  - It is very important to avoid confusion that can occur and to *NOT seek a tender point in tissues opposite the site of pain*.
  - The appropriate tender point will be located in the antagonists to the muscles *active in producing the painful or restricted movement – irrespective of where the pain is reported*.
  - Once located, the point would be used as a monitor – as in all SCS procedures.
- Any area of local tenderness identified during palpation most probably represents a response to some degree of imbalance, chronic strain or adaptive change. Using such a point as a monitor while local or general positioning is introduced to remove the sensitivity from the point, will almost certainly help to modify whatever stress pattern is causing or maintaining it, even if this has not been identified.

TENDER POINTS AND THE POSITION OF EASE

Jones's discovery that somatic dysfunction involves associated areas of palpable tenderness, that are frequently only tender when palpated or probed, led to the realization that when the joint or area is suitably positioned to ease tenderness in these points, associated hypertonia or spasm usually diminishes.

He called these points 'tender points' (see Chapter 1, Box 1.1).

Describing his methods, Jones (1981) states:

Finding the myofascial tender point, and the correct position of release, will probably take a few minutes at first. Watching a skilled physician find a tender point, in a few seconds, and a position of release in a few seconds more, may give a false impression of simplicity to the beginner.

It may take longer than a few minutes to locate tender points initially; however, accurate palpation methods, such as the 'drag' method, can usually be rapidly learned if practised regularly.

What happens next?

- Once located, the tense tender point should be palpated, with just less than sufficient pressure to cause pain in normal tissue.
- The pain/sensitivity should be apparent to both the physician and the patient.
- By careful guiding of the joint (or other tissue) while constantly palpating the tender point (or by intermittently probing it), a monitoring of progress towards the ideal neutral (reduced or no pain in the palpated point) position is eventually achieved.
- The practitioner senses and evaluates reducing (desirable) or increasing (undesirable) levels of tension/tone in the palpated tissues, as well as the patient's report of either increasing or diminishing levels of sensitivity/pain in the point.
- These indicators are used to guide ('fine-tuning') the practitioner/therapist to the position where eventually there is a feeling of relative ease in the soft tissues, together with markedly reduced pain in the tender point (by 70% at least, ideally).
- An absence of 'bind' and also, most importantly, the patient's report that pain has significantly lowered are the desired indicators.

Jones (1981) states:

The point of maximum relaxation accompanied by an abrupt increase in joint mobility, within a very small arc, is the mobile point.

After holding this position for 90 seconds (see Box 4.4), the practitioner/therapist slowly returns the area to its neutral position.

What are the tender points?

Jones equates tender points with trigger points (Simons et al. 1999; Travell & Simons 1992) and with Chapman's neurolymphatic reflexes (Owens 1982). However, this comparison cannot be strictly accurate, despite an inevitable degree of overlap in all reflexively active points on the body surface.

There are differences in the nature, if not in the feel, of these different point systems (Kuchera & McPartland 1997). For example, myofascial trigger points will refer sensitivity, pain or other symptoms to a target area when pressed, which is not usually the case with Chapman's (neurolymphatic) reflex points, which are found in pairs and not singly, as are Jones's tender points and most trigger points.

Schwartz (1986) – developer of facilitated positional release (FPR, see Chapter 5) noted that:

Generally, but not always, pressure on the tender point will cause pain at a site distant to the point itself.

That description could define such a point as a trigger point, as well as a tender point. Schwartz highlights the difference between SCS and other methods which use such points in treatment by saying:

Other methods invade the point itself, for example by needle in acupuncture, injection of lidocaine into the point, or the use of pressure or ultrasound to destroy the tender point.

Osteopathic physician, Eileen DiGiovanna (1991), summarizes the overlap:

Today many physicians believe there is a relationship among trigger points, acupuncture points and Chapman's reflexes. Precisely what the relationship may be is unknown.

She quotes from prestigious osteopathic pioneer, George Northrup (1941), who stated:

One cannot escape the feeling that all of the seemingly diverse observations [regarding reflex patterns of surface 'points'] are but views of the same iceberg, the tip of which we are beginning to see, without understanding either its magnitude or its depth of importance.

Felix Mann, one of the pioneers of acupuncture in the West, has entered the controversy as to the existence, or otherwise, of acupuncture meridians (and indeed acupuncture points). In an effort to alter the emphasis which traditional acupuncture places on the specific charted positions of points, he stated (Mann 1983):

McBurney's point, in appendicitis, has a defined position. In reality it may be 10 cm higher/lower, to the left or right. It may be 1 cm in diameter, or occupy the whole of the abdomen, or not occur at all. Acupuncture points are often the same, and hence it is pointless to speak of acupuncture points in the classical traditional way. Carefully performed electrical resistance measurements do not show alterations in the skin resistance to electricity corresponding with classical acupuncture points. There are so many acupuncture points mentioned in some modern books, that there is no skin left which is not an acupuncture point. In cardiac disease, pain and tenderness may occur in the arm; however, this does not occur more frequently along the course of the heart meridian than anywhere else in the arm.

Hence, Mann appears to conclude, meridians do not exist, or – more confusingly perhaps – that the whole body is an acupuncture point! Leaving aside the validity of Mann's comment, it is true to say that if all the multitude of points described in acupuncture, traditional and modern, together with those points described by Travell and colleagues, Chapman and Jones, were to be placed together on one map of the body surface, we would all soon come to the conclusion that the entire body surface is a potential acupuncture point.

The discussion in Chapter 2 on the evolution of soft-tissue dysfunction in general (along with the tight–loose concept), and trigger points in particular, offers a representation in which some areas are seen to become short, tight and bunched, while others become lax, stretched or distended.

If the broad guideline of 'exaggerating the distortion' (see Chapter 1) is brought into consideration in such situations, this suggests that whatever is short, tight and bunched is likely to benefit by having these characteristics amplified, reinforced and held/supported, as part of a treatment approach that attempts to offer these tissues an opportunity to change, to release.

Using a tender point (whether or not it is also a trigger point or plays some other role in relation to reflex activity) to guide the tissues towards the precisely balanced degree of crowding, folding and compression describes SCS methodology simplistically but accurately.

Are *ah-shi* points and tender points the same?

It is worth remembering that, in acupuncture, there exists a phenomenon known as the 'spontaneously sensitive point'. These 'points' arise in response to trauma, or joint dysfunction, and are regarded, for the duration of their existence, as 'honorary' acupuncture points (Academy of Traditional Chinese Medicine 1975).

Most acupuncture points that receive treatment by means of needling, heat, pressure, lasers, etc. are clearly defined and mapped. The only exception to this rule relates to these spontaneously arising (ah-shi) points, associated with joint problems, which become available for treatment for the duration of their sensitivity.

In an earlier text (Chaitow 1991), I make the following comment:

Local tender points in an area of discomfort may be considered as spontaneous acupuncture points. The Chinese term these ah-shi points, and use them in the same way as classical points, when treating painful conditions.

It is worth recalling that in Chinese medicine, as well as use of acupuncture, manual acupressure of ah-shi points is also considered an appropriate form of treatment.

It would seem that Jones's points are in many ways the same, if not identical, to ah-shi points.

Is the muscle weak or strong?

Goodheart suggested a simple test to identify a tender point's usefulness as a monitor of the counterstrain procedure.

- If the muscle containing the tender point tests is weak following a maximal 3-second isometric contraction, it will probably benefit from counterstrain (Walther 1988).
- When a counterstrain is successful, this same protocol suggests that the muscle will no longer weaken after a short, strong, isometric contraction.

Different focus

Whereas Jones's use of counterstrain is largely focussed towards treatment of painful conditions, Goodheart has focussed on improving the neuromuscular function of muscles, even if no pain is present.

Goodheart's associate, David Walther, notes that:

Neuromuscular dysfunction that responds to strain/counterstrain technique may be from recent trauma, or be buried in the patient's history.

Goodheart and Walther agree with the interpretation of the role of neurological imbalance, which Jones and Korr (Korr 1975) have described as a key factor leading to many forms of soft-tissue and joint dysfunction, in which antagonistic muscles fail to return to neurological equilibrium following acute or chronic strain.

When this happens, an abnormal neuromuscular pattern is established that benefits from being held in 'ease' during a positional release treatment. The muscles that have shortened in the process of strain, and *not* those that were stretched (where pain is commonly noted), are the tissues to be used in the process of rebalancing.

> *Understanding that the cause of the continued pain … is usually not at the location of pain, but in an antagonistic muscle, is the most important step in solving the problem.*
>
> (Walther 1988)

The tender point might lie in muscle, tendon or ligament but the perpetuating factor is the imbalance in the spindle cell mechanisms. Since the patient can usually easily describe which movements increase the pain (or which are restricted), the search sites for tender areas are easily decided.

Positioning to find ease

As we have seen, Jones discovered a further use for tender points, apart from pressing or puncturing them.

Maintaining a sufficient degree of pressure on such a point allows the patient to be able to report on the level of pain being produced as the joint is (re)positioned, becoming a monitor and guide for the practitioner. The disappearance, or at least marked reduction of pain noted on pressure, after holding the joint in the position of ease for the prescribed period, is instant evidence as to the success of the procedure.

The holding, or periodic probing, of the point during the 90-second period recommended by Jones, leads to a further question; one which Jones acknowledges as being asked of him quite frequently. This queries whether the pressure on the tender point is not in itself therapeutic? Jones answered:

> *The question is asked whether the repeated probing of the tender point is therapeutic, as in acupressure, or Rolfing techniques (or ischemic compression as used in neuromuscular technique). It is not intentionally therapeutic, but is used solely for diagnosis and guidance of accuracy of treatment.*

This answer could be thought of as being equivocal for it does not address the possibility of a therapeutic end-result from the use of pressure on the tender point, but states only the intention of such pressure.

It may be assumed that some therapeutic effect does indeed derive from sustained inhibitory (also known as

> **Box 4.6 Some of the effects of sustained compression**
>
> - Ischaemia is reversed when pressure is released (Simons et al. 1999).
> - Neurological 'inhibition' results from sustained efferent barrage (Ward 1997).
> - Mechanical stretching occurs as 'creep' of connective tissue commences (Cantu & Grodin 1992).
> - Piezoelectric effects modify hardened 'gel-like' tissues, towards a softer more 'sol-like' state (Barnes 1997).
> - Mechanoreceptor impulses resulting from applied pressure interfere with pain messages ('gate theory') (Melzack & Wall 1988).
> - Analgesic endorphin and enkephalins are released in local tissues and the brain (Baldry 1993).
> - 'Taut bands' associated with trigger points release due to local biochemical modifications (Simons et al. 1999).
> - Traditional Chinese medicine concepts associate digital pressure with altered energy flow.
> - In the use of acupuncture there is clear evidence of a pain-reducing effect when pressure methods are applied to acupuncture points.

'ischaemic') pressure on such a spontaneously arising tender point, for the reasons described in Box 4.6.

Applied pressure and positioning

Since acupuncture authorities both in China and the West include spontaneously tender (ah-shi) points (which seem to be in every way the same as Jones's points) as being suitable for needling or pressure techniques, the avoidance of a clear answer on this point by Jones may be taken to indicate that he has not really addressed himself to the possibility that the applied pressure aspect of SCS contributes to the results.

That his method has other mechanisms which achieve release of pain and spasm in injured joints seems highly probable. The total effect of SCS would seem to derive from a combination of the positioning of the joint in a neutral position, and the pressure on the tender point.

The process of positioning used in SCS is similar, but not identical, to that described in functional technique by Harold Hoover (see Chapter 5). Hoover's methods involved the positioning of a joint or tissues which display a limited range of motion in what he called a 'dynamic neutral' position. He sought a position in which there was a balance of tensions, fairly near the anatomical neutral position of the joint.

Jones also aims at a position of ease, but he relates more to the identical position in which the original strain occurred, or by exaggeration of existing distortions.

By combining the position of ease, in which the shortened muscle(s) are able to release themselves, while simultaneously applying pressure (which, despite Jones's doubts, appears to involve a therapeutic effect), improvements in severe and painful conditions are possible.

Jones's conclusions regarding joints

Jones came to a number of conclusions as a result of his work, which may be summarized as follows:

- The pain in joint dysfunction is related very much to the position in which the joint is placed – varying from acute pain in some positions, to a pain-free position, which would be almost directly opposite the position of maximum pain.
- The dysfunction in a joint that has been strained is the result of something which occurs in response to the strain – a reaction to it. The palpable evidence of this is found by searching not in the tissues that were placed under strain, but by searching for tenderness in the (usually shortened) antagonists of these overstretched tissues.
- These painful structures in joint problems are usually not those which were stretched at the time of the injury, but which were in fact shortened, and which have remained so.
- It is in these shortened tissues that the tender points will be found.

Jones's technique

Jones described the use of 'tender points' as follows:

A physician skilled in palpation techniques will perceive tenseness and/or edema as well as tenderness. The tenderness, often a few times greater than that for normal tissue, is for the beginner the most valuable sign.

Jones suggested maintaining the palpating finger over the tender point, to monitor expected changes in tenderness, while with the other hand, he positioned the patient into a posture of comfort and relaxation.

Jones reported that he might proceed successfully just by questioning the patient as to comfort, reduction in pain, etc., as he probed intermittently, while moving towards the position of ease. If the correct position is arrived at, the patient would report diminished tenderness in the palpated area.

By intermittent deep palpation, as he fine-tuned the positioning, he monitored the tender point, seeking the ideal position at which there was at least a 70% reduction in tenderness. This degree of pressure stimulus is similar to that applied in the treatment of similar tender points by acupressure or Japanese 'tsubo' techniques.

The key to successful normalization by means of these methods seems to be the achievement of the position of maximum ease of the joint, in which the tender point becomes markedly less sensitive to palpation pressure.

Most importantly, the subsequent return to the neutral resting position, after the maintenance of the joint in this position of ease for not less than 90 seconds, is achieved very slowly. Without this slow repositioning, the likelihood exists of a sudden return to a shortened state of the previously disturbed structures.

THE GEOGRAPHY OF SCS

Tender points, relating to acute and chronic strain, can be found in almost all soft-tissue locations which have come under adaptation stress.

Although Simons et al. (1999) indicate that trigger points close to attachments are the ones most likely to benefit from positional release methods, D'Ambrogio & Roth (1997) observe:

Tender points are found throughout the body, anteriorly, posteriorly, medially, and laterally on muscle origins or insertions, within the muscle belly, over ligaments, tendons, fascia and bone.

Jones has identified a large number of conditions that are related to predictable tender points and from his vast clinical experience, and a lengthy process of trial and error, he has concluded that when tender points are found on the anterior surface of the body they are (with a few exceptions) indicative of the associated joint requiring a degree of forward-bending during its treatment (see Box 4.3). The location (in this case on the anterior aspect of the body) also indicates that the joint was probably initially injured in a forward-bending position.

Thus, information as to the original injury position (or observation of the direction in which adaptation is directing distortion) helps to direct the search for the tender points to the likeliest aspect of the body.

The exception to this rule is that the tender point related to the fourth cervical vertebra, when injured in flexion, is not necessarily treated with the neck in flexion, but may require side-bending and rotation, away from the side affected. Reduction in pain from the tender point during positioning and fine-tuning, will produce the guide to the most suitable position.

Tender points found on the posterior aspect of the body indicate joint dysfunction, which calls for some degree of backward-bending in the treatment (see Box 4.3). There are also exceptions to this rule, notably involving the piriformis muscle and the third and fifth cervical vertebrae. These exceptions may involve a degree of flexion on treatment.

Maps

Figure 4.4 will guide the reader to the most common tender point positions, as noted by Jones. Proprioceptive skills, and the use of careful palpation, will enable the required technique to be acquired. Reading of Jones's (1981) book, or that of D'Ambrogio & Roth (1997) is suggested for greater detail and understanding of his approach and for those who wish to work in this structured, somewhat formulaic, manner.

The examples that follow are adapted from Jones's text (Jones 1981) and are not recommendations but are for general information only.

Settings in which SCS/positional release might ideally be applied are given in Box 4.2.

The suggested positions of ease relate to the findings of Jones and his followers over many years, and while they are largely accurate, the author is critical of formulae that prescribe a set protocol for any given joint or muscular strain, and encourages the use of 'Goodheart's guidelines', described earlier in this chapter, as well as the development of palpation skills that allow for sensing of ease in the tissues, rather than reliance on verbal feedback from the patient as to the current level of discomfort as tissues are being positioned and repositioned.

Reminder about positioning

(see Box 4.3)

Remember that when positioning/fine-tuning the body as a whole or just the part in question (elbow, knee, etc.), it is normally found that tender points on the anterior aspect of the body require flexion, and those on the posterior aspect require extension as a first part of the process of easing pain or excessive tone.

The more lateral the point is from the midline the greater the degree of additional side-bending and/or rotation required to achieve ease.

Notes on prioritizing points for treatment

(see Box 4.5)

When selecting a tender point for use as a monitor in SCS treatment, there are often a confusing number of possibilities. The consensus among clinicians (McPartland & Klofat 1995) experienced in the use of SCS is that choice should be based on the following priorities:

- First, the most sensitive point found in the area with the largest accretion of tender points should be treated.
- If there are a number of similarly tender points, the most proximal and/or medial of these should be chosen.
- If there exists an apparent 'line' of points, one close to the centre of the chain should be chosen to 'represent' the others.
- Clinical experience suggests that no more than five points should be treated at any one session to avoid adaptive overload, and that one treatment weekly is usually adequate.

These 'guidelines' are based on experience rather than research.

An example might be where tender points of similar intensity are noted in the low back as well as the hip region. A point in the low back would receive primary attention (i.e. the most proximal point treated first). However, if tender points were found in the low back and hip, but the hip point was more sensitive, this would receive primary attention (i.e. most sensitive point treated first). If a row of points was noted between the low back and the hip and these were equally sensitive, the most central point in the row would receive primary attention (i.e. treat middle of a line of points first).

Notes on patient feedback

In order to have instant feedback as to the degree of pain/sensitivity/discomfort being felt as the tender point is palpated, it is useful to ask the patient to 'grade' the pain out of 10 (0 = no pain) and to give frequent reports as to the 'value' of the pain being noted during the process of fine-tuning.

A reduction to a score of 2 or 3 (approximately 70% reduction in pain) is regarded as adequate to achieve the release required.

In the USA, a method commonly suggested is to say to the patient, *'The amount of pain you feel when I press this point is a dollar's worth. I want you to tell me when there is only 30 cents worth of pain'.*

Whichever approach is chosen, it is important to instruct the patient that a conversation is not what is needed, but simple indications as to the benefits or otherwise, in terms of pain felt in the point being palpated and monitored, of the various changes in position that are being made.

Continued on p. 75

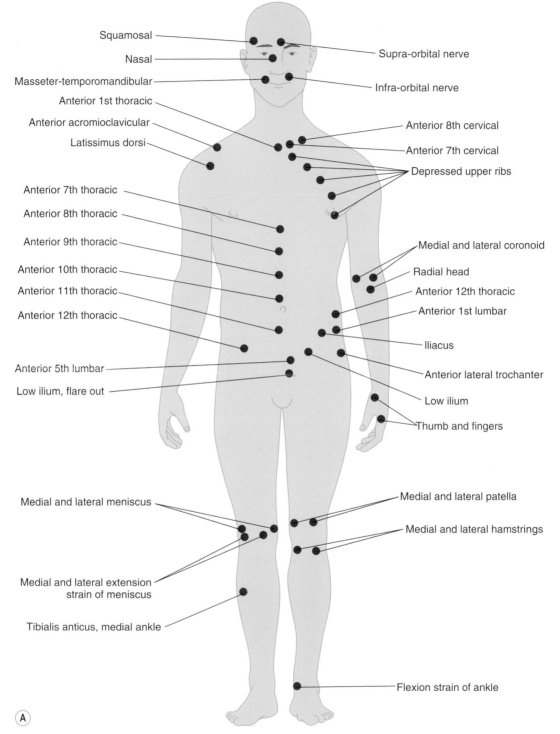

Figure 4.4 Note that although the most likely location of tender points may be bilateral they are shown on only one side of the body in these illustrations. The point locations are approximate, and vary within the indicated area, depending upon the specific mechanics and tissues associated with the particular trauma or strain, according to Jones.

(A) Common locations of Jones's tender points on the anterior body surface, commonly relating to flexion strains.

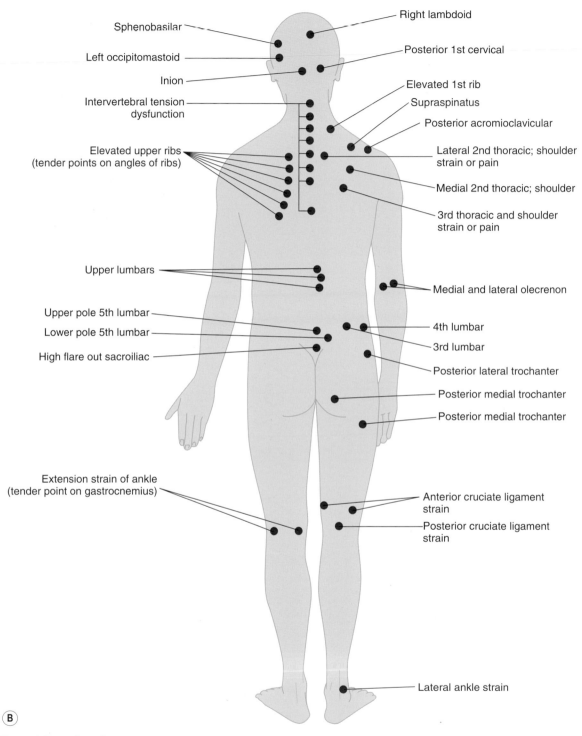

Sphenobasilar
Left occipitomastoid
Inion
Intervertebral tension dysfunction
Elevated upper ribs (tender points on angles of ribs)
Upper lumbars
Upper pole 5th lumbar
Lower pole 5th lumbar
High flare out sacroiliac
Extension strain of ankle (tender point on gastrocnemius)

Right lambdoid
Posterior 1st cervical
Elevated 1st rib
Supraspinatus
Posterior acromioclavicular
Lateral 2nd thoracic; shoulder strain or pain
Medial 2nd thoracic; shoulder
3rd thoracic and shoulder strain or pain
Medial and lateral olecrenon
4th lumbar
3rd lumbar
Posterior lateral trochanter
Posterior medial trochanter
Posterior medial trochanter
Anterior cruciate ligament strain
Posterior cruciate ligament strain
Lateral ankle strain

B

Figure 4.4, continued
(B) Common locations of Jones's tender points on the posterior body surface, commonly relating to extension strains.

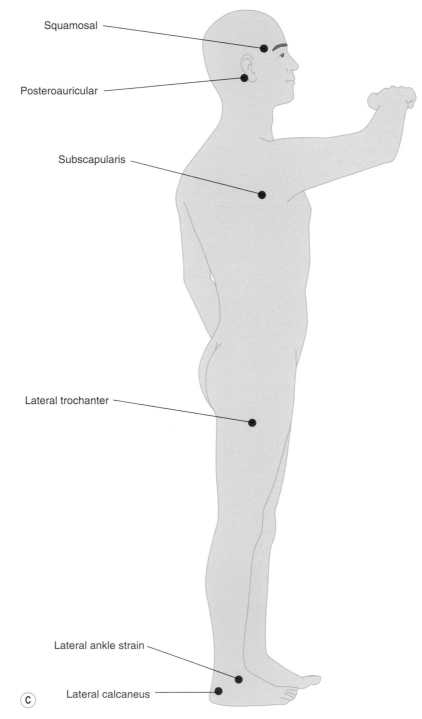

Squamosal

Posteroauricular

Subscapularis

Lateral trochanter

Lateral ankle strain

Lateral calcaneus

(C)

Figure 4.4, continued

(C) Common locations of Jones's tender points on the lateral body surface, commonly relating to strains involving side-flexion or rotation.

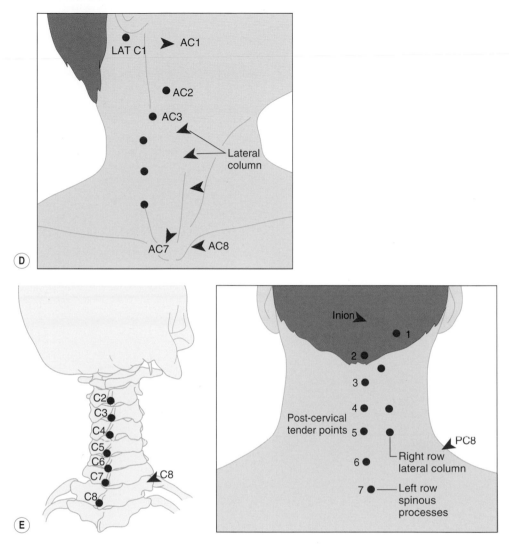

Figure 4.4, continued

(D) Common locations of anterior cervical tender point sites.

(E) Common locations of posterior cervical tender point sites.

Notes on fine-tuning the ease position

A crowding of the tissues to induce slackness in the affected tissues is a usual final aspect of the 'fine-tuning' once initial pain reduction has been achieved.

Additional ease can often be achieved by asking the patient to fully inhale or exhale to evaluate which phase of the breathing cycle reduces pain (or which reduces increased tone) the most.

Eye movements (visual synkinesis) can also be used in this way, always allowing the patient's report of pain levels and/or your palpation of a sense of ease in the tissues to guide you towards the 'comfort zone' (Lewit 1999).

Tips and comments about positioning into ease

1. There should be NO increase in pain elsewhere in the body during the treatment process.
2. It is not necessary to maintain possibly painful pressure on the tender point.

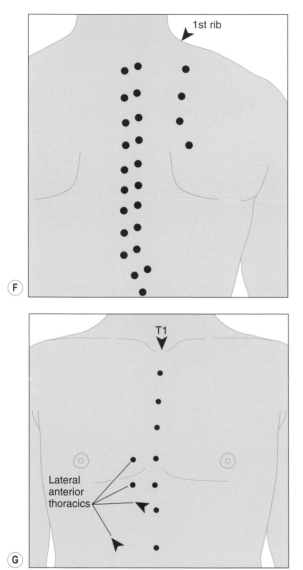

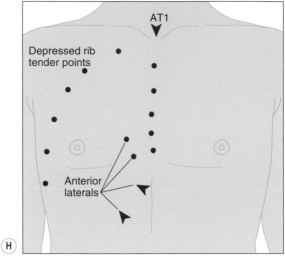

Figure 4.4, continued
(F) Common locations of posterior thoracic spine extension strain tender point sites.
(G) Common locations of anterior thoracic spine flexion strain tender point sites.
(H) Common locations of tender points relating to depressed upper ribs (2–7).

3. Intermittent pressure applied periodically, to evaluate the effects of a change in position in order to ascertain the degree of sensitivity still present, is the preferred Jones method.
4. The amount of time the position of ease should be maintained is discussed in Box 4.4.

After the 90-second hold

- It is necessary for a slow return to be made to the neutral start position, in order to avoid ballistic proprioceptors firing, and restoring the dysfunctional pattern that has just released.

- The patient should be advised to avoid strenuous activity over the following days.
- If the treatment has been helpful, reassessment of the tender point should indicate that a reduction in previous sensitivity of at least 70% has taken place.
- Post-treatment soreness is a common phenomenon and the patient should be warned that this may occur and that it should pass over the next 48 hours or so without further attention.

Advice and choices

The listings that follow in this chapter describe the main sites of tender points relative to particular strain patterns, as identified by Jones (1981), and also give the most usual directions of ease as presented in his writings and teachings. It is suggested that these should not be taken as absolute, for the reasons explained above, and should be used as a starting point in guiding you towards identifying the desired position of ease.

If ease (as judged by pain reduction in the palpated tender point) is not achieved in the position suggested by Jones, then that which emerges by careful fine-tuning is the 'correct' position. The body and its tissues, in other words, are being 'consulted' during the positioning phase, and the answer comes in the form of a reduction in pain in the palpated point.

As will become clear in Chapter 5, which describes functional technique and facilitated positional release, the use of pain in a point as a guide to the state of 'ease' is not the only way of arriving at the point of tissue balance – palpated reduction in 'bind' can be used as an equally clear message from the tissues to indicate that 'ease' is being approached.

Pressure – constant or intermittent?

It is suggested that at times, it may be useful to maintain pressure on the tender point throughout the repositioning process, rather than using the intermittent probing urged by Jones. The reasoning for this is explained in Box 4.6.

Patient's assistance

A final variation worth restating, involves, where convenient, asking the patient to apply pressure to the tender point sufficient to register pain.

In many instances, especially in intercostal areas, this has proved very useful, allowing freedom of movement for the practitioner/therapist as the positioning process is carried out and, in some instances more significantly, allowing pressure to be applied to areas of extreme sensitivity by the patient, when he or she was unable to tolerate practitioner/therapist application of pressure.

Contraindications and indications

There are very few contraindications to the use of SCS, but those that are suggested are listed in Box 4.7.

Box 4.8 lists major indications for the use of SCS (in combination with other modalities or on its own).

What does SCS treatment do?

- Where should treatment start?
- What should be treated first?
- Is there a way of prioritizing areas of dysfunction and choosing 'key' locations for primary attention?

Box 4.7 SCS: contraindications and cautions

- Particular care should be taken in application of SCS in cases of malignancy, aneurysm and acute inflammatory conditions.
- Skin conditions may make application of pressure to the tender point undesirable.
- Protective spasm should not be treated unless the underlying conditions are well considered (osteoporosis, bone secondaries, disc herniation, fractures).
- Recent major trauma or surgery precludes anything other than gentle superficial positional release methods (see later in this chapter for details concerning SCS in hospital settings).
- Infectious conditions call for caution and care.
- Any increase in pain during the process of positioning shows that an undesirable direction, movement or position is being employed.
- Sensations, such as numbness or aching may arise during the holding of the position of ease, and as long as this is moderate and not severe, the patient should be encouraged to relax and view the sensation as transient and part of the desirable changes taking place.
- Caution should be exercised when placing the neck into extension. It is important to maintain verbal communication with the patient at all times and to ask them to keep the eyes open, so that any signs of nystagmus are observable.

The notes on selecting and prioritizing points for treatment given earlier in this chapter (see Box 4.5), as well as the discussion on soft-tissue dysfunction in Chapter 2, should offer some general guidelines as to how and when dysfunctional tissues should be selected for treatment.

The author, to a large extent, works with a model of care that attempts to achieve one of two objectives (and sometimes both) when treating general or local (e.g. soft tissue) dysfunction.

It can be argued that all potentially beneficial therapeutic interventions depend on the manifestation of that benefit on the response of the body and tissues being treated. In other words, the treatment (involving any technique whatsoever) has a catalytic influence, but is of itself not capable of 'curing' anything.

The objectives relating to the two areas of influence, within which all therapeutic interventions operate, can be summarized as follows:

- Reduction of the adaptive load to which the organism as a whole, or the local tissues, are adapting (or failing to adapt), i.e. the objective is to 'lighten the load' and to 'down-regulate' a sensitized nervous system.

- Enhancement of the ability of the organism as a whole, or of the local tissues, to adapt to whatever stress load is being coped with, i.e. the objective is to 'enhance homeostatic self-regulating functions'.

As an additional emphasis: 'Don't make matters worse', by overloading adaptive functions even more.

The decision, therefore, as to which and how many points to treat at a given time using PRT methods, as well as whether to combine this with other methods of treatment, depends on individual characteristics, including age, vulnerability, the chronicity or acuteness of the condition, as well as the specific objectives in the individual case, with all these considerations being related to assessment findings and therapeutic objectives.

Scanning and mapping

Clinicians such as D'Ambrogio & Roth (1997), who have developed a counterstrain variant known as 'positional release therapy' (PRT), argue for a 'scanning evaluation' (SE) that records tender points, as well as their severity, in which the entire body is evaluated.

Just as a postural evaluation will provide a number of pointers that might relate to the patient's symptoms, or the palpation and eliciting of active trigger points might show patterns that explain the pain being experienced by the patient, or testing for shortness, weakness or malcoordination in muscles might correlate with somatic dysfunction, so might a grid or map of areas of tenderness ('tender points') – and their severity – be seen to contribute to the formulation of a plan of therapeutic action.

A major element in this mapping approach is the identification of what have been termed 'dominant tender points' (DTPs), the deactivation of which, it is claimed, can lead to a chain reaction in which less tender areas will normalize. This concept is not dissimilar to that of Simons et al. (1999) who maintain that chains of active trigger points can be 'switched off', if a primary trigger can be identified.

As D'Ambrogio & Roth (1997) explain:

> *Several patients may have the same complaint (e.g. knee pain, shoulder pain, or low back pain) but the source of the condition, as revealed by the scanning evaluation (and the 'dominant tender points'), may be different for each. By identifying the location of key dysfunctions and treating restrictive muscular and fascial barriers, the pain may begin to subside.*

For details of the complex mapping and charting exercise, as recommended by D'Ambrogio & Roth (1997), the reader is referred to their book.

The mapping and charting exercise is a useful procedure, albeit time-consuming; for busy therapists the guidelines offered earlier in this chapter (see Box 4.5) may suffice, and should provide good clinical results.

A number of exercises are described below that offer the reader a chance to experiment with SCS methodology, and to become familiar in a 'hands-on' way with the mechanics of its use. These exercises are followed by a series of descriptions of SCS in clinical use, covering a variety of the muscles and joints of the body.

SCS EXERCISES

1. The SCS 'box' exercise

(Woolbright 1991)

Colonel Jimmie Woolbright (1991), Chief of Aeromedical Services at Maxwell Airforce Base, Alabama, devised a

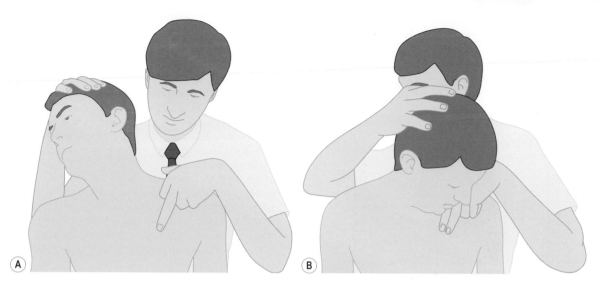

Figure 4.5 (A) The second head/neck position of the 'box' exercise as pain and tissue tension is palpated and monitored (in this instance in the left upper pectoral area). (B) The fourth and final head/neck position of the 'box' exercise as pain and tissue tension is palpated and monitored.

teaching tool that enables SCS skills to be acquired and polished. This is not designed as a treatment protocol but is an excellent means of acquiring a sense of the mechanisms involved.

'Box' exercise guidelines

Note: As the head and neck are positioned during this exercise (Figs 4.5, 4.6), no force at all should be used.

- Each position adopted is not the furthest the tissues can be taken in any given direction but rather it is where the first sign of resistance is noted.
- Thus, an instruction to take the patient/model's head and neck into side-bending and rotation to the right would involve the very lightest of guidance towards that position, with no force and no effort, and no strain or pain being noted by the patient/model.
- As each position described below in this 'box' exercise is achieved, three key elements require consideration:
  1. Is the patient/model comfortable and unstressed by this position? If not, too much effort is being used, or they are not relaxed.
  2. In this position, are the palpated tissues (in this exercise those on the upper left thoracic area) less sensitive to compression pressure in this particular head/neck position?
  3. In this position, are the palpated tissues reducing in palpated tone, feeling more at 'ease', with less evidence of 'bind'?

The information derived by the palpating hand (left hand in this example) should, at the end of the exercise, allow the practitioner/therapist to judge which of the various head/neck positions offered the most 'ease' to the palpated tissues (Fig. 4.5).

It will be found that while only one position of the head and neck (in this particular application of the exercise) offers the greatest reduction in palpated tension or reported pain, there are other secondary positions that also offer some reduction in these two key elements (pain and palpated hypertonicity), just as a number of the positions adopted during application of the 'box' exercise will demonstrably *increase* tension and/or pain.

Woolbright (1991) notes that there are what he terms 'mirror-image' points which are 'directly diagonally across from the anticipated position of release', and that these may at times offer a better position of ease than that designated as the likeliest by virtue of Jones's research.

Method

When the each position is reached you should pause to evaluate the tissue response to the position, as well as inquiring of the patient/model what the 'score' is for the pain/discomfort being produced by the palpating digit. Try to be constantly vigilant to changes in tone as the head and neck move through the sequence of positions around the 'box'.

- The patient/model is seated with the practitioner/therapist standing behind.

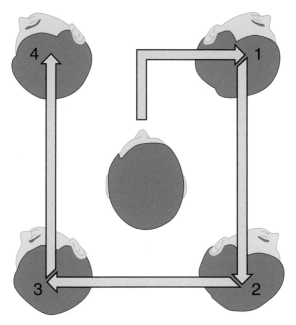

Figure 4.6 Box exercise. The head is taken into four positions: flexion with side-bending and rotation right (1); extension with side-bending and rotation right (2); extension with side-bending and rotation left (3); flexion with side-bending and rotation left (4). As these positions are gently adopted, tenderness and/or tissue tension is monitored.

- The practitioner/therapist's right hand rests **very lightly** on the crown of the patient/model's head (palm on head, fingertips touching forehead, or the hand can be transversely placed on the head so that the heel of the hand is on one side and the fingertips on the other), while the left hand/fingertips palpate an area of tenderness and tension a little below the left clavicle, in the pectoral muscles (Fig. 4.5).
- Sufficient pressure should be applied for a report to be made by the patient/model of discomfort or pain.
- This is given a value of '10' and it is explained that whenever a request is made for the level of pain to be reported, a number (up to '10', where '10' is the greatest pain) should be given.
- The discomfort/pain will change as the head and neck alter their positions, and it is the primary objective of the exercise that you should be able to sense – by virtue of changes in the palpated tension in the tissues – whether the 'score' is going to go up or down.
- As the patient/model exhales, the head should be guided, *with minimal effort*, into flexion and it is then

gently side-flexed and rotated to the right to go to position 1 (Fig. 4.6).

- Pausing momentarily to assess changes in the palpated tissues and/or to obtain feedback as to reduction or otherwise in sensitivity, the practitioner/therapist then takes the head out of right rotation (while maintaining a slight right side-bend) and as the patient inhales, the practitioner/therapist introduces a slight pressure on the brow which allows the head to 'float' up out of flexion and into slight extension.
- When the easy limit of extension is reached, rotation to the right is again introduced taking it to position 2 (Fig. 4.5A, 4.6(2)).
- After a brief pause for evaluation of both tone and reported levels of pain/discomfort, the head is then moved gently to the left, back to a neutral position.
- Next, side-bending and finally some rotation to the left should be introduced, to an easy end-point, as the head comes to rest in position 3, still in slight extension (Fig. 4.6(3)).
- The head/neck is then, after a momentary pause, eased out of left rotation and into flexion (during an exhalation), while left side-bending is maintained.
- Rotation to the left is again introduced as the head/neck comes to rest in flexion, as in position 4 (Figs 4.5B, 4.6(4)).
- Taking the head back to the right and losing the side-bending/rotation at the midline returns it to the starting, neutral, position.
- Continuation to the right past the midline, again introducing flexion side-bending and subsequent rotation to the right, takes it back to position 1.
- The head and neck are moved around the box (as described above) a number of times, in order to assess for any additional relaxation (or increased bind) in the tissues under the palpating and monitoring hand.
- It is useful to try to note whether additional assistance to the process can be gained by having the patient/model, with eyes closed, 'look' up or down or sideways in the direction in which the head is moving, as it moves.
- Very often, experimenting with eye movements in this way allows for increased ease to be achieved, if the direction in which the eyes are looking is synchronized with the direction of movement.
- It is suggested that the practitioner/therapist can make the process of moving the model/patient around the box more fluid by duplicating the movements of the patient's eyes and breathing, as well as by leaning in the direction, and at

the speed, of the movement that the patient is being directed to follow, by the hand on the head.

- The whole exercise should be repeated a number of times (with different people) until the practitioner/therapist feels comfortable in using the 'box' approach to palpation of a specific tender point – noting the changes in tissue tone and reported discomfort under the listening/monitoring/palpating hand/finger.

- When palpating a posterior (extension) tender point, the 'box' should be entered from neutral by first going into extension (on inhalation) with the addition of side-bending and rotation towards the side of the tender point followed by progressing around the box.

- When palpating an anterior (flexion) tender point, the 'box' should be entered from neutral by flexing the head/neck (on exhalation) and then side-bending and rotating away from the side being palpated, before progressing around the box.

Note: Before continuing with this series of exercises and clinical treatment protocols, it is suggested that you review all the text boxes of information in this chapter, particularly Box 4.3 (Counterstrain positioning guidelines), which describes the general guidelines regarding positioning, derived from the clinical experience of Jones and many others, including the author.

2. SCS cervical flexion exercise

- The patient/model is supine and the practitioner/therapist sits or stands at the head of the table.

- An area of local dysfunction is sought using an appropriate form of palpation, such as a 'feather-light', single-finger, stroking touch on the skin areas overlying the tips of the transverse processes of the cervical spine.

- Using this method, a feeling of 'drag' is being sought for, which indicates increased sudomotor (sympathetic) activity and therefore a likely site of dysfunction, local or reflexively induced (Lewit 1999), as described in Chapter 2.

- When drag is noted, light compression is introduced to identify and establish a point of sensitivity, a tender point, which in this area represents (based on Jones's findings) an anterior (forward-bending) strain site.

- The patient is instructed in the method required for reporting a reduction in pain during the positioning sequence which follows.

- The author's approach is to say, 'I want you to score the pain caused by my pressure, before we start moving your head (in this example) as a "10" and to

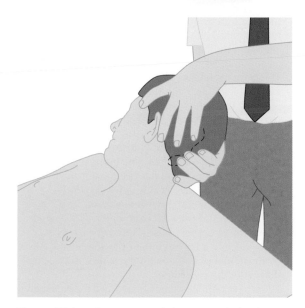

Figure 4.7 Learning to use strain/counterstrain for the treatment of a cervical flexion strain.

not speak apart from giving me the present score (out of 10) whenever I ask for it'.

- The aim is to achieve a reported score of 3 or less before ceasing the positioning process.

- In the example illustrated in Figure 4.7, an area of sensitivity/pain will have been located just anterior to the tip of a transverse process, on the right, and this is being palpated and monitored by the practitioner/therapist's right thumb.

- The head/neck is then taken lightly into flexion until some degree of ease is achieved based on the score reported by the patient. At this stage of the process this is being constantly compressed.

- When a reduction of the pain score of around 50% is achieved, fine-tuning is commenced, introducing a very small degree of additional positioning (side-flexion, rotation, etc.) in order to find the position of maximum ease, at which time the reported 'score' should be reduced by at least 70%.

- Remember that in Box 4.3, the guidelines for SCS suggest that anteriorly situated pain requires (as a rule, but not always) flexion, together with side-flexion and rotation toward the side of pain.

- Once relative 'ease' has been achieved, the patient may be asked to inhale fully and exhale fully, while observing for changes in the level of pain, in order to evaluate which phase of the cycle reduces it still more.

- The phase of the breathing cycle in which the individual senses the greatest reduction in sensitivity is maintained for a period that is tolerable (holding the breath in or out or at some point between the two extremes), while the overall position of ease continues to be maintained, and the tender/tense area monitored.

- This position of ease is held for 90 seconds in Jones's methodology, although there exist mechanisms for reducing this, which will be explained later in this chapter.
- During the holding of the position of ease, the direct compression can be reduced to a mere touching of the point, along with a periodic probing to establish that the position of ease has been maintained.
- After 90 seconds, the neck/head is very slowly returned to the neutral starting position. This slow return to neutral is a vital component of SCS, since the neural receptors (muscle spindles) may be provoked into a return to their previously dysfunctional state if a rapid movement is made at the end of the procedure.
- The tender point/area may be retested for sensitivity at this time and should be found to be considerably less hypertonic.

3. SCS cervical extension exercise

- With the patient/model in the supine position and with the head clear of the end of the table, fully supported by the practitioner/therapist, areas of localized tenderness are sought by light palpation alongside or over the tips of the spinous processes of the cervical spine.
- When a point that is unusually tender is located, compression is applied to elicit a degree of sensitivity or pain.
- The model/patient is asked to ascribe a score of '10' to this tenderness.
- The head/neck is then very slowly taken into light extension, along with side-bending and rotation, as in (Fig. 4.8) (usually away from the side of the pain – see guidelines for positioning in Box 4.3), until a reduction of at least 50% is achieved in the reported sensitivity.
- The compression can be constant or intermittent, with the latter being preferable, if sensitivity is great.
- Once a reduction in sensitivity of at least 70% has been achieved, inhalation and exhalation are monitored by the patient/model to see which phase reduces sensitivity even more, and this is maintained for a comfortable period.
- If intermittent compression of the point is being used, this needs to be applied periodically during the 90-second holding period, in order to ensure that the position of ease has been maintained.
- After 90 seconds, a very slow and deliberate return to neutral is performed and the patient is rested for several minutes.

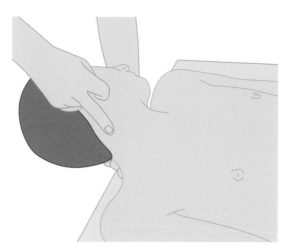

Figure 4.8 Learning to use strain/counterstrain for the treatment of a cervical extension strain.

- The tender point should be re-palpated for sensitivity, which may have reduced markedly, as should excessive hypertonicity in the surrounding tissues.

4. SCS 'tissue tension' exercise

(Chaitow 1990)

- SCS exercises 2 and 3 should be performed again; however, this time, instead of relying on feedback from the patient as to the degree of sensitivity being experienced in the tender point and using this feedback as the guide which takes the practitioner/ therapist towards the ideal position of ease, the practitioner/therapist's own palpation of the tissues and their movement towards ease becomes the guide.
- A light contact should be maintained on the previously treated tender point, while positioning of the head and neck is carried out, to achieve maximum 'ease'.
- Ideally, a final position should be achieved which closely approximates the position in which reduction of the pain was achieved in the previous exercises.
- This is an exercise that begins a process of palpatory skill acquisition and enhancement, which will be carried further in exercises involving functional technique described in Chapter 5.

5. SCS exercise involving compression

- Exercises 1, 2 and 3 should be performed again, but this time when pain/sensitivity and/or hypertonicity have reduced by 70% by means of positioning, and after the breathing element has been carried out to aid this process, a light degree of 'crowding' or compression is introduced by means of pressure onto the crown of the head through the long axis of the spine.

- No more than 1 lb (0.5 kg) of pressure – more often usually less than half of that – should be involved.
- This can be achieved by use of pressure from the practitioner/therapist's abdomen, or from the hands that are holding and supporting the neck and head.
- This additional element of crowding/slackening the tissues should not increase the sensitivity from the palpated point or cause pain anywhere else.
- If the addition of crowding does cause any additional pain/discomfort, it should be abandoned.
- The more usual response is for the patient to report an even greater degree of pain relief, and for the practitioner/therapist to sense greater 'ease' in the palpated tissues.
- This addition of crowding to the procedures reduces the time required during which the position of ease needs to be held, and mimics a major feature of facilitated positional release (FPR, see Chapter 5).
- The time-scale for SCS when crowding is a feature is commonly given as between 5 and 20 seconds.

These first five exercises – starting with the 'box' exercise – offer an initial opportunity to become familiar with SCS methodology.

The skills that should be enhanced by use of these exercises include:

1. A greater sense of the delicacy of the SCS process.
2. The ability to locate tender points and, depending on their location, to be able to position the area into flexion plus fine-tuning (anterior aspect) or extension plus fine-tuning (posterior aspect) until sensitivity reduces, or palpated tone reduces, by at least 70%.
3. A sense of the changes that occur in response to light 'crowding' of the tissues once they have been taken into their initial ease position.

Before moving on to a series of clinically useful examples of SCS, two more exercises will be described, and should be practised.

These involve:

- A low back exercise (exercise 6).
- A small joint (elbow) exercise (exercise 7).

In both of these, processes such as those used in the 'box' exercise (above) will be described.

Note that, although these are 'training exercises', meant to familiarize you with SCS assessment and treatment

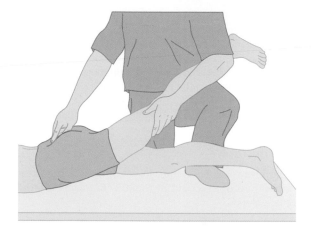

Figure 4.9 SCS low back/lower limb exercise.

methodology, they are in fact perfectly usable in clinical settings to treat the areas being focussed upon.

These are authentic SCS protocols.

6. SCS low back/lower limb exercise

- With the patient prone, one of the lower limbs can be used as a 'handle' with which to modify tone and tension and/or tenderness in the low back, as an area of this is palpated (Fig. 4.9).
- The practitioner palpates an area of the lumbar musculature as a systematic evaluation is carried out of the effects of moving the *ipsilateral* and then the *contralateral* limb into (slight) extension, adduction and internal rotation.
- Once the effects of these different positions have been assessed, take the limb to a neutral position and introduce abduction and external rotation, while still in extension.
- A further experiment to assess the effects on low back tenderness (palpating a tender point) and hypertonicity should involve taking the abducted limb into flexion (over the edge of the table) and then introducing external rotation.
- Following this, with the hip still in flexion, remove the rotation and take the limb into adduction and, at its easy end-of-range, introduce a little internal rotation.
- In this way, an approximation of a 'box' movement will have been created while a low back area is palpated for changes in perceived pain or modifications of tone.
- Assess which positions offer the greatest ease in low back areas as this sequence is repeated several times.

- Evaluate whether greater influence is noted in the tissues being palpated when the ipsilateral or contralateral leg is employed as a lever.
- Repeat these processes but this time, at the end of the fine-tuning, add long-axis compression, by easing the limb towards the pelvis using no more than 1 lb (0.5 kg) of pressure.
- Evaluate the effects of this on tenderness and tone.

Best position?

According to SCS theory and clinical experience, the likeliest positions of 'ease' will be found with the *contralateral leg in extension*.

Other variables will influence which parts of the low back eases most when the limb is adducted or abducted, and internally or externally rotated. Refer to Box 4.3, which provides the model that should produce optimal results.

As the limb is eased into extension (but only a very small amount – avoiding hyperextension of the spine), and is adducted and slightly rotated, a tender point on the *right low back area* would be placed into its greatest degree of ease when there is:

- extension of the contralateral (left) leg
- adduction of that limb (so rotating the lumbar spine slightly to the left, i.e. away from the side of palpated pain on the right side of the posterior aspect of the patient)
- some fine-turning involving rotation of the limb one way or the other to achieve 70% reduction in tenderness or tone
- long-axis compression.

7. SCS upper limb (elbow) exercise

- The concept and methodology of the 'box' exercise can be used to introduce a series of movements, while palpating tenderness and tension in the lateral epicondyle area.
- The patient lies supine while one hand palpates an area of tenderness on the lateral epicondyle.
- The other hand holds the wrist as the elbow is placed into extension with side-bending and rotation towards the side of the palpated tender point (i.e. externally rotated).
- Assess changes of palpated tone and reported pain with the arm in this position, and then introduce side-bending and rotation internally (still in extension).
- Now introduce flexion, and while in flexion assess the changes in palpated tone and reported discomfort and then introduce first internal and then external rotation with side-bending to assess

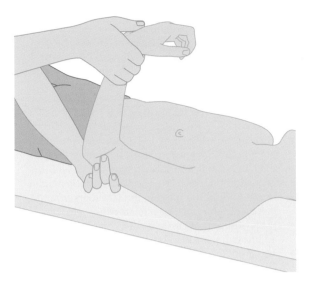

Figure 4.10 The lateral epicondyle is palpated as various positions of the lower arm (flexion, extension, rotation) are introduced to evaluate their influence on the palpated tissues.

changes in reported sensitivity, and changes in tissue tone.
- Identify the position in which the greatest reduction in tone and sensitivity is achieved.
- Then introduce long-axis compression, from the wrist towards the elbow, using no more than a few ounces (grams) of pressure (Fig. 4.10).

The most probable position of ease for an anterior lateral epicondyle tender point is flexion with side-bending and external rotation. However, as in all tender points, the particular mechanisms involved in the dysfunctional strain pattern can make such predictions inaccurate. In the end, it is the position that achieves the maximum degree of ease which is likely to produce the most beneficial effects.

This and the previous exercises offer a useful starting point for anyone new to SCS.

SCS TECHNIQUES

Much of the remainder of this chapter comprises descriptions of recommended protocols for the treatment of many of the joints and muscles of the body.

Some descriptions are derived from the work of Jones (1981), while others are either modifications developed by the author or are modifications of protocols described by Deig (2001) or D'Ambrogio & Roth (1997).

The descriptions of these clinical applications of SCS will follow a descending pathway, starting at the neck and working inferiorly to the feet (with the exception of descriptions of cranial and temporomandibular joint (TMJ) methods that can be located in Chapter 5).

Cervical flexion strains

(see Fig. 4.4D)

Anterior strain of C1:

- The tender point for anterior strain in a C1 joint is found in a groove between the styloid process and angle of the jaw.
- Treatment usually involves rotation of the head of the supine patient away from the side of dysfunction, either maintaining pressure or repetitively probing Jones's point (Fig. 4.11).
- Fine-tuning is usually by side-flexing away from the painful side.

An alternative or second point for C1 flexion strain lies ½ inch (1 cm) anterior to the angle of the mandible. This is usually treated by introducing flexion and rotation, approximately 45° away from the side of pain.

Remaining *cervical anterior (flexion) strain tender points* are located on or about the tips of the transverse processes of the involved vertebrae (Fig. 4.12).

- These spinal segments are usually treated by positioning into forward-bending and rotation, to remove pain from the tender point.

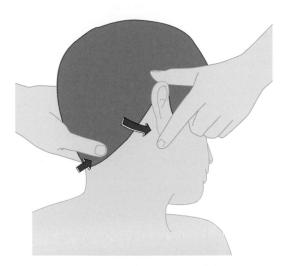

Figure 4.11 First cervical flexion strain tender point commonly lies between the styloid process and the angle of the jaw. A likely position of ease is as illustrated. However, alternative positions of ease can sometimes involve movement of the head and neck into different positions.

- In general, the more cephalad the palpated tender point the more rotation away from it is needed in fine-tuning (Fig. 4.12A).
- The more caudad the point the more flexion, and the less rotation, is usually required.

Note: Whenever the suggestion is given that rotation should be towards the tender point, this is the *likeliest* beneficial direction that will take the area towards ease; however, if this fails to achieve results, it is quite possible that rotation away from the side of pain would provide greater ease.

In the end, each strain pattern is unique, and while guidelines as to likely directions of positioning are usually accurate, this is not always so, and the feedback from palpated tissues and the patient is the true guideline.

Cervical side-flexion strains

Tender points relating to side-flexion strains of the cervical spine are located as follows:

- for C1 side-flexion restriction – tip of transverse process of C1
- for C2–C6 side-flexion restriction – on the lateral aspects of the articular processes, close to the spinous process (Fig. 4.13).

Treatment involves pressure being applied to the tender point and side-flexion *towards or away from* the side being treated, depending on the tissue response and patient's reports as to pain levels.

Fine-tuning might involve slight increase in flexion, extension or rotation.

Clinical tip: Do not forget to use drag palpation in order to *rapidly* identify localized areas of dysfunction (hyperalgesic skin zones) – as described in Chapter 2.

Suboccipital strains

(see Fig. 4.4B,E)

The tender points associated with upper cervical/suboccipital strains are located on the occiput, or in the muscles attaching to it, such as rectus capitis anterior, obliquus capitis superior and rectus capitis posterior major and minor.

Treatment involves either localizing cranial flexion or cranial extension to the C1 area, while applying precisely focussed flexion or extension procedures that markedly reduce the tenderness from the palpated tender point.

For example:

- If a tender point is located on rectus capitis anterior, just medial to the insertion of semispinalis capitis, inferior to the posterior occipital protuberance, it is said by Jones (1981) to relate to flexion strain of the region.

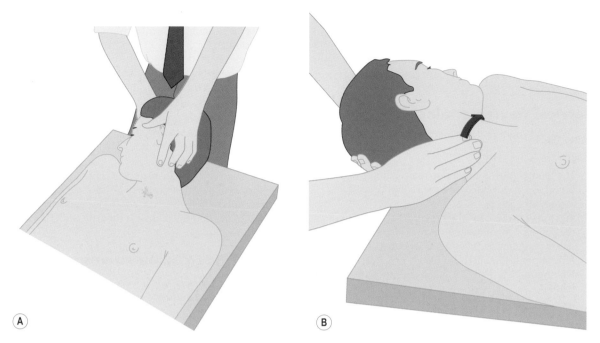

A   B

Figure 4.12 (A,B) A flexion strain of a mid to lower cervical vertebra, with the tender point close to the tip of a transverse process. The position of ease is often as illustrated – flexed and rotated away from the side of palpated pain – however, as noted in the text, alternative positioning may be called for.

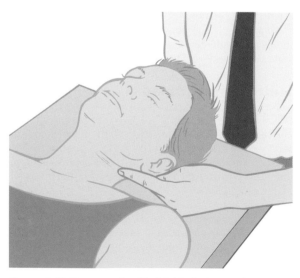

Figure 4.13 Treatment for C2–C6 side-flexion strain.

- The ease position involves localized flexion of the suboccipital region.
- The patient is supine with the practitioner seated or standing at the head of the table.
- One hand palpates the tender point while simultaneously applying light distraction to the occiput, in a cephalad direction.
- The other hand rests on the frontal bone and applies *light* caudad pressure, inducing upper cervical flexion, bringing the chin close to the trachea (Fig. 4.14), until an appropriate tissue response is noted, accompanied by a reduction in perceived tenderness.
- Fine-tuning may also be required, possibly involving rotation towards and side-flexion away from the treated side.

Alternatively:

- If a tender point is located on obliquus capitis superior, approximately 1.5 cm medial to the mastoid process, it is said by Jones (1981) to relate to an extension strain of the region.
- The ease position involves localized extension of the tissues.
- The patient is supine and the practitioner is at the head of the table with one hand supporting the

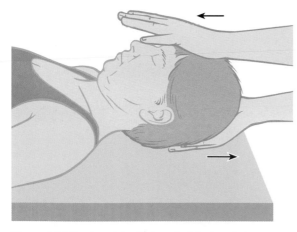

Figure 4.14 Treatment for first cervical flexion strain.

head, and with one finger of that hand localizing the tender point (Fig. 4.15).
- The other hand is on the crown of the head applying light pressure to induce upper cervical extension (as the occiput extends on C1).
- This position, together with fine-tuning involving side-flexion and/or rotation, should establish the position of ease.

Or:

- If a tender point is located on the occiput (when cephalad and medial pressure is applied), just lateral to the insertion of semispinalis capitis, or on the superior surface of the second cervical transverse process, the dysfunctional tissues may involve rectus capitis posterior major or minor (commonly traumatized through whiplash injuries or stressed through a forward-head posture).
- The ease positions for either point involve upper cervical extension.
- The treatment position is almost identical to that suggested in the previous description (Fig. 4.15).

Other cervical extension strains

These tender points are found on or about the spinous processes (see Fig. 4.4D).

Treatment should commence by introduction of increased extension.

- Extension strains in the lower cervical and upper thoracic areas are usually treated by taking the pain out of the palpated tender point, by means of extension of the head on the neck.

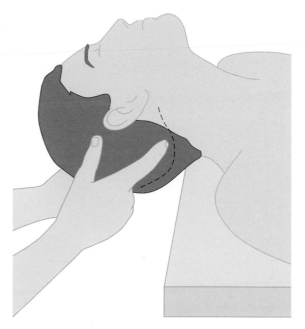

Figure 4.15 First cervical extension strain. The position of ease requires extension of the neck and (usually) rotation away from the side of pain.

- In a bed-bound patient, the patient lies on the side with the painful side uppermost, so that fine-tuning can be accomplished by means of slight side-bending and rotation towards the side of the dysfunction (Fig. 4.16A). (See Chapter 6 for Schwartz's (1986) suggestions regarding treating these points in a bed-bound patient.)
- Exceptions to the positioning suggestions given above include those applying to C3/4 extension strains, which can usually be treated in either flexion or extension.
- C8 extension strain may also need to be treated in slight extension, with marked side-bending and rotation away from, rather than towards, the side of strain (C8 point lies on the transverse process of C7).

Extension strains of the lower cervical and upper thoracic spine

(see Fig. 4.4B,E)

The patient should be prone. Jones states:

> *The head is supported by the doctor's left hand holding the chin. The practitioner/therapist's left forearm is held along the right side of the patient's*

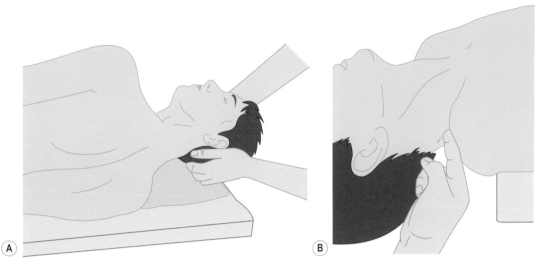

Figure 4.16 (A,B) Extension strains of the lower cervical and upper thoracic spine usually require extension and slight side-bending, and rotation away from the painful side.

head for better support. The right hand monitors tender points on the right side of the spinous processes. The forces applied are mostly extension, with slight side-bending and rotation left (Fig. 4.16B).

The tender points of the posterior thorax are located interspinally, paraspinally and at the rib angles, when there exist extension dysfunctions of intervertebral joints, side-bending dysfunction and ribs that are more comfortable when elevated.

The simplicity of Jones's methods is obvious.

- The shortened fibres relate to the areas where tender points are to be found, and the positioning is such as to increase the already existing shortening, while palpating the tender point(s).
- 90 seconds of holding the position of ease is suggested.
- The skill required lies in locating and localizing the tender point, and identifying and duplicating the nature of the original strain or injury.
- There are few exceptions to Jones's directions in this region, for extension strains.

Treating bed-bound patients

Recommendations for use of SCS methodology in hospital or home (bed-bound) situations, are given in Chapter 6, where additional functional approaches that may be useful for fragile patients, or in acute situations, are also outlined.

Clinical tip: Be aware that it is commonly necessary to use alternative positions to achieve ease, if the directions given in this text fail to produce ease and relief from pain in the tender point.

The Spencer shoulder sequence protocol

Note: The Spencer sequence is extremely useful clinically as either an assessment or a treatment approach.

It should be obvious that instead of positional release methods, as described below, muscle energy techniques (MET), or other modalities can also be used to good effect.

The Spencer sequence derives from osteopathic medicine in the early years of the 20th century (Spencer 1916), and is taught at all osteopathic colleges in the USA. Over the years it has been modified to include treatment elements other than the original intent to achieve articulation and mobilization.

Research evidence

(Knebl 2002)

A study involved 29 elderly patients with pre-existing shoulder problems. The patients were randomly assigned to a Spencer sequence osteopathic treatment or a control group.

The placebo group were placed in the same seven positions as those receiving the active treatment, but without MET ('corrective force') as part of the protocol.

Over 14 weeks, there were a total of eight 30-minute treatment sessions, during which time both groups demonstrated significantly increased ranges of motion and a decrease in perceived pain. However, following the end of the treatment period: 'Those subjects who had received OMT demonstrated continued improvement in ranges of motion, while that of the placebo group decreased'.

Choice

What has become clear in clinical practice is that the Spencer sequences, can not only be transformed from assessment and articulation into a muscle energy approach, but also into a positional release (SCS or functional) method, as the situation demands.

One key factor that would determine the choice of using articulation, and/or MET and/or SCS, would be the relative acuteness of the condition, and the relative sensitivity of the patient. The more acute, and the more fragile and sensitive the individual, the more the choice would tilt towards SCS or functional positional release methodology.

Spencer sequence method

A number of the Spencer positions are described below (shoulder flexion, extension, internal rotation, circumduction – with compression and with distraction, as well as adduction and abduction).

Note: There is no specific description of external rotation of the shoulder in these notes, although this movement is a part of the adduction sequence.

Method

(Patriquin 1992)

- When assessing and treating the shoulder, the scapula is fixed firmly to the thoracic wall to focus humeral movement to the glenoid fossa, as a variety of movements are introduced.
- In all Spencer assessment and treatment sequences, the patient is side-lying, with the side to be assessed uppermost, arm lying at the side with the elbow (usually) flexed.
- In all assessments, the practitioner stands facing the patient, at chest level or, if preferred, stands behind the side-lying patient.

Assessment and PRT treatment of shoulder extension restriction

- The practitioner's cephalad hand cups the shoulder, firmly compressing the scapula and clavicle to the thorax while the patient's flexed elbow is held by the practitioner's caudad hand, as the arm is taken into passive extension towards the optimal 90° (Fig. 4.17).

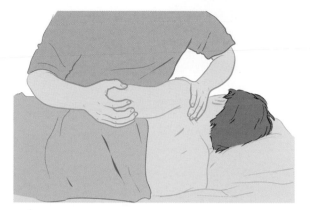

Figure 4.17 Spencer sequence treatment of shoulder extension restriction.

- Any restriction in range of motion is noted, ceasing movement *at the first indication of resistance* or if any pain is reported resulting from the movement.
- When restriction is noted during movement towards extension of the shoulder joint, the soft tissues implicated in maintaining this dysfunction could be the shoulder flexors – anterior deltoid, coracobrachialis and the clavicular head of pectoralis major.
- Palpation of these (using drag or other evaluation methods) should reveal areas of marked tenderness.
- The most painful tender point (painful to digital pressure) elicited by palpation is then used as a monitoring point.
- Digital pressure on the point, sufficient to allow the patient to give this a value of '10', is followed by the arm being moved into a position that reduces that pain by not less than 70% – without creating any additional pain elsewhere.
- This position of ease usually involves some degree of flexion and fine-tuning to slacken the muscle housing the tender point.
- This ease state should be held for 90 seconds (or less if compression is added), before a slow return to neutral and a subsequent re-evaluation of the range of motion.

Assessment and PRT treatment of shoulder flexion restriction

- The patient has the arm lying alongside the trunk, with the practitioner holding the wrist/forearm with one hand, while the other hand stabilizes the scapula and clavicle firmly to the chest wall.
- The practitioner slowly introduces passive shoulder flexion in the horizontal plane, as range of motion toward 180° is assessed, by which time the elbow is fully extended (Fig. 4.18).

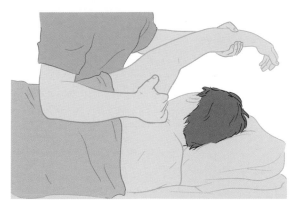

Figure 4.18 Spencer sequence treatment of shoulder flexion restriction, showing the position towards the end of range of motion assessment.

- At the very first indication of restriction (or a report of pain as a result of the flexion movement) the movement should cease.
- When a restriction towards flexion of the shoulder joint is noted, the soft tissues implicated in maintaining this dysfunction would probably be the shoulder extensors – posterior deltoid, teres major, latissimus dorsi, and possibly infraspinatus, teres minor and/or long head of triceps.
- Palpation of these (drag palpation or any other appropriate method) should reveal areas of marked tenderness.
- The most painful tender point (painful to digital pressure) elicited by palpation should then be used as a monitoring point by application of digital pressure that the patient registers as having a 'value' of '10'.
- The arm is then moved into a position that reduces the tender point pain by not less than 70%.
- This position of ease will probably involve some degree of extension and fine-tuning to slacken the muscle housing the tender point.
- This ease state should be held for 90 seconds (or less if compression is added) before a slow return to neutral and a subsequent re-evaluation of range of motion.

Shoulder articulation and assessment of circumduction capability with compression or distraction

- The patient is side-lying with elbow flexed while the practitioner's cephalad hand cups the shoulder firmly, compressing the scapula and clavicle to the thorax (Fig. 4.19).
- The practitioner's caudad hand grasps the elbow and takes the shoulder through a slow clockwise (and subsequently an anticlockwise) circumduction, while

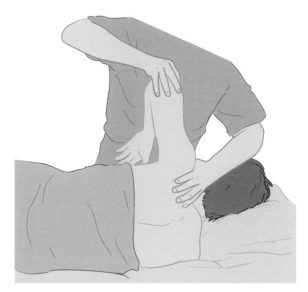

Figure 4.19 Spencer sequence assessment of circumduction capability with compression.

adding compression through the long axis of the humerus.
- Subsequently, the same assessment is made with light distraction being applied.
- If restriction or pain is noted in either of the sequences involving circumduction of the shoulder joint (clockwise and anticlockwise, utilizing compression or distraction), evaluate which muscles would be active if precisely the opposite movement were undertaken.
- For example, if on compression and clockwise rotation, a particular part of the circumduction range involves either restriction or discomfort/pain, cease the movement and evaluate which muscles would be required to contract in order to produce an active reversal of that movement (Chaitow 1996; Jones 1981; Walther 1988).
- In these antagonist muscles, palpate for the most 'tender' point and use this as a monitoring point as the structures are taken to a position of ease which reduces the perceived pain, or increased tone, by at least 70%.
- This is held for 90 seconds (or less if compression is added) before a slow return to neutral, and retesting.

Assessment and PRT treatment of shoulder abduction restriction

- The patient is side-lying as the practitioner cups the shoulder and compresses the scapula and clavicle to the thorax with his cephalad hand, while cupping the flexed elbow with his caudad hand.

- This position of ease will probably involve some degree of adduction and internal or external rotation, to slacken the muscle housing the tender point.
- This ease state should be held for 90 seconds (or less if compression is added), before a slow return to neutral and a subsequent re-evaluation of range of motion.

Assessment and PRT treatment of shoulder adduction (and external rotation) restriction

- The patient is side-lying and the practitioner cups the shoulder and compresses the scapula and clavicle to the thorax with his cephalad hand, while cupping the elbow with his caudad hand.
- The patient's hand is supported on the practitioner's cephalad forearm/wrist to stabilize the arm.
- The elbow is taken in an arc, anterior to the chest, so that the elbow moves both cephalad and medially as the shoulder adducts and externally rotates.
- The action is performed slowly and any signs of resistance, or discomfort, are noted.
- If there is a restriction towards adduction of the shoulder joint, the soft tissues implicated in maintaining this dysfunction would be the shoulder abductors – deltoid, supraspinatus.
- Since external rotation is also involved, other muscles implicated in restriction or pain may include internal rotators, such as subscapularis, pectoralis major, latissimus dorsi and teres major.
- Palpation of these, using drag palpation or another suitable method, should reveal areas of marked tenderness.
- The most painful tender point (painful to digital pressure) elicited by palpation should be used as a monitoring point.
- Apply digital pressure sufficient to allow the patient to ascribe a value of '10' to the discomfort.
- Then slowly move the arm into a position which reduces the tender point pain by not less than 70%.
- This position of ease will probably involve some degree of abduction together with fine-tuning involving internal rotation, to slacken the muscle housing the tender point.
- This ease state should be held for 90 seconds (or less if compression is added) before a slow return to neutral and a subsequent re-evaluation of range of motion.

Assessment and PRT treatment of internal rotation restriction of the shoulder

- The patient is side-lying and the arm is flexed in order to evaluate whether the dorsum of the hand can be painlessly placed against the dorsal surface of the ipsilateral lumbar area (Fig. 4.21).
- This arm position is maintained throughout the procedure.

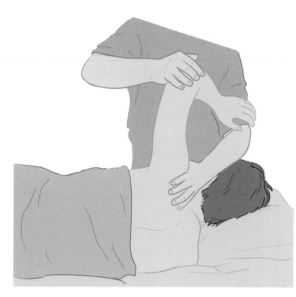

Figure 4.20 Spencer sequence assessment and treatment of shoulder abduction restriction.

- The patient's hand is supported on the practitioner's cephalad forearm/wrist to stabilize the arm (Fig. 4.20).
- The elbow is abducted towards the patient's head as range of motion (and/or discomfort relating to the movement) is assessed.
- Some degree of external rotation is also involved in this abduction.
- Pain-free easy abduction should be close to 180°.
- Note any restriction in range of motion, or report of pain/discomfort on movement.
- At the position of very first indication of resistance or pain, the movement is stopped.
- If there is a restriction towards abduction of the shoulder joint, the soft tissues implicated in maintaining this dysfunction would be the shoulder adductors – pectoralis major, teres major, latissimus dorsi, and possibly the long head of triceps, coracobrachialis, short head of biceps brachii.
- Palpation of these muscles (using drag palpation or another appropriate method) should reveal areas of marked tenderness.
- The most painful tender point (painful to digital pressure) elicited by this palpation should be used as a monitoring point by applied digital pressure, sufficient to allow the patient to ascribe a value of '10' to it.
- The arm is then moved and fine-tuned into a position that reduces the tender point pain by not less than 70%.

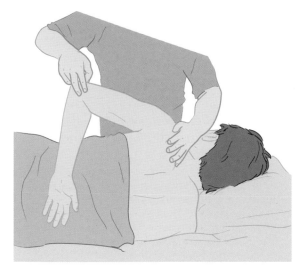

Figure 4.21 Spencer sequence assessment and treatment of internal rotation restriction.

- The practitioner cups the shoulder and compresses the scapula and clavicle to the thorax with his cephalad hand, while cupping the flexed elbow with the caudad hand.
- The practitioner slowly brings the elbow (ventrally) anteriorly, and notes any sign of restriction or reported pain resulting from the movement, as increasing internal rotation of the shoulder joint, proceeds.
- At the position of the very first indication of resistance, or reported pain, movement is stopped.
- If there is a restriction towards internal rotation, the soft tissues implicated in maintaining this dysfunction would be the shoulder external rotators – infraspinatus and teres minor – with posterior deltoid also possibly being involved.
- Palpation of these, using drag or other suitable assessment methods, should reveal areas of marked tenderness.
- The most painful tender point (painful to digital pressure) elicited by palpation should be used as a monitoring point.
- Digital pressure to the point should be sufficient to allow the patient to ascribe a value of '10' to the discomfort.
- The arm should then be moved into a position that reduces the tender point pain by not less than 70%.
- This position of ease will probably involve some degree of external rotation to slacken the muscle housing the tender point.
- This ease state should be held for 90 seconds (or less if compression is added) before a slow return to neutral and a subsequent re-evaluation of range of motion.

Note: All Spencer assessments should be performed passively in a controlled, slow, manner.

Specific muscle dysfunction – SCS applications

The description of SCS treatment methods for those muscles described below should be seen as representative, rather than comprehensive.

It is assumed that once the basic principles of SCS application have been understood, and the exercise methods already described in this chapter have been practised, the following selection of muscles should present few problems.

In all descriptions, it is assumed that a finger or thumb will be monitoring the tender point.

In some instances it is suggested that the practitioner should encourage the (intelligent and cooperative) patient to apply the monitoring pressure on the tender point, if two hands are needed by the practitioner to efficiently and safely position the patient into 'ease'.

The tender points may be used to treat the named muscles if these are hypertonic, painful or are in some way contributing to a joint dysfunction.

It is worth re-emphasizing that where chronic changes have evolved in muscles (e.g. fibrosis), positional release may be able to ease hypertonicity and reduce pain, but cannot of itself modify tissues which have altered structurally.

In all instances of treatment of muscle pain using SCS, the position of ease should be held for not less than 90 seconds, after which a very slow return is made to neutral.

No 'new' or additional pain should be caused by the positioning of the tender point tissues into ease.

Upper trapezius

The tender points are located approximately centrally in the posterior or anterior fibres (Fig. 4.22).

Method

- The supine patient's head is side-flexed towards the treated side while the practitioner uses the positioning of the ipsilateral arm to reduce reported tender point pain by at least 70%.
- The position of ease usually involves shoulder flexion, abduction and external rotation (Fig. 4.23).

Subclavius

The tender point lies inferior to the central portion of clavicle, on its undersurface (Fig. 4.24A).

See the fibre direction of the muscle, and the structural layout, in Figure 4.24 (Fig. 4.24B). This should offer

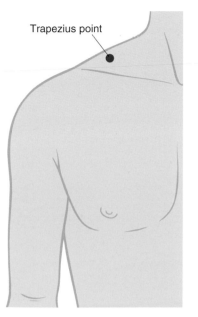

Figure 4.22 Common location of trapezius tender point.

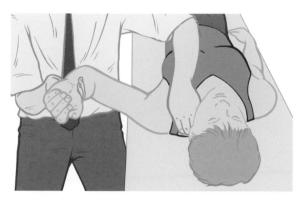

Figure 4.23 Treatment of trapezius tender point.

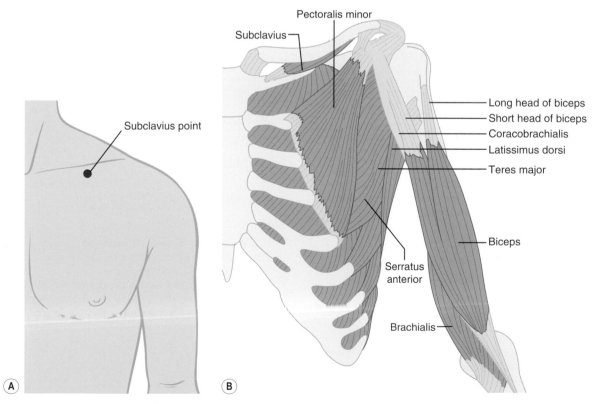

Figure 4.24 (A) Common location of subclavius tender point. (B) Deep muscles of the front of the chest and left arm. *(From Gray's Anatomy, 39th edn.)*

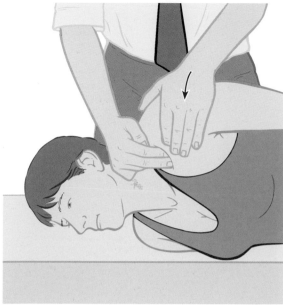

Figure 4.25 Treatment of subclavius tender point.

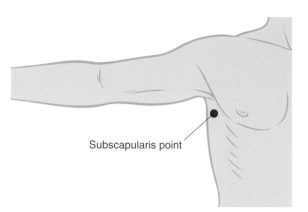

Figure 4.26 Common location of subscapularis tender point.

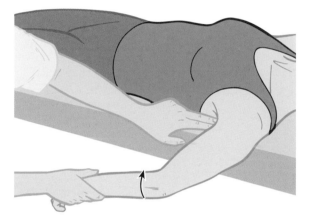

Figure 4.27 Treatment of subscapularis tender point.

an awareness of the way 'crowding' of the tissues, to ease tenderness in the palpated point, requires that the clavicle be taken inferiorly and medially. Consider also tensegrity factors, as described in Chapter 7, Box 7.1 (see also Fig. 4.49C).

Method
- The patient is side-lying, with ipsilateral shoulder in slight extension, forearm behind patient's back (or lying supine).
- The practitioner applies slight compression to the ipsilateral shoulder in an inferomedial direction, with fine-tuning possibly involving protraction until reported sensitivity in the palpated point drops by at least 70% (Fig. 4.25).

Subscapularis

The tender point lies close to the lateral border of the scapula, on its anterior surface (Fig. 4.26).

Method
- The patient lies close to the edge of the table with the arm held slightly (~30°) in abduction, extension and internal (sometimes external) rotation at the shoulder (Fig. 4.27).
- Slight traction on the arm may be used for fine-tuning, if this significantly reduces reported sensitivity.

Pectoralis major

The tender point lies on the muscle's lateral border close to the anterior axillary line (Fig. 4.28).

Method
- The patient lies supine as the ipsilateral arm is flexed and adducted at the shoulder, taking the arm across the chest (Fig. 4.29).
- Fine-tuning involves varying the degree of flexion and adduction, which can at times usefully be amplified by applied traction to the arm (but only if this reduces the reported sensitivity in the tender point).

Pectoralis minor

The tender point is just inferior and slightly medial to the coracoid process (and also on the anterior surfaces of ribs 2, 3 and 4 close to the mid-clavicular line) (Fig. 4.30).

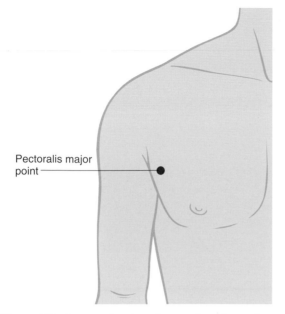

Figure 4.28 Common location of pectoralis major tender point.

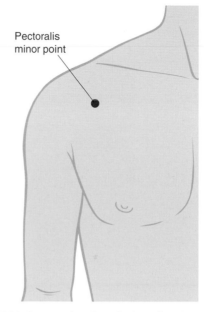

Figure 4.30 Common location of pectoralis minor tender point.

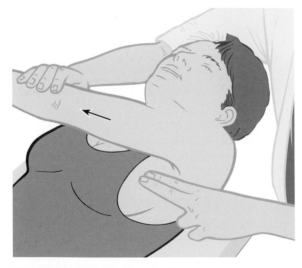

Figure 4.29 Treatment of pectoralis major tender point.

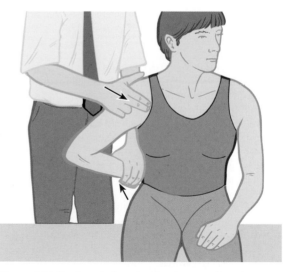

Figure 4.31 Treatment of pectoralis minor tender point.

Method

- The patient is seated and the practitioner stands behind. The patient's arm is taken into extension and internal rotation, bringing the flexed forearm behind the back (Fig. 4.31).
- The hand which is palpating the tender point is used to introduce protraction to the shoulder, while at the same time compressing it anteromedially to fine-tune the area and reduce reported sensitivity by at least 70%.

Rib dysfunction

Assessment of elevated first rib

Among the commonest rib dysfunctions is that of an elevated first rib (see Fig. 4.4B). Assessment of this is as follows:

- The patient is seated and the practitioner stands behind (Fig. 4.32A).

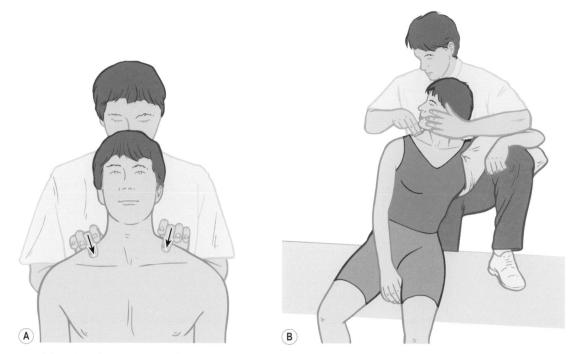

Figure 4.32 (A) Position for assessment of elevated first rib. (B) Position for treatment of elevated first rib.

- The practitioner places his hands so that the fingers can draw the upper trapezius fibres lying superior to the first rib, posteriorly.
- The tips of the practitioner's middle and index, or middle and ring fingers, should be eased caudally until they rest on the superior surface of the posterior shaft of the first rib.
- Symmetry should be evaluated as the patient breathes normally.
- The commonest dysfunction relates to one of the pair of first ribs becoming 'locked' in an elevated position (i.e. it is locked in, unable to fully exhale).
- The superior aspect of this rib will palpate as tender and attached scalene structures are likely to be short and tight (Greenman 1996). (The various ways in which rib dysfunctions are described are summarized in Box 4.9).

Or:

- The patient is seated and the practitioner stands behind.
- The practitioner places his hands so that the fingers can draw the upper trapezius fibres lying superior to the first rib, posteriorly.
- The tips of the practitioner's middle and index, or middle and ring fingers, should be eased caudally until they rest on the superior surface of the posterior shaft of the first rib.

Box 4.9 The semantics of rib dysfunction descriptions

A rib that is unable to move into full exhalation can be described as being:
- *locked in its inhalation phase*
- *elevated* – unable to move to its exhalation position
- an *inhalation restriction* (osteopathic terminology). Therefore, if one of a pair of ribs fails to descend as far as its pair on exhalation, it is described as an elevated rib, unable to move fully to its end of range on exhalation ('inhalation restriction' or 'restricted in inhalation').

A rib that is unable to move into full exhalation can be described as being:
- *locked in its exhalation phase*
- *depressed* – unable to move to its inhalation position
- an *exhalation restriction* (osteopathic terminology).

Therefore, if one of a pair of ribs fails to rise as far as its pair on inhalation, it is described as a depressed rib, unable to move fully to its end of range on inhalation ('exhalation restriction' or 'restricted in exhalation').

To avoid confusion, the two shorthand terms *elevated* and *depressed* are most commonly used to describe these two possibilities.

- The patient exhales fully, and shrugs his shoulders and as he does so the palpated first ribs should behave symmetrically.
- If they move asymmetrically (one moves superiorly more than the other), this suggests either that the side that moves most cephalad is elevated, or that the side that does not rise as far as the other is locked in a depressed (exhalation phase) position.
- The commonest restriction of the first rib is into elevation and the likeliest soft-tissue involvement is of shortness of the anterior and medial scalenes (Goodridge & Kuchera 1997).

Notes on rib dysfunction

- Unless direct trauma has been involved in the aetiology of dysfunctional rib restriction patterns, it is very unusual for a single rib to be either elevated or depressed.
- Most commonly, groups of ribs are involved in any dysfunctional situation of this sort.
- As a general rule, based on clinical experience, the most superior of a group of depressed ribs or the most inferior of a group of elevated ribs, is treated first.
- If this 'key rib' responds to treatment (using positional release or any other form of mobilization), the remainder of the group commonly release spontaneously.
- Positional release methods, as described in this chapter, are remarkably effective in normalizing rib restrictions, often within a matter of minutes.
- As with almost all musculoskeletal problems, whether such normalization is retained depends largely on whether the cause(s) of the dysfunction is ongoing (breathing pattern disorders, asthma, repetitively imposed stress – as examples) or not.

Treatment of elevated first rib

- The patient is seated and the practitioner stands behind with his contralateral foot on the table, patient's arm draped over practitioner's knee (Fig. 4.32B).
- The practitioner's ipsilateral hand palpates the tender point on the superior surface of the first rib.
- Digital pressure to the point should be sufficient to allow the patient to ascribe a value of '10' to the discomfort
- Using body positioning, the practitioner induces a side-shift (translation) of the patient *away* from the treated side.
- At the same time, using his contralateral hand, the practitioner eases the patient's head into slight extension, side-flexion away from, and rotation

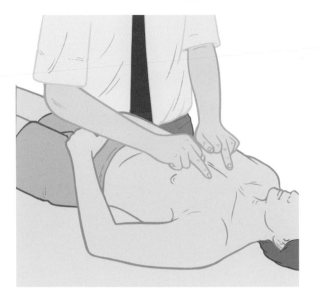

Figure 4.33 Position for assessment of rib status – ribs 2 to 10.

towards, the tender point, in order to fine-tune, until tenderness in the palpated point reduces by at least 70%.
- This is held for not less than 90 seconds.

Assessment and treatment of elevated and depressed ribs (ribs 2–12)

Identification of rib dysfunction is not difficult.

Restrictions in the ability of a given rib to move fully (as compared with its pair) during inhalation indicates a *depressed* status, while an inability to move fully (as compared with its pair) into exhalation indicates an *elevated* status as discussed in Box 4.9 (Fig. 4.33).

Assessment of rib status (ribs 2–10)

- The patient is supine or seated, and the practitioner places a single finger contact on the superior surfaces of one pair of ribs.
- The practitioner's dominant eye determines the side of the table from which he is approaching the observation of rib function – right eye dominant calls for standing on the patient's right side.
- The fingers are observed as the patient inhales and exhales fully (eye focus is on an area between the palpating fingers so that peripheral vision assesses symmetry of movement).
- If one of a pair of ribs fails to rise as far as its pair on inhalation, it is described as a depressed rib, unable to move fully to its end of range on inhalation ('exhalation restriction'). See Box 4.9.

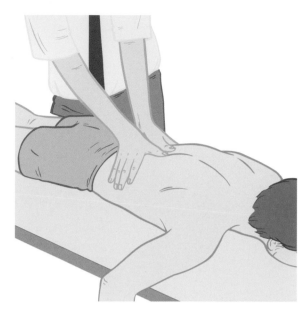

Figure 4.34 Position for assessment of rib status – ribs 11 and 12.

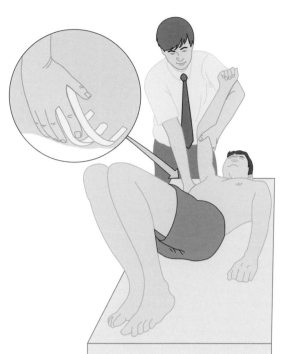

Figure 4.35 Positional release of an elevated rib while monitoring a tender point on the posterior surface close to the angle of the ribs in an interspace above or below the affected rib. The ease position may involve the flexed knees being allowed to fall to one side or the other, with fine-tuning involving positioning of the head, neck and/or the arms. Assessment of the influence of respiratory function on the tender point pain is also used.

- If one of a pair of ribs fails to fall as far as its pair on exhalation it is described as an elevated rib, unable to move fully to its end of range on exhalation ('inhalation restriction'). See Box 4.9.

Assessment of rib status (ribs 11 and 12)

- Assessment of the eleventh and twelfth ribs is usually performed with the patient prone, with a hand contact on the posterior shafts in order to evaluate the range of inhalation and exhalation motions (Fig. 4.34).
- The eleventh and twelfth ribs usually operate as a pair, so that if any sense of reduction in posterior motion is noted on one side or the other, *on inhalation*, the pair are regarded as depressed, unable to fully inhale ('exhalation restriction'). See Box 4.9.
- If any sense of reduction in anterior motion is noted on one side or the other, *on exhalation*, the pair are regarded as elevated, unable to fully exhale ('inhalation restriction'). See Box 4.9.
- Depressed rib strains produce points of tenderness on the anterior thorax, commonly close to the anterior axillary line while elevated ribs produce points of tenderness posteriorly, in the intercostal spaces close to the angles of the ribs.

Treatment of elevated ribs (ribs 2–10)

(see Fig. 4.4B,F)

- Elevated ribs produce tender points on the posterior thorax, commonly in the intercostal space above or

below the affected rib, at the angle of the ribs posteriorly (see Fig. 4.4B).

- In order to gain access to these for palpation or treatment purposes, the scapula requires distraction or lifting.
- This is done by the arm of the affected side of the supine patient being pulled across the chest, or the shoulder being raised by a pillow (Fig. 4.35).
- The practitioner/therapist stands on the side of the disorder, and palpation of the tender point, once identified, is continuous, as positional change is engineered.
- The patient's knees should be in a flexed position during treatment of elevated ribs, and should be allowed to move toward the side of the dysfunction.
- If this fails to achieve ease (perceived either as palpated change or a reduction in sensitivity of the palpated tender point), the knees are moved towards the opposite side, in order to evaluate the effect on palpated pain and tissue tone.

- As a rule, reported pain from the tender point will reduce by around 50% as the knees fall to one side or the other.
- The head may then be turned towards, or away, from the affected side to further fine-tune and release the stress in the palpated tissues.
- Additional fine-tuning for elevated ribs may be accomplished by raising the arm or shoulder cephalad, in effect exaggerating the positional deformity.
- The influence of respiratory function should also be used to evaluate which stage of the breathing cycle reduces discomfort (in the tender point) most.
- If identified the patient is asked to maintain that phase for as long as is comfortable.

Treatment of depressed ribs (ribs 2–10)

- The tender points for a depressed rib are located in the intercostal spaces above or below the affected rib, on the anterior axillary line (see Fig. 4.4A,H).
- For treatment of depressed ribs, the patient may be supine or in a partially seated, recumbent position.
- If supine, the knees are flexed and falling to one side or the other, whichever produces better release in the tissues being palpated at the anterior axillary line.
- Depending on the response of the tissues and the reported levels of discomfort in the tender point, the head may be turned towards, or away from, the affected side to further fine-tune and release the stress in the palpated tissues.
- For additional fine-tuning, the practitioner/therapist stands on the side of dysfunction and draws the patient's arm, on the side of dysfunction, caudad until release is noted.
- In some cases, the other arm may need to be elevated, and even have traction applied, to enhance release of tender point discomfort (Fig. 4.36).
- Once the tender point being monitored reduces in intensity by 70% or more, this is held for not less than 90 seconds.

Alternatively:

- The patient may be seated (Fig. 4.37) and resting against the support offered by the practitioner's flexed leg (foot on table) and trunk.
- The practitioner palpates the tender point with one hand and uses the other to support the head, guiding it into rotation for fine-tuning, as a combination of flexion and side-flexion/rotation is encouraged by modification of the position of the supporting leg.
- Once the tender point being monitored reduces in intensity by 70% or more, this is held for not less than 90 seconds.

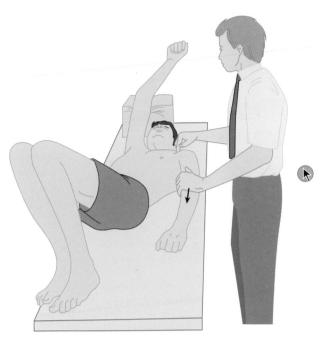

Figure 4.36 Positional release of a depressed rib involves the monitoring of a tender point on the anterior axillary line, in an interspace above or below the affected rib. Ease is achieved by positioning of flexed legs, head and/or arms, as well as use of the respiratory cycle, until a position is found in which the palpated pain eases by at least 70%, or vanishes from the tender point.

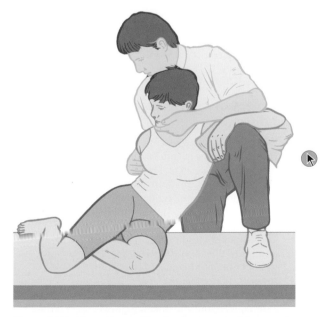

Figure 4.37 Alternative position for treatment of depressed ribs (see text).

- A notable improvement in respiratory function is commonly noted after this simple treatment method, with an obvious increase in the excursion of the thoracic cage and subjective feelings of 'ease of breathing' being reported.

Interspace dysfunction

(see Fig. 4.4G,H)

- Tender points for strains of the interspace tissues lie between the insertions of the contiguous ribs into the cartilages, close to the sternum.
- Ribs may be noted to be over-approximated, and the pain reported when the tender points are palpated may be very strong.
- The more recent the strain (frequently a sequel of excessive coughing), the more painful the points.
- Oedema and induration may be palpable.
- In chronic conditions, pressure on these soft tissues produces a reactivation of the extreme tenderness noted in more recent strains.
- These strains are found in costochondritis, the persistent pain noted in cardiac patients.
- Tenderness in these points may well relate to respiratory dysfunction, and their release assists (together with breathing pattern rehabilitation) in normalization.
- These areas of tenderness are common in people with asthma and following bronchitis, as well as the all-too-common pattern of upper chest breathing relating to patent or incipient hyperventilation, which produces major stress of the intercostal structures and the likelihood of such tender points being located on palpation (Perri & Halford 2004; Sachse 1995).

Treatment of interspace dysfunction and discomfort

- Treatment involves placing the patient supine while the tender point is contacted by the practitioner/ therapist, *or the patient* (Fig. 4.38).
- The practitioner/therapist should be on the side of dysfunction with his caudad hand providing contact on the point, unless the patient is performing this function.
- The cephalad hand cradles the patient's head/neck and flexes this, and eases it towards the side of dysfunction, at an angle of approximately 45° towards the foot of the bed.
- If fine-tuning is efficient, the pain on palpation will ease rapidly, and the position of ease should then be maintained for 90 seconds.

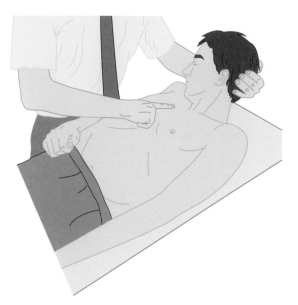

Figure 4.38 Treatment of interspace dysfunction involves flexion of the head and neck and usually the thoracic spine towards the palpated tender point, which lies close to the sternum. A seated position (not illustrated) offers an alternative for achieving this positioning.

Alternatively:

- This same procedure for release of interspace dysfunction tender points can be achieved in a seated position, and can be taught as a home treatment to the patient.
- The point is located and the patient – on her own, or with assistance – is flexed gently towards the side of pain until it vanishes.
- This position is held for 90 seconds, after which another point can be located and treated.

It is hard to envisage a simpler protocol.

A note on induration technique (a derivative of SCS)

Texan chiropractor Marsh Morrison (1969) recommended gentle palpation, using extremely light touch, as a means of feeling a 'drag' sensation (see Chapter 2 and notes on palpation in other chapters) alongside the spine – as lateral as the tips of the transverse processes.

Drag palpation identifies areas of increased hydrosis, a physiological response to increased sympathetic activity, a seemingly invariable feature in skin overlying trigger points and other forms of reflexively active myofascial areas ('hyperalgesic skin zones') (Lewit 1999).

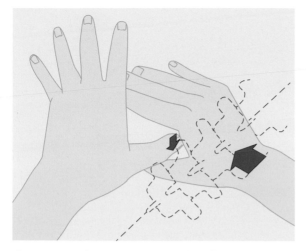

Figure 4.39 Induration technique method for paraspinal soft tissue dysfunction – described fully in the text.

Once drag is noted, pressure into the tissues normally results in a report of pain.

- The practitioner/therapist stands on the side of the prone patient opposite the side in which pain has been identified in paraspinal tissues.
- Once located, tender or painful points (lying no more lateral than the tip of the transverse process) are palpated for the degree of their sensitivity to pressure.
- Once confirmed as painful, pressure is maintained by firm thumb pressure while, with the soft thenar eminence of the other hand, the tip of the spinous process most adjacent to the pain point is very gently eased towards the pain (ounces/grams of pressure only), effectively crowding and slackening the tissues being compressed by the thumb, until pain reduces by at least 70% (Fig. 4.39).
- Direct pressure of this sort (lightly applied) towards the pain should lessen the degree of tissue contraction as well as sensitivity.
- If it does not do so, then the angle of push on the spinous process towards the painful point should be varied slightly so that, somewhere within an arc embracing a half circle, a direction is identified that largely abolishes the pain as well as lessening the subjective feeling of tissue-tension.
- This position is held for 20 seconds, after which the next point is treated.
- A spinal treatment is possible using this extremely gentle approach which incorporates the same principles as SCS and functional technique, the achievement of 'ease' along with pain reduction as the treatment focus.

That method can usefully accompany the various SCS treatment applications for spinal dysfunction described in this chapter.

Flexion strains of the thoracic spine

- According to Jones et al. (1995), the tender point for a flexion strain of the first thoracic segment is located on the superior surface of the manubrium, on the midline (see Fig. 4.4G).
- Tender points for flexion strains of the second to the sixth thoracic segments lie on the sternum approximately $\frac{1}{2}$ to $\frac{3}{4}$ of an inch (1–2 cm) apart (see Fig. 4.4G).
- Anterior T7 point lies close to the midline, bilaterally under the xiphoid. Other anterior T7 tender points are found on the costal margin close to the xiphoid.
- T8–T11 anterior (flexion strain) dysfunction produces tender points which lie in the abdominal wall, approximately 1 inch (2.5 cm) lateral to the midline (see Fig. 4.4A).
- A horizontal line $\frac{1}{2}$ inch (1 cm) below the umbilicus locates the tenth thoracic anterior (flexion) strain tender point.
- 1 and 3 inches (2.5–7.5 cm) above T10 lie the points for T9 and T8, respectively.
- $1\frac{1}{2}$ inches (3 cm) below the T10 point is T11.
- The T12 point lies on the crest of the ilium at the mid-axillary line (see Fig. 4.4A).

Note: In a rotation strain of the mid-thoracic region, it is possible for extension and flexion strains to coexist, say flexion (anterior) strain on the left and extension (posterior) strain on the right.

Treatment for anterior thoracic flexion strains

Upper thoracic flexion strains, semi-seated or supine:

- Treatment of upper thoracic flexion strains (T1–T6) may be carried out with the patient semi-seated or supine on the treatment table.
- The patient should be supported by cushions to enhance upper thoracic flexion, while the tender point is monitored by one hand, and the practitioner's other hand assists in fine-tuning to the position of ease (Fig. 4.40A).

Alternatively:

- If treated without cushions for support, the supine patient's head is flexed towards the chest while the tender point is contacted as a monitor of ease. (This is a very similar position to that used to treat interspace dysfunction, see Fig. 4.38.)
- Fine-tuning is usually by slight rotation of the head/neck towards or away from the side of

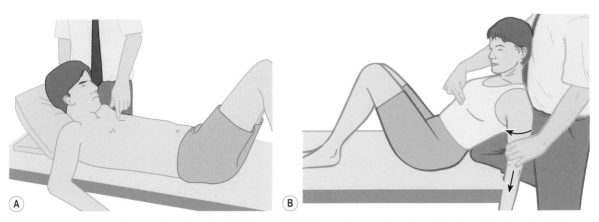

Figure 4.40 Treatment of upper thoracic spinal flexion strain. (A) Fine-tuning may involve positioning of the head–neck in rotation and or side-flexion in addition to flexion. (B) Semi-seated position for assessment and treatment of T2–T6 flexion strain.

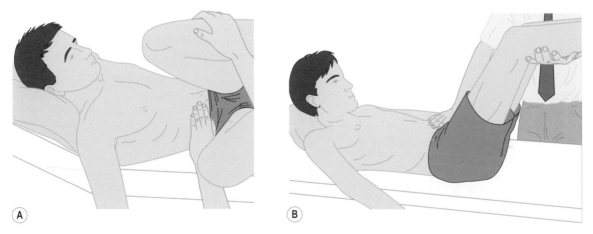

Figure 4.41 (A,B) Lower thoracic flexion strains involve positioning the supine patient into flexion while the tender point on the abdominal wall is palpated.

dysfunction. The head may be supported in flexion by the practitioner/therapist's thigh for the necessary 90 seconds of release time.

Semi-seated:

- Jones's method for dealing with flexion strain of the upper thoracic spine, in non-bed-bound patients, had the patient seated on a treatment table, leaning back onto the practitioner/therapist's chest/abdomen, so that forced flexion of the upper body can easily be achieved as shown in Figure 4.40B.
- A variety of changes in the position of the patient's arms may then be used as part of the fine-tuning process in order to introduce 'ease' into different thoracic segments.
- The practitioner palpates the tender point with one hand and utilizes the other to add fine-tuning variations.

Lower thoracic flexion strains:

- For treatment of lower thoracic flexion strains (Fig. 4.41), a pillow should be placed under the supine patient's neck and shoulders.
- If helpful in reducing sensitivity in the tender point, another pillow should be placed under the buttocks, allowing the lower spine to move into flexion, or the patient's knees should be flexed and supported by the practitioner/therapist's (hand or thigh), standing at waist level while palpating the tender point.
- Fine-tuning is achieved by movement into side-bending and/or rotation, one way or the other, using the patient's legs as a lever (for treatment of T8).
- T9–T12 flexion strains involve the same position – patient's head and buttocks on a pillow, or the

patient's flexed knees supported by the practitioner/ therapist, while the practitioner's caudad hand palpates the abdominal tender point.

- Fine-tuning is by means of a movement that introduces slight side-bending, or which slightly alters the degree of flexion (Fig. 4.41).
- The tender point should be constantly monitored and tenderness should reduce by at least 70%.
- T12 treatment requires more side-bending than other thoracic strains.
- Once a position has been found where tenderness reduces by 70% or more, this is maintained for 90 seconds.

See Chapter 6 for suggestions regarding treating these points in a bed-bound patient.

Jones et al. (1995) describe the treatment of lower thoracic flexion strains as follows:

This one procedure is usually effective for any of this group. To permit the supine patient to flex at the thoracolumbar region, a table capable of being raised at one end is desirable [Fig. 4.41A]. A flat table may be used if a large pillow is placed under the patient's hips, raising them enough to permit flexion to reach the desired level of the spine. With the patient supine, the physician raises the patient's knees and places his own thigh below those of the patient [as in Fig. 4.43]. By applying cephalad pressure on the patient's thighs, he produces marked flexion of the patient's thoracolumbar spine. Usually, the best results come from rotation of the knees moderately towards the side of tenderness. These joint dysfunctions account for many low-back pains that are not associated with tenderness of the vertebrae posteriorly. The pain is referred from the anterior dysfunction, into the low lumbar, sacral and gluteal areas. Treatment directed to the posterior pain sites of these dysfunctions, rather than to the origins of the pain, has been disappointing.

To summarize:

- Treatment for flexion strains involving the ninth thoracic to first lumbar level is usually achieved by placing the patient supine in flexion, using a cushion for the upper back and flexing the knees and hips, which are usually rotated towards the side of dysfunction (see Figs 4.41, 4.42).
- Tender points will be found close to the abdominal midline, or slightly to one side (see Fig. 4.4A), and should be palpated during this manoeuvre.

- The practitioner/therapist's cephalad hand palpates the tender point while the patient's position is modified until tenderness in the point reduces by 70% or more.
- This position is held for 90 seconds, after which a slow return is made to a neutral position.
- The position of ease usually involves marked flexion through the joint, as well as appropriate side-bending and rotation, resulting in reduction of sensitivity in the tender points on the anterior body surface.

Extension strains of the thoracic spine

- These strains are treated in a similar manner to that used for extension strains of the cervical spine.
- Tender points are usually found on, or close to, the spinous processes, bilaterally, or in the lateral paravertebral muscle mass.
- It is usual to find that the lower the strain, the closer is the tender point to the transverse process (see Fig. 4.4F).
- Direct extension (backwards-bending) is the usual method used for SCS treatment of this region, with the patient side-lying, seated, supine or prone.

Prone:

- Figure 4.42A illustrates SCS treatment of an extension strain in the upper thoracic region, with the patient prone.

Side-lying:

- If the patient is side-lying the patient's arms should be placed resting on a pillow to avoid rotation of the spine (Fig. 4.42B).
- See Chapter 6 for Schwartz's (1986) suggestions regarding treating these points in relation to a hospitalized or bed-bound patient.
- For the T5–T8 thoracic spine levels the arms are usually placed slightly above head level, to increase extension.

Seated:

- Any thoracic spine extension strains may be treated with the patient seated, either on the treatment table or on a stool, with the therapist standing to one side (Fig. 4.42C).
- Ideally, the patient's feet should be on the floor for stability.
- One of the practitioner's hands palpates the tender point located in relation to a particular segmental strain area, while the other hand fine-tunes the patient into a position where 'ease' is

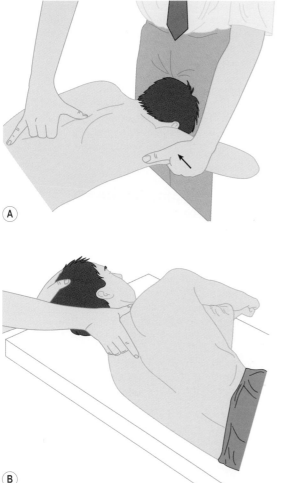

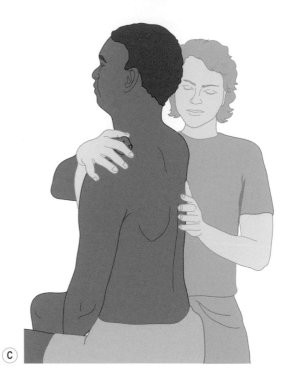

Figure 4.42 (A) Position of ease for tender points relating to extension strains of the upper thoracic region of the spine when treating the prone patient. (B) Side-lying position for treatment of thoracic extension strains. (C) Seated patient with practitioner to one side.

achieved, and tenderness in the point drops by at least 70%.

- After 90 seconds a slow return to a neutral position should be made.

Flexion strains of the lumbar spine

- Gross positioning is virtually the same as for thoracic flexion strains, with tender points on the anterior surface (abdomen mainly) and the ease position involving taking the patient into flexion (see Fig. 4.4A for the positions of these points).
- L1 has two tender points: one is at the tip of the anterior superior iliac spine and the other on the medial surface of the ilium just medial to the anterior superior iliac spine (ASIS).

- The tender point for second lumbar anterior strain is found lateral to the anterior inferior iliac spine (AIIS).
- The tender point for L3 is not easy to find but lies on the lateral surface of the AIIS, pressing medially.
- L4 tender point is found at the insertion of the inguinal ligament on the ilium.
- L5 points are on the body of the pubes, just to the side of the symphysis.

SCS method

- Treatment for all of these points is similar to that used for thoracic flexion strains except that the patient's knees are placed together (Fig. 4.43).
- In bilateral strains both sides should be treated.

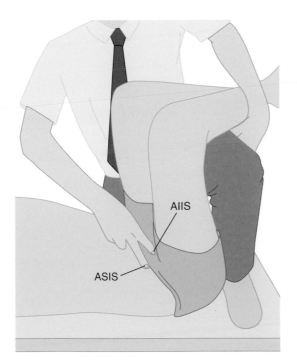

Figure 4.43 Position of ease for flexion strain of segments from T9 to the lower lumbar regions usually require positioning into flexion, side-bending and rotation, until ease is achieved in the monitored tender point on the lower abdominal wall or the ASIS area. AIIS, anterior inferior iliac spine; ASIS, anterior superior iliac spine.

- L3 and L4 usually require greater side-bending in the fine-tuning process.

Extension strains of the lumbar spine

See also various treatment options for this region, described in Chapter 6.

L1, L2

- L1 and L2 tender points are located close to the tips of the transverse processes of the respective vertebrae (see Fig. 4.4B).
- Extension strains relating to these joints may be treated with the patient prone, seated or side-lying, using the tender points to monitor changes of discomfort as the ease position is sought.

Prone (Fig. 4.44A):

- If the patient is prone, the practitioner/therapist stands on the side opposite the strain, grasping the leg on the side of the dysfunction/tender point, just above the knee, bringing it into extension and

adducting it towards the practitioner/therapist, in a scissor-like movement.

Side-lying (Fig. 4.44B):

- If the patient is side-lying, with the side of dysfunction uppermost, the upper leg can be extended to introduce extension into the region of the strain, while fine-tuning is accomplished by slightly adducting or abducting the leg.
- When an ease position has been established with the palpated tender point less painful by at least 70%, or when a marked degree of tissue change is noted, this should be maintained for 90 seconds, before a slow return to neutral.

See Chapter 6 for Schwartz's (1986) suggestions regarding treating these points in a bed-bound patient. Side-lying alternative (Fig. 4.44C):

- In some cases of low-back dysfunction relating to extension strains, a tender point is located on the sacral sulcus (see Fig. 4.4B).
- Rather than using hip extension (as in Fig. 4.44A,B) hip flexion may be helpful in achieving ease (Fig. 4.44C).
- Fine-tuning to achieve ease may involve adduction or abduction of the leg, or altering the degree of rotation in the upper body.

L3, L4

- The tender point for extension strain of L3 is found about 3 inches lateral to the posterior superior iliac spine, just below the superior iliac spine. L4 tender point lies an inch or two lateral to this following the contour of the crest (see Fig. 4.4B).
- Treatment of L3 and L4 extension strains is accomplished with the patient prone, practitioner/therapist on the side of dysfunction, or in side-lying (Fig. 4.44A–C).
- The practitioner/therapist's knee or thigh can be usefully placed under the raised thigh of the patient to hold it in extension while fine-tuning it, accomplished usually by means of abduction and external rotation of the foot.
- This procedure can also be performed with the patient side-lying, dysfunction side uppermost.
- The practitioner/therapist's foot should be placed on the heel behind the patient's lower leg.
- The patient's uppermost leg is raised and the extended thigh of this leg can then be supported on the practitioner/therapist's thigh.
- Rotation of the foot and positioning of the patient's leg in a more anterior or posterior plane, always in a degree of extension, is the fine-tuning mechanism to reduce or remove pain from the palpated tender point during this process.

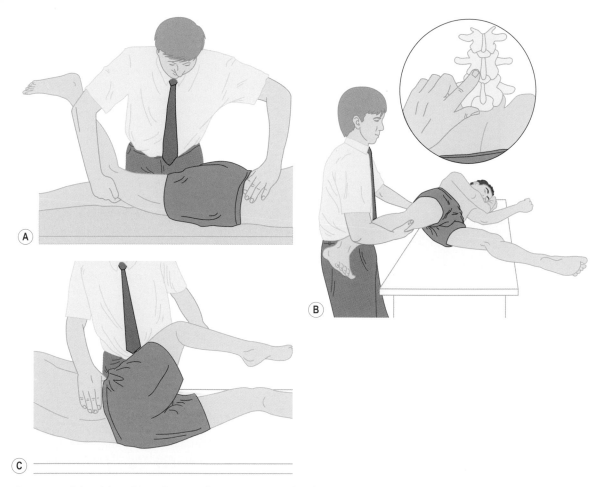

Figure 4.44 (A) Position of ease for a tender point associated with an extension strain of the lumbar spine usually requires use of the legs of the prone patient as means of achieving extension and fine-tuning. (B) Side-lying position for treatment of lumbar extension strains. (C) Some lumbar extension strains, where, for example, the tender point lies in the superior sacral sulcus, may ease if the hip is flexed in the side-lying position as illustrated.

L5

- There are various L5 tender points for extension strain as shown in Figure 4.4B.
- These are all treated as in extension strains of L1 and L2 (Fig. 4.44A–C) using scissor-like extension of the prone patient's leg on the side of the dysfunction, and fine-tuning by variation in position (or treated in side-lying).
- In some cases, the contralateral leg may be placed in flexion (over the edge of the table) to achieve ease of the tender point.
- As in all SCS protocols, once a 70% reduction in sensitivity of the tender point has been achieved, this should be held for 90 seconds before slowly returning to neutral.

SCS for psoas dysfunction (and for recurrent sacroiliac joint problems)

- The tender point for iliopsoas is located approximately 2 inches (5 cm) medial, and slightly inferior, to the anterior superior iliac spine.
- The practitioner stands on the side contralateral to that being treated.
- With the widely separated knees of the supine patient (Fig. 4.45) flexed, and the ankles crossed, the limbs are raised by flexing the hips – supported by the practitioner's leg.
- The process involves finding the amount of hip flexion that reduces palpated pain in the tender point markedly, at which time fine-tuning is

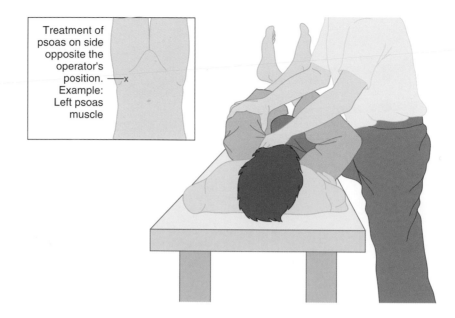

Treatment of psoas on side opposite the operator's position. —x Example: Left psoas muscle

Figure 4.45 Positional release for psoas dysfunction. *(After Vleeming.)*

introduced in which small amounts of side-flexion or rotation are introduced to assess the effects on tenderness.

• When tenderness drops by at least 70% the position is maintained for not less than 90 seconds, before slowly returning the patient to neutral.

Jones et al. (1995) report:

Any time there is a knee complaint place that leg's foot on top (in the leg crossing stage). This treatment produces flexion, marked external rotation and abduction of the femoral joint. Whenever you have a patient with a sacro-iliac problem that keeps recurring, be sure to check for this dysfunction. It is also common when there are no sacro-iliac dysfunctions.

Sacral tender points and low back pain

In 1989, osteopathic physicians Ramirez and colleagues identified a series of 'new' tender points, collectively known as medial sacral tender points. These tender points were found to relate directly to low back and pelvic dysfunction and were found to be amenable to very simple SCS methods of release (Ramirez et al. 1989).

A few years later, Cislo et al. (1991) described additional sacral foramen tender points, which they identified as being related to sacral torsions. Cislo et al. have provided clear guidelines as to the usefulness of these in the treatment of low back pain associated with sacral torsion, using counterstrain methods.

The original identification of the 'new' medial sacral points occurred when a patient with chronic low back pain and pelvic hypermobility was being treated (Ramirez et al. 1989). Use of counterstrain methods was found to be efficient using anterior and posterior lumbar tender points; however, despite relative comfort, the patient was left with 'tender points in the middle of the sacrum, associated with no problems'. These were originally ignored but when the patient's back pain recurred, the sacral points were re-evaluated and a number of release positions were attempted. Recognizing that the usual 'crowding' or 'folding' of tissue to induce ease in tender points was impossible in the mid-sacral area, the researchers then experimented with application of pressure to various areas of the sacrum.

Ramirez et al. (1989) explained their progress from then on:

In the 3 weeks following this initial encounter with the unnamed sacral tender points, 14 patients with the presenting complaint of low back (sacral or lumbar, with or without radicular) pain demonstrated tenderness at one or more of the new sacral tender points. Ultimately we found six new tender points, all of which were relieved by positional release techniques to the sacrum.

107

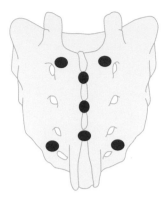

Figure 4.46 Common location of positions of tender points relating to sacral and low back dysfunction.

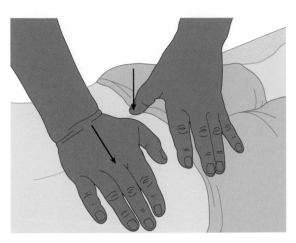

Figure 4.47 SCS treatment of medial sacral tender points relating to sacral and low back dysfunction.

Location of the new sacral medial tender points

Collectively known as the 'medial sacral tender points', these are located as follows:

- There are two possible cephalad tender points that lie just lateral to the midline, approximately 1.5 cm medial to the inferior aspect of the posterior superior iliac spine (PSIS) bilaterally, and they are known as PS1 (for posterior sacrum). See Figure 4.46 where these two points (left and right) are identified by the letter A.
- The caudad two tender points are known as PS5 and may be located approximately 1 cm medial and 1 cm superior to the inferior lateral angles of the sacrum, bilaterally. See Figure 4.46, where these two points (left and right) are identified by the letter E.
- The remaining two tender points may be located on the midline: one (PS2) lies between the first and second spinous tubercles of the sacrum, identified as being involved in sacral extension, and the other (PS4) lies on the cephalad border of the sacral hiatus, which is identified as a sacral flexion point. See Figure 4.46, where these two points (superior and inferior) are identified by the letters B and D.
- Schwartz identified a seventh point lying between the second and third sacral tubercles (PS3), which relates to sacral extension. See Figure 4.46, where this point is identified by the letter C.

How to identify medial sacral tender points

Cislo et al. (1991) note that when they first started trying to identify the precise locations of the sacral tender points they used drag palpation, as described earlier in this chapter, and more fully in Chapter 2.

However, they state:

> We have found that when these tender points occur in groups the associated sudomotor change is frequently confluent over the mid-sacrum. For this reason, we have begun to check all six points on all patients with low back pain, even in the absence of sudomotor changes.

They report that this process of localization can be rapid if the bony landmarks are used during normal structural examination.

Treatment of medial sacral tender points

(Fig. 4.47)

- With the patient prone, pressure on the sacrum is applied according to the location of the tender point being treated.
- Pressure is always straight downwards, in order to induce rotation around a perceived transverse or oblique axis of the sacrum.
- The PS1 tender points require pressure to be applied at the corner of the sacrum *opposite the quadrant in which the tender point lies*, i.e. left PS1 requires pressure at the right inferior lateral angle of the sacrum.
- The PS5 tender points require pressure to be applied *near the sacral base, on the contralateral side*, i.e. a right PS5 point requires downward – to the floor – pressure on the left sacral base just medial to the sacroiliac joint.
- The release of PS2 (sacral extension) tender point requires downwards pressure (to the floor) *at the apex of the sacrum in the midline*.

- The lower PS4 (sacral flexion) tender point requires pressure to *the midline of the sacral base.*
- Schwartz tender point PS3 (sacral extension) requires the same treatment as for PS2 described above.
- In all of these examples it is easy to see that the pressure is attempting to *exaggerate the existing presumed distortion* pattern relating to the point, which is in line with the concepts of SCS and positional release as explained earlier.

Jones (1995, p. 84) is on record as describing his approach to the use of the sacral tender points identified by Ramirez et al. (1989):

> *To keep this simple and practical, I search for the tender points. When one is found I press on the sacrum as far away from the tender point as possible.*

What if medial sacral points are too sensitive?

From time to time, pressure on the sacrum itself was found to be too painful for particular patients, and a refinement of the techniques of SCS was therefore devised for the medial points (not the midline points).

- The patient is placed on a table, prone, with head and legs elevated (an adaptable McManus-type table can achieve this, as can appropriately sited pillows and bolsters), inducing extension of the spine, which usually relieves the palpated pain by approximately 40%.
- Different degrees of extension (and sometimes flexion) are then attempted to find the position which reduces sensitivity in the point(s) most effectively.
- When this has been achieved, side-bending the upper body or the legs away from the trunk is carefully introduced, to assess the effects of this on the palpated pain.
- As in all SCS procedures, the final position is held for 90 seconds once pain has been reduced by at least 75% in the tender point(s).

Identification of sacral foramen tender points

Additional tender points were later identified as a result of problems attempting to treat a difficult patient (Cislo et al. 1991) (Fig. 4.48).

A patient with low back pain, with a recurrent sacral torsion, was being treated using SCS methods with poor results. When muscle energy procedures were also found to be inadequate, a detailed survey was made of the region, and an area of sensitivity that had previously been ignored was identified in one of the sacral foramina.

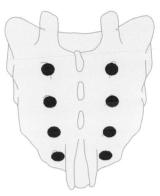

Figure 4.48 Sacral foramen tender points as described in the text.

Experimentation with various release positions for this tender point resulted in benefits and also in the examination of this region in other patients with low back pain and evidence of sacral torsion.

All the patients (who were examined) demonstrated tenderness at one of the sacral foramina, ipsilateral to the engaged oblique axis (of the sacrum) (Cislo et al. 1991).

These foramen tender points have been named according to their anatomical position and are to be differentiated from sacral border tender points previously identified by Jones, and from the medial tender points as discussed above.

Clinically, these tender points are located by their positions relative to the posterior superior iliac spine.

- The most cephalad of the points (SF1, sacral foramen tender point 1) is 1.5 cm (1 inch) directly medial to the apex of the PSIS.
- Each successively numbered sacral foramen tender point (SF2, SF3, SF4) lies approximately 1 cm below the preceding tender point location.

Locating sacral foramen tender points

Evaluation of the sacral foramina should be a fairly rapid process.

- If a sacral torsion is identified, the foramina on the ipsilateral side should be examined by palpation and the most sensitive of these is treated as described below.
- A left torsion (forward or backward) involves the foramina on the left side.
- Alternatively, palpation of the foramina using the skin-drag method (see Chapter 2) may reveal dysfunction, even if the precise nature of that dysfunction is unclear.
- If there is obvious skin-drag over a foramen, and if compression of that foramen is unduly painful,

some degree of sacral torsion is suggested – on the same side as the tender foramen.

Treatment protocol for sacral foramen points

For treatment of a tender point located over a left-side sacral foramen (Fig. 4.49A):

- The patient lies prone with the practitioner/therapist on the side of the patient contralateral to the foramen tender point to be treated – right side in this example.
- The right leg (in this example) is abducted to about 30°.
- The practitioner/therapist, applies pressure to the sensitive foramen with his left hand (in this example) with the patient ascribing a value of '10' to the resulting discomfort.
- The practitioner/therapist then applies pressure to the ilium a little lateral to the patient's right PSIS, directed anteromedially, using his right forearm or hand (in this example). This should reduce reported levels of sensitivity from the tender point.
- Variations in angle of pressure and slight variations in the position of the right leg are used for fine-tuning.
- The degree of reduction of sensitivity in the palpated sacral foramen tender point should achieve 70%.
- The position of ease is held for 90 seconds before a slow return to neutral (leg back to the table, contact released) is passively brought about.
- Whether the sacral torsion is on a forward or backward axis, it should respond to the same treatment protocol as described.

Tensegrity and the pelvis

When envisaging the internal biomechanics of the effects of treating medial sacral points, or sacral foramen points, as described above, it may be helpful to keep the balance between compression and tension forces and other tensegrity concepts in mind (Figs 4.49B,C). See Figure 4.49C for a tensegrity structure.

Pubococcygeus dysfunction

The tender point for pubococcygeus dysfunction lies on the superior aspect of the lateral ramus of the pubis, approximately a thumb width from the symphysis (Fig. 4.50).

Method

- The patient lies supine as the ipsilateral leg is flexed (Fig. 4.51) until sensitivity in the palpated point drops by at least 70%.

- Long-axis compression through the femur towards the pelvis may be useful as part of fine-tuning.

Coccygeal ('filum terminale cephalad') lift

Goodheart described a method that relies on the crowding or slackening, of spinal dural tissues, with the coccyx being used as the means of achieving this.

Startling results in terms of improved function and release of hypertonicity in areas some distance from the point of application are claimed (Goodheart 1985). Goodheart's term for this is a 'filum terminale cephalad lift': it is proposed that this be shortened to 'coccygeal lift', at least in this text.

This method focusses on normalizing flexion/extension dysfunction between the spinal column and the spinal cord, despite the spiral nature of the manner in which the spine copes with forced flexion (Illi 1951).

Goodheart and Walther report that there is frequently a dramatic lengthening of the spinal column after application of this procedure, with Goodheart mentioning specifically that, in good health, there should be no difference greater than about half an inch in the measured length of the spinal column sitting, standing and lying, using a tapeless measure which is rolled along the length of the spine.

Goodheart quotes from the work of Upledger and of Breig in order to substantiate physiological and pathological observations which he makes relating to the dura, its normal freedom of movement, and some of its potential for problem-causing when restricted (Breig 1978; Upledger & Vredevoogd 1983).

Breig states that, using radiography, microscopic examination and mechano-elastic models, it has been shown that there are deforming forces, which relate to normal movements of the spine, impinging on the spinal cord and meninges, from the brainstem to the conus medullaris and the spinal nerves.

Upledger, in discussion of the physiological motion of the central nervous system, recalls that, when assisting in neurosurgery in 1971, in which extradural calcification was being removed from the posterior aspect of the dural tube in the midcervical region, his task was to hold the dura with two pairs of forceps during the procedure. However, he states:

> *The membrane would not hold still, the fully anaesthetized patient was in a sitting position and it became apparent that the movement of the dural membrane was rhythmical, independent of the patient's cardiac or respiratory rhythms.*

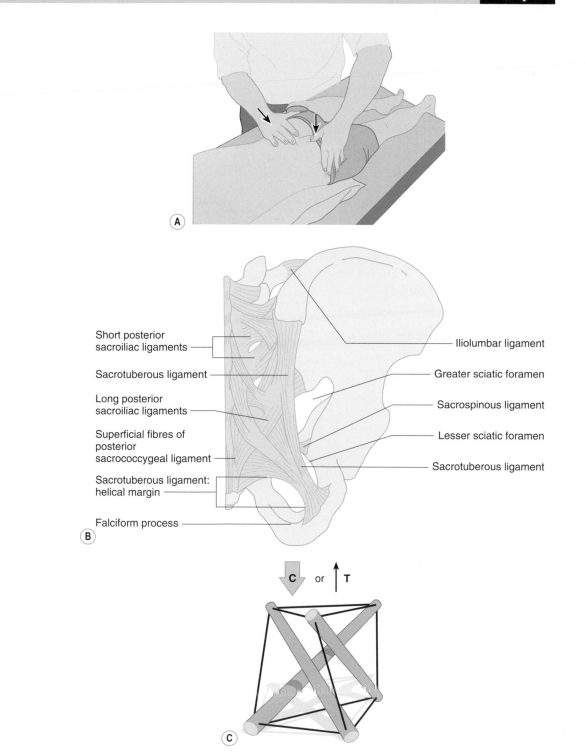

Figure 4.49 (A) SCS treatment of sacral foramen tender points relating to sacral torsion dysfunction. (B) Joints and ligaments on the posterior aspect of the right half of the pelvis and fifth lumbar vertebra. (C) A simple model of a tensegrity structure in which internal tensions 'T' and externally applied compression 'C' forces are absorbed by the component solid and elastic structures by adaptation of form. *(B from Gray's Anatomy, 38th edn.; C from Chaitow 1999.)*

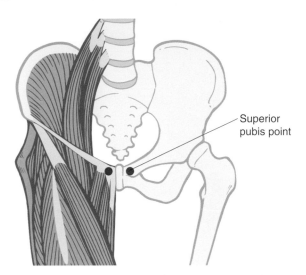

Superior pubis point

Figure 4.50 Common location of pubococcygeus tender point.

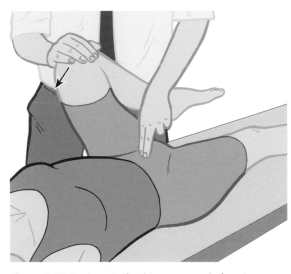

Figure 4.51 Treatment of pubococcygeus dysfunction.

Goodheart states:

Tension can be exerted where the foramen magnum is attached to the dura, and also at the 1st, 2nd and 3rd cervicals, which if they are in a state of fixation can limit motion. The dural tube is completely free of any dural attachment all the way down to the 2nd anterior sacral segment where finally the filum terminale attaches to the posterior portion of the

1st coccygeal segment. The release which comes from the coccygeal lift cannot be just a linear longitudinal tension problem. The body is intricately simple and simply intricate and once we understand the closed kinematic chain and the concept of the finite length of the dura, we can see how spinal adjustments can sometimes allow compensations to take place.

What may be happening during this 'lift'?

The anatomy of what is happening and the process of using this procedure is suggested to be as follows (Sutherland 1939; Williams & Warwick 1980):

- The dura mater attaches firmly to the foramen magnum, axis and third cervical vertebrae, and possibly to the atlas, with a direct effect on the meninges.
- Its caudad attachments are to the dorsum of the first coccygeal segment by means of a long filament, the filum terminale.
- Flexion of the spine alters the length of the intervertebral canal, while the cord and the dura have a finite length (the dura being approximately 2.5 inches longer than the cord, allowing some degree of slack when the individual sits), which Goodheart reasons requires some form of 'arrangement' between the caudal and the cephalad attachments of the dura, a 'take-up' mechanism to allow for maintenance of proper tension on the cord.
- Measurement of the distance between the external occipital protuberance to the tip of the coccyx shows very little variation from the standing to the sitting and lying positions.
- However, if all the contours between these points are measured in the different positions, a wide variation is found: the greater the degree of difference the more likely there is to be spinal dysfunction and, Goodheart postulates, dural restriction and possible meningeal tension.
- Tender areas of the neck flexors or extensors are used as the means of monitoring the effect of coccygeal lift procedure, to judge whether the palpated pain and/or hypertonicity eases, so indicating the ideal degree of lift.

Method as described by Goodheart (1985)

See below for modifications that simplify application:

- With the patient prone, the practitioner stands at waist level.
- After palpation and identification of the area of greatest discomfort and/or hypertonicity in the cervical spinal musculature with the practitioner's cephalad hand, the index finger of the caudad hand is placed so that the tip of the index or middle finger

is on the very tip of the coccyx, while the hand and fingers follow precisely the contours of the coccyx and sacrum (Fig. 4.52).

- This contact slowly and gently takes out the available slack as it lifts the coccyx, along its entire length including the tip, directly towards the painful contact on the neck, using anything up to 15 lb (7 kg) of force.

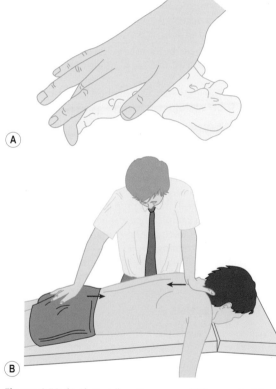

Figure 4.52 (A,B) Goodheart's coccygeal lift – see text for full descriptions.

- If the painful monitoring point does not ease dramatically, the direction of lift is altered (by a few degrees only) slightly towards one shoulder or the other.
- Once the pain has been removed from the neck point, *and without inducing additional pain in the coccyx*, this position is maintained for up to 1 minute.
- Additional ease to the restricted or torsioned dural sleeve can be achieved by using the hand palpating the cervical structures to impart a gentle caudal traction by holding the occipital area in such a way as to lightly compress it, while easing it towards the sacrum (so moving the upper three cervical segments inferiorly) as the patient exhales.
- This hold is maintained for four or five cycles of breathing.

Goodheart and others report dramatic changes in function following use of this procedure, including lengthening of the spine so that it measures equally in all positions, reduction in cervical dysfunction, removal of chronic headaches and release of tension in psoas and piriformis.

Coccygeal lift variation

The author has commonly found that the following variations make application of the coccygeal lift less difficult to achieve (Fig. 4.53):

- Once identified, the patient can be requested to apply the compressive force to the cervical tender point being used as a monitor until ease is achieved.
- This frees the practitioner so that positioning and application of the coccygeal lift is less stressful.
- The position described above, as advised by Goodheart and Walther, can be awkward if the practitioner is slight and the patient tall.
- A side-lying position of the patient allows for a less uncomfortable application of the procedure, for the practitioner.
- In this instance, the patient monitors the pain in the cervical area.

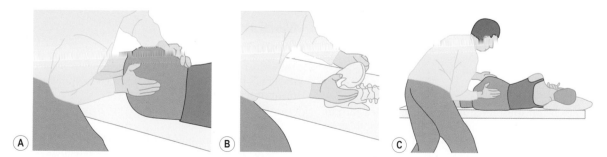

Figure 4.53 (A–C) Coccygeal lift variation – see text for full descriptions.

- The practitioner stands at upper thigh level, behind the side-lying patient, and makes contact along the whole length of the coccyx (the tip of which is cushioned in the hyperthenar eminence, see Fig. 4.53 A-C), with the elbow braced against his own hip/abdomen area.
- The force required to achieve the lift is applied by means of the practitioner leaning into the hand contact, while the caudad hand stabilizes the anterior pelvis of the patient.
- As in Jones's SCS methods, the patient reports on the changes in palpated pain levels until a 70% reduction is achieved.

Morrison's 'inguinal lift'

American chiropractor Marsh Morrison was responsible for popularizing a number of methods that bear a close resemblance to SCS, and which certainly fall into the context of positional release methods.

Morrison maintained that most women who periodically wear high heels present with a degree of what he termed 'pelvic slippage' that is associated with undue pelvic and low back stress (Morrison 1969).

The use of the inguinal lift is meant to enable low back manipulation and mobilization methods to be more effective, by balancing ligamentous and muscular tension patterns (see Chapter 8 for variations on this theme). Morrison recommended its application when low back problems failed to respond to more usual methods, since he maintained that the pelvic imbalance could act to prevent the normalization of spinal dysfunction.

Method

- The patient lies supine with legs slightly apart.
- The superior margin of the pubis should be palpated, close to the inguinal area.
- Pain will be found on the side of 'slippage'.
- This painful site is palpated *by the patient* who reports a numerical value for the pain, where '10' is the greatest pain imaginable, with the objective of reducing pain during the procedure, from a starting level of 10, by at least 70%.
- The patient (if male) should be asked to hold the genitals towards the non-treated side.
- Whether the patient is male or female, a second person should be in the room, since the practitioner is in a vulnerable position when contacting the inguinal area.
- The practitioner stands to the side of the patient, just below waist level on the side to be treated, and places the flat table-side hand on the inner thigh so that the web between finger and thumb comes into contact with the tendon of gracilis, at the ischiopubic junction.

- It is important, in order to minimize the potential sensitivity of the region, that the contact hand on the gracilis tendon should be relaxed, not rigid, with the 'lift' effort being introduced via a whole-body effort, rather than by means of pushing with that hand.
- Light pressure, superiorly directed, is then introduced to assess for discomfort.
- If the pressure is tolerable, the hemipelvis on the affected side is 'lifted' towards the shoulder on that side until pain reduces adequately in the palpated tender point, and this position is held for 30 seconds.
- The author has found that by supporting the ischial tuberosity with the non-tableside hand during the 'lift' a greater degree of pain reduction in the palpated point may be achieved.

Morrison described 'multiple releases' of tension in supporting soft tissues, as well as a more balanced pelvic mechanism.

The author suggests that this method may be usefully applied to lower abdominal 'tension' as well as to pelvic imbalances.

By removing the tension from highly stressed ligamentous and other soft tissues in the pelvis, some degree of rebalancing normalization may occur. Whether this involves the same mechanisms as are thought to occur when SCS is applied, or whether it relates directly to Goodheart's coccygeal lift method, remains for further evaluation. It is an example of positional release, involving a palpated pain point being used as a monitor, and so fits well with SCS methodology.

See Chapter 9 for discussion and illustration of a number of similar ligament balancing methods.

Gluteus medius

The commonest tender point for gluteus medius dysfunction lies laterally, on the posterior superior iliac spine.

Method

- The prone patient's ipsilateral leg is extended at the hip and abducted (Fig. 4.54), until reported pain reduces by at least 70%.

Medial hamstring (semimembranosus)

The tender point for the medial hamstrings is located on the tibia's posteromedial surface on the tendinous attachment of semimembranosus (Fig. 4.55).

Method

- The patient lies supine, with the affected leg off the edge of the table, so that the thigh is extended and slightly abducted, and the knee is flexed (Fig. 4.56).

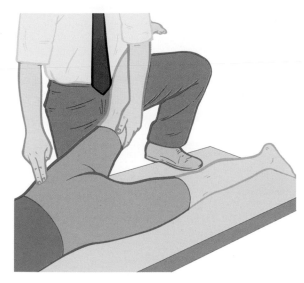

Figure 4.54 Common location of gluteus medius tender point and treatment position.

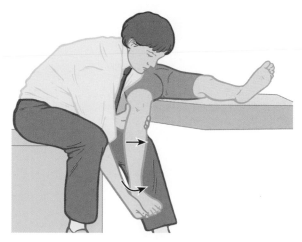

Figure 4.56 Treatment of medial hamstrings using the tender point as a monitor of discomfort.

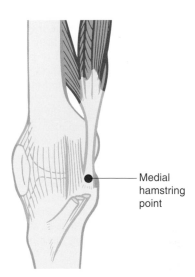

Figure 4.55 Common location of medial hamstring tender point, and treatment position.

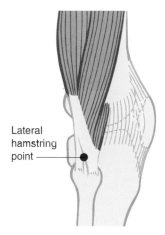

Figure 4.57 Common location of lateral hamstring tender point.

- Internal rotation of the tibia is applied for fine-tuning to reduce reported sensitivity in the tender point by at least 70%.

Lateral hamstring (biceps femoris)

The tender point for the lateral hamstring is found on the tendinous attachment of biceps femoris on the posterolateral surface of the head of the fibula (Fig. 4.57).

Method

- The patient lies supine, with the affected leg off the edge of the table so that the thigh is extended and slightly abducted, and the knee is flexed (Fig. 4.58).
- Adduction or abduction, as well as external or internal rotation of the tibia, is introduced for fine-tuning, to reduce reported sensitivity in the tender point by at least 70%.

Tibialis anterior

The tender point for tibialis anterior is found in a depression on the talus, just medial to the tibialis anterior tendon, anterior to the medial malleolus (Fig. 4.59).

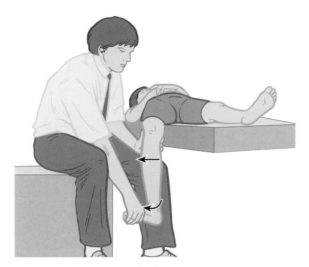

Figure 4.58 Treatment of the lateral hamstring using the tender point as a monitor of discomfort.

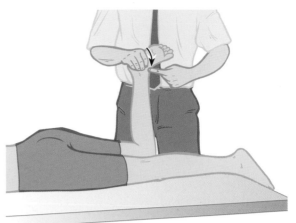

Figure 4.60 Treatment of tibialis anterior using the tender point as a monitor of discomfort.

SIDE-EFFECTS AND REACTIONS

(McPartland 1996)

Despite the extreme gentleness of the methods involved in the application of all positional release in general, and SCS in particular, in about one-third of patients there is likely to be a reaction in which soreness, or fatigue may be experienced, just as in more strenuous therapeutic measures.

This reaction is considered to be the result of homeostatic adaptation processes in response to the treatment, and is a feature of many apparently very light forms of treatment. Since the philosophical basis for much body-work involves the concept of the treatment itself acting as a catalyst, with the normalization or healing process being the prerogative of the body itself, the reaction described above is an anticipated part of the process.

It is logical and practical to request that the patient refrain from excessive activity for some hours following SCS treatment to avoid disturbing any 'resetting' of tone that may have occurred.

McPartland (1996) notes that between one-quarter and one-third of patients treated by SCS have some reaction, despite the gentleness of these approaches.

Very occasionally there are extensive 'muscle release' reactions. These are usually transitory and seldom last more than a few hours. However, patients should be fore-warned of the possibility, to allay anxiety. No treatment is needed for the reaction if it occurs, as it is itself merely evidence of an adaptation process and passes rapidly.

In relation to positional release methods applied to the cranium (see Chapter 5) it is important to highlight a report on iatrogenic effects from inappropriately applied cranial treatment (most of which involves positional release methodology) (McPartland 1996). This report

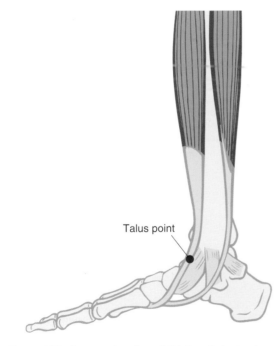

Talus point

Figure 4.59 Common location of tibialis anterior tender point.

Method

- The prone patient's ipsilateral knee is flexed as the foot is inverted and the ankle internally rotated to fine-tune (Fig. 4.60), until reported sensitivity in the palpated tender point reduces by at least 70%.

presented nine illustrative cases, of which two involved intra-oral treatment. All cases seemed to involve excessive force being used, and this highlights the need for care and gentleness in all cranially applied treatment, particularly when working inside the mouth.

CLINICAL REASONING

With the information in this and subsequent chapters, and using the basic principle of identifying areas of tenderness in shortened structures, and easing these by positioning, it should be possible for the reader to become familiar with the clinical possibilities offered by PRT in general and SCS in particular, without becoming bound by rigid formulaic procedures.

At its simplest, SCS suggests the following procedures if tissues are restricted or painful, with some tissues displaying 'tightness' and others, 'looseness':

- Consider the tight structures as primary sites for tender point location (see Chapter 2).
- Locate the most tender local point using simple palpation, such as 'drag' (see Chapter 2).
- Monitor this point while positioning and fine-tuning the tissues to reduce the perceived pain by not less than 70%.
- Hold the position of comfort/ease for up to 90 seconds.
- Slowly return to neutral, and reassess.
- Anticipate an instant functional improvement (e.g. greater range of motion) and some reduction in pain/discomfort that should commonly continue over the coming hours and days.

The reader is urged to re-visit the various text boxes in this chapter that cover different aspects of clinical decision-making:

- Box 4.1: Ideal settings for application of SCS/PRT
- Box 4.2: SCS application guidelines
- Box 4.3: Counterstrain positioning guidelines
- Box 4.4: Timing and SCS
- Box 4.5: Which points to treat first?
- Box 4.6: Some of the effects of sustained compression
- Box 4.7: SCS: contraindications and cautions

- Box 4.8: Indications for SCS (alone or in combination with other modalities)
- Box 4.9: The semantics of rib dysfunction descriptions.

SCS and other positional release methods are most appropriate in acute and subacute settings. They can also offer benefits in chronic conditions, but by their noninvasive, indirect, nature are not capable of modifying structural changes (fibrosis, etc.).

The end-result of such positioning, if painless, slowly performed and held for an appropriate length of time (Box 4.4), is:

- A reduction in sensitivity of the neural structures
- A resetting of these to painlessly allow a more normal resting length of muscle to be achieved
- Reduced nociceptor activity (see Chapter 1)
- Enhanced circulation as hypertonicity decreases.

Hopefully, the explanations in this chapter will have produced sufficient awareness to allow experimentation with the principles involved, in clinical settings, involving both the areas presented and others.

As long as the guiding principles of producing no additional pain, while also relieving pain from the palpated tender point during the positioning and fine-tuning, are adhered to, no damage can result, and a significant degree of pain relief and functional improvement is possible.

The following chapter explores different models of positional release – functional and facilitated positional release for example, where tissues are guided to their 'ease' positions using palpated features of modified tone, rather than relying on patient feedback, as in counterstrain.

THIS CHAPTER

This chapter has offered a detailed overview of the use of counterstrain, including the modified Goodheart model.

Mechanisms, guidelines and exercises provide a comprehensive foundation for the safe clinical application of this versatile methodology.

NEXT CHAPTER

The next chapter details functional (including cranial) and facilitated positional release methods.

REFERENCES

Academy of Traditional Chinese Medicine, 1975. An Outline of Chinese Acupuncture. Foreign Language Press, Peking.

Bailey, M., Dick, L., 1992. Nociceptive considerations in treating with counterstrain. Journal of the American Osteopathic Association 92, 334–341.

Baldry, P., 1993. Acupuncture, Trigger Points and Musculoskeletal Pain. Churchill Livingstone, Edinburgh.

Barnes, M., 1997. The basic science of myofascial release. Journal of Bodywork and Movement Therapies 1, 231–238.

Breig, A., 1978. Adverse Mechanical Tension in the CNS. John Wiley, New York.

Cantu, R., Grodin, A., 1992. Myofascial Manipulation. Aspen Publications, Gaithersburg, MD.

Chaitow, L., 1990. Palpatory Literacy. Thorsons/Harper Collins, London.

Chaitow, L., 1991. Acupuncture Treatment of Pain. Healing Arts Press, Rochester, VT.

Chaitow, L., 1996. Palpation Skills. Churchill Livingstone, Edinburgh.

Chaitow, L., 1999. Cranial Manipulation: Theory and Practice. Churchill Livingstone, Edinburgh.

Chaitow, L., 2003. Palpation and Assessment Skills. Churchill Livingstone, Edinburgh.

Chaitow, L., 2009. Editorial. Journal of Bodywork and Movement Therapies 13, 115–116.

Cislo, S., Ramirez, M., Schwartz, H., 1991. Low back pain: treatment of forward and backward sacral torsion using counterstrain technique. Journal of the American Osteopathic Association 91, 255–259.

D'Ambrogio, K., Roth, G., 1997. Positional Release Therapy. Mosby, St Louis.

Deig, D., 2001. Positional Release Technique. Butterworth Heinemann, Boston.

DiGiovanna, E., 1991. An Osteopathic Approach to Diagnosis and Treatment. Lippincott, Philadelphia.

Dodd, J.G., Good, M., Nguyen, T.L., et al., 2006. In vitro biophysical strain model for understanding mechanisms of osteopathic manipulative treatment. Journal of the American Osteopathic Association 106 (3), 157–166.

Dyhre-Poulsen, P., Krogsgaard, M.R., 2000. Muscular reflexes elicited by electrical stimulation of the anterior cruciate ligament in humans. Journal of Applied Physiology 89, 2191–2195.

Goodheart, G., 1985. Applied Kinesiology. Workshop Procedure Manual, twenty-first ed. Privately published, Detroit.

Goodridge, J., Kuchera, W., 1997. Muscle energy techniques for specific areas. In: Ward, R. (Ed.), Foundations for Osteopathic Medicine. Williams and Wilkins, Baltimore, MD.

Greenman, P., 1996. Principles of Manual Medicine, second ed. Williams and Wilkins, Baltimore, MD.

Howell, J.N., Cabell, K.S., Chila, A.G., et al., 2006. Stretch reflex and Hoffmann reflex responses to osteopathic manipulative treatment in subjects with Achilles tendinitis. Journal of the American Osteopathic Association 106, 537–545.

Illi, F., 1951. The Vertebral Column. National College of Chiropractics, Chicago.

Jacobson, E., Lockwood, M.D., Hoefner, V.C. Jr., et al., 1989. Shoulder pain and repetition strain injury to the supraspinatus muscle: etiology and manipulative treatment. Journal of the American Osteopathic Association 89, 1037–1045.

Jones, L., 1964. Spontaneous release by positioning. The Doctor of Osteopathy 4, 109–116.

Jones, L., 1966. Missed anterior spinal dysfunctions – a preliminary report. The Doctor of Osteopathy 6, 75–79.

Jones, L., 1981. Strain and Counterstrain. Academy of Applied Osteopathy, Colorado Springs.

Jones, L., Kusunose, R., Goering, E., 1995. Jones Strain-Counterstrain. Jones Strain-Counterstrain Inc., Boise, IN.

Jones, L.H., 1995. Strain-counterstrain. Jones Strain-Counterstrain Inc., IN.

Klingler, W., Schleip, R., Zorn, A., 2004. European Fascia Research Project Report. 5th World Congress Low Back and Pelvic Pain, Melbourne.

Knebl, J., 2002. The Spencer sequence. Journal of the American Osteopathic Association 102, 387–400.

Korr, I., 1947. The neural basis of the osteopathic dysfunction. Journal of the American Osteopathic Association 48, 191–198.

Korr, I., 1975. Proprioceptors and somatic dysfunction. Journal of the American Osteopathic Association 74, 638–650.

Korr, I., 1976. Collected Papers of I M Korr. American Academy of Osteopathy, Newark, OH.

Krogsgaard, M.R., Dyhre-Poulsen, P., Fischer-Rasmussen, T., 2002. Cruciate ligament reflexes. Journal of Electromyography and Kinesiology 12, 177–182.

Kuchera, M.L., McPartland, J.M., 1997. Myofascial trigger points: an introduction. In: Ward, R. (Ed.), Foundations for Osteopathic Medicine. Williams and Wilkins, Baltimore, MD.

Lewis, C., Flynn, T., 2001. The use of strain-counterstrain in the treatment of patients with low back pain. Journal of Manual and Manipulative Therapy 9, 92–98.

Lewit, K., 1999. Manipulative Therapy in Rehabilitation of the Locomotor System, third ed. Butterworths, London.

McPartland, J., 1996. Side effects from cranial treatment. Journal of Bodywork and Movement Therapies 1, 2–5.

McPartland, J.M., Klofat, I., 1995. Strain and Counterstrain. Technik Kursunterlagen. Landesverbände der Deutschen Gesellschaft für Manuelle Medizin, Baden, Germany.

Mann, F., 1983. International Conference of Acupuncture and Chronic Pain. September 1983. New York.

Mathews, P., 1981. Muscle spindles – their messages and their fusimotor supply. In: Brookes, V. (Ed.), Handbook of Physiology. American Physiological Society, Bethesda, MD.

Meltzer, K.R., Cao, T.V., Schad, J.F., et al., 2010. In vitro modeling of repetitive motion injury and myofascial release. Journal of Bodywork and Movement Therapies 14, 162–171.

Melzack, R., Wall, P., 1988. The Challenge of Pain, second ed. Penguin, London.

Morrison, M., 1969. Lecture Notes Presentation/Seminar. Research Society for Naturopathy, British College of Osteopathic Medicine, London.

Northrup, T., 1941. Role of the reflexes in manipulative therapy. Journal of the American Osteopathic Association 40, 521–524.

Owens C. 1982. An Endocrine Interpretation of Chapman's Reflexes. Academy of Applied Osteopathy, Colorado Springs.

Patriquin, D., 1992. Evolution of osteopathic manipulative technique: the Spencer technique. Journal of the American Osteopathic Association 92, 1134–1146.

Perri, M., Halford, E., 2004. Pain and faulty breathing – a pilot study. Journal of Bodywork and Movement Therapies 8, 237–312.

Ramirez, M., Hamen, J., Worth, L., 1989. Low back pain: diagnosis by six newly discovered sacral tender points and treatment with counterstrain. Journal of the American Osteopathic Association 89, 905–913.

Rathbun, J., Macnab, I., 1970. Microvascular pattern at the rotator cuff. Journal of Bone and Joint Surgery 52, 540–553.

Sachse, J., 1995. The thoracic region's pathogenetic relations and increased muscle tension. Manuelle Medizin 33, 163–172.

Schiowitz, S., 1990. Facilitated positional release. Journal of the American Osteopathic Association 90, 145–156.

Schleip, R., Duerselen, L., Vleeming, A., et al., 2012. Strain hardening of fascia: static stretching of dense fibrous connective tissues can induce a temporary stiffness increase accompanied by enhanced matrix hydration. Journal of Bodywork Movement Therapies 16, 94–100.

Schwartz, H., 1986. The use of counterstrain in an acutely ill in-hospital population. Journal of the American Osteopathic Association 86, 433–442.

Simons, D., Travell, J., Simons, L., 1999. Myofascial Pain and Dysfunction: the Trigger Point Manual, vol. 1, second ed. Williams and Wilkins, Baltimore, MD.

Solomonow, M., 2009. Ligaments: a source of musculoskeletal disorders. Journal of Bodywork and Movement Therapies 13, 136–154.

Solomonow, M., Lewis, J., 2002. Reflex from the ankle ligaments of the feline. Journal of Electromyography and Kinesiology 12, 193–198.

Spencer, H., 1916. Shoulder technique. Journal of the American Osteopathic Association 15, 2118–2220.

Standley, P., Meltzer, K., 2007. Modeled repetitive motion strain and indirect osteopathic manipulative techniques in regulation of human fibroblast proliferation and interleukin secretion. Journal of the American Osteopathic Association 107, 527–536.

Standley, P., Meltzer, K., 2008. In vitro modeling of repetitive motion strain and manual medicine treatments: potential roles for pro- and anti-inflammatory cytokines. Journal of Bodywork and Movement Therapies 12, 201–203.

Sutherland, W., 1939. The Cranial Bowl. Free Press Co., Mankato, MN.

Travell, J., Simons, D., 1992. Myofascial Pain and Dysfunction, vol. 2. Williams and Wilkins, Baltimore, MD.

Upledger, J., Vredevoogd, J., 1983. Craniosacral Therapy. Eastland Press, Seattle, WA.

Van Buskirk, R., 1990. Nociceptive reflexes and somatic dysfunction. Journal of the American Osteopathic Association 90, 792–809.

Walther, D., 1988. Applied Kinesiology. SDC Systems, Pueblo, CO.

Ward, R.C. (Ed.), 1997. Foundations for Osteopathic Medicine. Williams and Wilkins, Baltimore.

Weiselfish, S., 1993. Manual Therapy for the Orthopedic and Neurologic Patient. Regional Physical Therapy, Hertford, CT.

Williams, P., Warwick, R., 1980. Gray's Anatomy. WB Saunders, Philadelphia, PA.

Woolbright, J., 1991. An alternative method of teaching strain/counterstrain manipulation. Journal of the American Osteopathic Association 91, 370–376.

Wong, C.K., Abraham, T., Karimi, P., et al., 2014. Strain counterstrain technique to decrease tender point palpation pain compared to a control condition: a systematic review with meta-analysis. Journal of Bodywork Movement Therapies 18, 165–173.

Chapter | 5 |

Functional and facilitated positional release approaches, including cranial methods

ORIGINS OF FUNCTIONAL TECHNIQUE

There is a long tradition in manipulative medicine in general, and osteopathy in particular, of positional release methods. Variations on the theme of movement towards 'ease' and away from 'bind' or pain, in non-osteopathic contexts, include McKenzie's exercise protocols, Mulligan's *mobilisation with movement*, kinesio-taping methods that 'unload' tissues, Chiropractic's *sacro-occipital technique* (SOT) and more.

Hoover (1969a) quotes the words used by two osteopaths who had been students of the founder of osteopathy in the late 19th century, Andrew Taylor Still. They individually responded to a question as to what it was that they were doing while treating a patient, with the words, 'I am doing what the body tells me to do' moving tissues into situations that are 'comfortable', 'easy'. It can be seen that osteopathic positional release methods go back to its very origins. As Dr Hruby makes clear in Chapter 8 on Balanced ligamentous tension techniques, the developers of that functional positional release approach were 'merely applying Still's original principles'.

All the words in the world cannot substitute for actually *feeling* what happens when these methods are applied, and for this reason, exercises later in this chapter have been included in order to help bring to life the meaning and feeling of the explanations for what is, in essence, the most simple and yet one of the most potent of manipulative methods; one that creates a situation in which dynamic homeostatic balance of the affected tissues is created; one in which self-regulating repair mechanisms have an enhanced opportunity to operate.

The term 'functional technique' grew out of a series of study sessions held in the New England Academy of Applied Osteopathy in the 1950s, under the general heading of 'A *functional approach to specific osteopathic manipulative problems*' (Bowles 1955, 1956, 1957).

As indicated, the methods being explored in those sessions derived from traditional methods that dated back to the origins of osteopathy in the 19th century, but which had never been formalized or scientifically evaluated.

It was only in the 1950s and 1960s that research, most notably by Korr (1947), coincided with a resurgence of interest in these approaches, largely as a result of the clinical and teaching work of Hoover, with the result that, '*functional technique has become quite comfortable in today's scientific climate, as well as streamlined and highly effective in practice*' (Bowles 1981).

Essential difference between counterstrain and functional methods

When considering the methodology of functionally orientated techniques, one distinctive difference stands out when compared with most other positional release methods – and with strain/counterstrain (SCS) in particular.

In functional work, palpation for a 'position of ease' involves a subjective appreciation of tissues, as these are brought through a process of positioning, towards ease, to a state of 'dynamic neutral' (see Chapter 1). In complete contrast to counterstrain methods, there is no reliance on feedback from the patient as to reduction in pain during the process of positioning and fine-tuning. Instead all positioning decisions are based on practitioner perception of changes in tissue tension/tone.

Theoretically (and usually in practice), the palpated position of maximum ease (reduced tone) in the distressed tissues should closely approximate the position that would have been found if pain was being used as a guide, as in Jones's or Goodheart's approaches, as described in Chapters 4.

Similarly, if the principle of 'exaggeration of distortion' or 'replication of position of strain' were employed, the same end-position ('dynamic neutral') should be achieved, irrespective of whether functional or counterstrain methods were being used (see Chapters 1 and 4).

Example (Bowles 1956):

> A patient has an acute low back and walks with a list. A structural diagnosis is made and the fingertips palpate the most distressed tissues, within the area of most distress. The operator begins tentative positioning of the patient, preferably sitting. The fingertips pick up a slight change toward a dynamic neutral response, a little is gained, not much, but a little. A little, but enough so the original segment is no longer the most distressed area within the area of general distress. The fingers then move to what is now the most acute segment. A feeling of dynamic neutral is obtained here as far as is possible. Being temporarily satisfied with slight improvements here and there, this procedure continues until no more improvement is detectable. That is the time to stop. Using tissue response to guide the treatment the operator has step-by-step eased the lesioning (dysfunctional area) and corrected the structural imbalance to the extent that the patient is on the way to recovery.

Note: Chapter 8, Balanced ligamentous tension, techniques describes a specialized variant of functional technique.

FUNCTIONAL OBJECTIVES

Hoover (1957) summarized the key elements of functional technique in diagnosis and treatment:

- Diagnosis of function involves passive evaluation as the part being palpated responds to physiological demands for activity made by the operator or the patient.
- Functional diagnosis determines the presence or absence of normal activity of a part which is required to respond as a part of the body's activities (say respiration, or the introduction of passive or active flexion or extension).
- If the participating part has free and 'easy' motion, it is normal. However, if it has restricted or 'binding' motion, it is dysfunctional.
- The degree of ease and/or bind present in a dysfunctional site when motion is demanded is a fair guide to the severity of the dysfunction.
- The most severe areas of observed or perceived dysfunction are the ones to treat initially.
- The directions of motion which induce ease in the dysfunctional sites indicate precisely the most desirable pathways of movement.
- Use of these guidelines automatically precludes undesirable manipulative methods, since an increase in resistance, tension or 'bind' would result from any movement towards directions of increased tissue stress.
- Treatment using these methods is seldom, if ever, painful and is well received by patients.
- The application requires focussed concentration on the part of the operator and may be mentally fatiguing.
- Functional methods are suitable for application to the very ill, the extremely acute and the most chronic situations.

FUNCTIONAL EXERCISES

The exercises described in this chapter are variously derived from the work of the pioneers of these methods: Johnston (1964, 1988a,b); Johnston, Stiles and colleagues (Johnston et al. 1969); Greenman (1989); Hoover (1969b) and Bowles (1955, 1964, 1981).

Bowles (1981) is precise in his instructions to those attempting to learn to use their palpating contacts in ways that allow the application of functional methods:

1. The palpating contact ('listening hand') must not move.
2. It must not initiate any movement.

3. Its presence in contact with the area under assessment/treatment is simply to derive information from the tissue beneath the skin.
4. It needs to be tuned into whatever action is taking place beneath the contact and must temporarily ignore all other sensations, such as 'superficial tissue texture, skin temperature, skin tension, thickening or doughiness of deep tissues, muscle and fascial tensions, relative positions of bones and range of motion'.
5. All these signs should be assessed and evaluated and recorded separately from the functional evaluation, which should be focussed single-mindedly on tissue response to motion: 'It is the deep segmental tissues, the ones that support and position the bones of a segment, and their reaction to normal motion demands, that are at the heart of functional technique specificity' (Bowles 1981).

Terminology

Bowles (1964) explains the shorthand use of these common descriptive words:

Normal somatic function is a well-organized complexity and is accompanied by an easy action under the functionally-orientated fingers. The message from within the palpated skin is dubbed a sense of 'ease' for convenience of description. Somatic dysfunction could then be viewed as an organized dysfunction and recognized under the quietly palpating fingers as an action under stress, an action with complaints, an action dubbed as having a sense of 'bind'.

In addition to the 'listening hand' and the sensations it is seeking, of *ease* and *bind*, Bowles suggests we develop a 'linguistic armament', which will allow us to pursue the subject of functional technique without 'linguistic embarrassment' and without the need to impose quotation marks around the terms each time they are used.

He therefore asks us to become familiar with the additional terms, 'motive hand', which indicates the contact hand that directs motion (or fingers, or thumb or even verbal commands for motion – active or assisted), and also 'normal motion demand', which indicates what it is that the motive hand is asking of the body part. The motion could be any normal movement such as flexion, extension, side-bending, rotation or combination of movements – the response to which will be somewhere in the spectrum of ease and bind, which will be picked up by the 'listening hand' for evaluation.

At its simplest, functional technique sets up a 'demand–response' situation, which allows for the identification of dysfunction – as bind is noted – and which also allows for therapeutic intervention as the tissues are guided towards ease.

Bowles's summary of functional methods

In summary, whatever region, joint or muscle is being evaluated by the listening hand, the following results might occur:

1. The motive hand makes a series of motion demands (within normal range), which includes all possible variations. If the response noted in the tissues by the listening hand is *ease* in all directions, then the tissues are functioning normally.

2. However, if/when any of the directions of movement produce *bind* when the demand is within normal physiological ranges, the tissues are responding dysfunctionally.

3. For therapy to be introduced in response to an assessment of bind (dysfunction), relating to any motion demand, the listening hand's feedback is required so that, as the motion(s) which produced bind are reintroduced, movement is modified so that the maximum possible degree of ease is achieved: 'Therapy is monitored by the listening hand and fine-tuned information as to what to do next is then fed back to the motive hand. Motion demands are selected that give an increasing response of ease and compliance under the quietly palpating fingers' (Bowles 1964).

4. The results can be startling, as Bowles (1964) explains: *'Once the ease response is elicited it tends to be self-maintaining in response to all normal motion demands. In short, somatic dysfunctions are no longer dysfunctions. There has been a spontaneous release of the holding pattern'.*

1. Bowles's functional self-assessment exercise

(Bowles 1964)

- Stand up and place your fingers on your own neck muscles paraspinally, so that the fingers lie – very lightly, without pressing, but constantly 'in touch' with the tissues – approximately over the transverse processes.
- Start to walk for a few steps and try to ignore the skin and the bones under your fingers by concentrating all your attention on the deep supporting and active tissues as you walk.
- After a few steps, stand still and then take a few steps walking backwards, all the while evaluating the subtle yet definite changes under your fingertips.
- Repeat the process several times, once while breathing normally and once while holding the breath in, and again holding it out.

- Standing still, take one leg at a time backwards, extending the hip and then returning it to neutral before doing the same with the other leg.
- What do you feel in all these different situations?

This exercise should help to emphasize the 'listening' role of the palpating fingers and their selectivity as to what they wish to listen to.

The listening hand contact should be 'quiet, nonintrusive, non-perturbing' in order to register the compliance of the tissues, in order to evaluate whether there is a greater or lesser degree of 'ease' or 'bind' on alternating steps, and under different circumstances, as you walk.

2. Johnston and colleagues 'palpatory literacy' exercises

(Johnston et al. 1969)

Exercise 2(a) The time suggested for this exercise is 3 minutes.

- Have someone sit as you stand behind them resting your palms and fingers over their upper trapezius muscle, between the base of the neck and shoulder.
- The object is to evaluate what happens under your hands as your partner inhales deeply.
- This is not a comparison of inhalation with exhalation, but is meant to help you assess the response of the areas being palpated – to inhalation. Do they stay easy, or do they bind?
- You should specifically *not* try to define the underlying structures or their status in terms of tone or altered tissue status; simply assess the impact, if any, of inhalation on the tissues.
- Do the tissues resist, restrict, 'bind' or do they stay relaxed?
- Compare what is happening under one hand with what is happening under the other during inhalation.

Exercise 2(b) The time suggested for this exercise is 5–7 minutes.

- Go back to the starting position where you are palpating someone who is seated, with you standing behind.
- The objective this time is to map the various areas of 'restriction' or 'bind' in the thorax, anterior and posterior, as your partner inhales.
- In this exercise, try not only to identify areas of bind, but to assign what you find into 'large' (several segments) and 'small' (single segment) categories.
- To commence, place a hand, mainly fingers, on (say) the upper left thoracic area, between scapula and the spine, and have your partner inhale deeply several times, first when seated comfortably, hands on lap, and then with the arms folded on the chest (exposing more the costovertebral articulation).

- After several breaths with your hand in one position, re-situate the hand a little lower, or more medially or laterally, until the entire back has been 'mapped' in this way.
- Remember that you are not comparing how the tissues feel on inhalation compared with exhalation, but how different regions compare (in terms of ease and bind) *with each other*, in response to inhalation.
- Map the entire back – for locations of areas of bind. Also, note the 'size' of these area(s).
- Go back to any 'large' areas of bind and see whether you can identify any 'small' areas within them, using the same contact with inhalation as the active component.
- Individual spinal segments can also be mapped by sequentially assessing them one at a time as they respond to inhalations.
- Ask yourself how you would normally use the information you have uncovered via this functional assessment:
  - ▪ Would you try in some way to mobilize what appears to be restricted, and if so, how?
  - ▪ Would your therapeutic focus be on the large areas of restriction or the small ones?
  - ▪ Would you work on areas distant from, or adjacent to, the restricted areas?
  - ▪ Would you try to achieve a release of the perceived restriction by trying to move it mechanically towards and through its resistance barrier, or would you rather be inclined to try to achieve release by some indirect approach, moving away from the restriction barrier?
  - ▪ Or, would you try a variety of approaches, mixing and matching until the region under attention was free or improved?

There are no correct or incorrect answers to these questions; however, the various exercises in this section (and elsewhere in the book) should open up possibilities for other ways being considered, ways that do not impose a solution, but that allow one to emerge.

Exercise 2(c) The time suggested for this exercise is 5–7 minutes.

- With someone seated, arms folded on the chest, and with you standing behind, place your listening hand/fingertips onto the upper left thorax, in the scapula area.
- Your motive hand is placed at the cervico-dorsal junction, so that it can indicate your 'request' to move the head and upper torso anteriorly (in the coronal plane), not into flexion but in a manner that carries the head and upper torso forward.
- The repetitive movement forwards, into the position described, and back to neutral, is initiated by your motive hand, while the listening hand evaluates the changes created by this in different areas of the posterior thorax.
- In effect, you are comparing one palpated area with another, in response to this normal (anterior translation) motion demand.
- As Johnston and colleagues (1969) state: '*It is not anterior direction of motion compared with posterior direction, but rather a testing of motion into the anterior compartment only, comparing one area with the ones below, and the ones above, and so on*'.
- Your listening hand is asking the tissues whether they will respond easily or with resistance to the motion demanded of the trunk.
- In this way, try to identify those areas, large and small, that *bind* as the movement forward is carried out.
- Compare these areas with those identified when the breathing assessment was used in Exercise 2(b).

Implications

Ways of using the information gathered during Exercise 2(c):

> *In this particular testing what you have been doing is changing the positional relationship of the shoulders and the hips.*
>
> *Clues about this shoulder-to-hips relationship, elicited at the restricted area in this way, can become criteria for you in picking the technique you may want to use to effectively change the specific dysfunction being tested …. We feel that a better chance of 'correction' may be established if you use a technique which will take the dysfunctional area and deal not only with the flexion–extension component, the side-bending and the rotation, but also see that the shoulders are properly positioned in relation to the hips.*
>
> Johnston et al. 1969

Note: The patterns elicited in Exercise 2(c) involved movement initiated by you, whereas the information derived from 2(a) and 2(b) involved intrinsic motion, initiated by respiration. Johnston et al. have, in these simple exercises, taken us through the initial stages of palpatory literacy in relation to how tissues respond to motion that is self-initiated or externally induced.

Hoover's experimental exercises

Hoover (1969b) poses a number of questions in the following exercises (he calls them 'experiments'), the answers to which should always be 'yes'.

If your answers are indeed positive at the completion of the exercise, then you are probably sensitive enough in palpatory skills to be able to use functional technique effectively in clinical settings.

3. Hoover's functional clavicle exercise

(Hoover 1969a)

Exercise 3(a) Suggested time for this exercise is 5 minutes.

The question posed in this part of the exercise is: 'Does the (healthy) clavicle move in a definite and predictable manner?'

- Stand facing someone and place the pads of the fingers of your right hand (listening hand) onto the skin, above the right acromioclavicular joint.
- With your left hand, hold the right arm just below the elbow.
- Ensure the individual – and the shoulder/arm is relaxed and that you have the full weight of the arm and that there is no attempt to assist or hinder in any way, as the exercise is carried out. This can be tested by raising and lowering the arm several times (Fig. 5.1).
- Slowly and deliberately take the arm back from the midline, just far enough to sense a change in the tissues under your palpating hand, and then return it to neutral.
- Avoid quick movements, so that the sensations being palpated are accurately noted.
- Repeat this movement several times, so that the influence of this single movement can be assessed.
- Recall the question posed by Hoover for consideration, as you make this passive movement of the arm: 'Does the (healthy) clavicle move in a definite and predictable manner?'
- Now take the arm forward of the midline, until you sense a tissue change under your listening hand's fingertips.
- Repeat this single movement several times, forward and back to neutral, repeat and repeat, assessing as you do so.
- Introduce abduction of the arm from its neutral position, and then return it to neutral several times, assessing as you do so.
- Then introduce adduction – bringing the arm across the front of the trunk slightly – before returning it to neutral. Repeat this several times, assessing as you do so.
- In a similar manner, starting from and returning to neutral, assess the effect on *ease* and *bind* of a slowly introduced degree of internal and then external rotation, conducted individually.
- What was the response of individual physiological movements to the question: 'Does the clavicle move in a definite and predictable manner?'

The answer to the question posed should be that the clavicle does indeed move in a definite and predictable manner when demands for motion are made upon it – and that you can perceive the tissue changes that result.

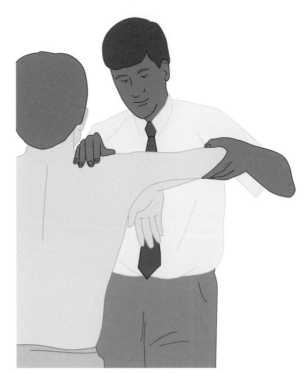

Figure 5.1 Assessing for positions that induce ease or bind in the acromioclavicular joint. The fully supported arm is passively moved in various directions. *(Hoover 1969b.)*

Exercise 3(b) Suggested time for this exercise is 5 minutes.

The question posed in this exercise is: 'Are there differences in ease of motion, and palpated feelings, when the clavicle is caused to move in different physiological motions?'

- Adopt the same starting position as in Exercise 3(a) and then move the person's arm backwards into extension, very slowly as you palpate tissue change at the lateral end of the clavicle.
- Compare the feelings of ease and bind as you then take the arm into flexion, bringing it forward of the body.
- Then compare the feelings of ease and bind as you abduct and adduct the arm sequentially, passing through neutral as you do so.
- Now compare the ease and bind sensations as you internally and externally rotate the arm.
- In this exercise, instead of motion demands assessed individually, you have the chance to evaluate what happens, in the tissues being palpated, as opposite motions are introduced, sequentially, without a pause.
- The question posed asks that you decide whether there were directions of motion that produced altered feelings of ease in the tissues.
- The answer should be that, usually, there are indeed identifiable differences or aberrations of motion and

tissue texture, when the clavicle is caused to move in the different physiological motions.

Exercise 3(c) Suggested time for this exercise is 5 minutes.

The question posed in this exercise is: 'Can the differences of ease of motion and tissue texture be altered by moving the clavicle in certain ways?'

- Repeat the introductory steps and commence by *flexing* the arm, and bringing it forwards of the midline until you note the clavicle beginning to move and the texture under palpation changing to bind.
- Then move the flexed arm backwards into *extension* until the clavicle starts to move and the sensation of bind is again noted.
- Between these two extremes lies a position of maximum ease, a position of physiological balance, in this plane of motion (forward and backward of the midline).
- This is the point of balance (*ease*) that you need to establish when using functional technique.
- Starting from this first *balanced point of ease*, use the same guidelines for assessing the point at which maximal 'ease' is noted in the acromioclavicular tissues, as you seek a point of balance between *abduction and adduction* of the arm.
- When you find the combined position of maximal ease, having previously explored flexion/extension and now abduction/adduction, you will effectively have 'stacked' one position of ease onto another.
- Starting from that combined position of ease, you now need to find the point of ease between the extremes where clavicular movement involves internal and *external rotation*.
- Once this third combined position of ease has been established, you will have achieved a reciprocal balance between the arm and the clavicle involving the most common movement patterns of the shoulder.
- For completeness, time allowing, you could also add the testing of tissue responses to: compression–distraction; inhalation–exhalation – each time commencing from the stacked/combined positions of ease previously identified.
- If you were treating dysfunction in these tissues/structures, you would maintain that combined ('stacked') position of ease for around 90 seconds.

In this process you should have effectively answered the question posed in Exercise 3(c), since it should now become clear that aberrations of motion and tissue texture/tension can be changed by motion of the clavicle.

The experiment continues

Starting from the position of reciprocal balance, reassess, as you did in the first part of the whole exercise, all the individual directions of motion of the arm (flexion, abduction, etc.).

Unlike the first part of the Exercise 3(a), you will not be starting from the position in which the arm hangs at the side, but rather from a point of dynamic balance, in which the tissues are at their most relaxed.

What you are seeking now are single motions of the arm/clavicle that exhibit the greatest degrees of freedom, the least sense of bind, starting from this balanced position.

When such a motion is identified (Hoover 1969a):

> *This one motion is continued slowly and gently as long as the sensory hand reports improving conditions, if a state is reached in which movement in that one direction increases bind and does not make movement more easy and tissue texture more normal, the sequence of physiological motions are again checked.*

What Hoover (1969a) is taking us towards in this exercise is the point at which we no longer impose action on the body, but follow it – where we allow the tissues to guide us towards their most desired directions of motion and positional ease.

In effect, what he has done, if we can follow his instructions up to this point, is to bring us to the start of using functional technique clinically.

The process described above, of finding physiological, dynamic balance and then seeking the pathways of greatest ease for the tissues, is functional technique in action.

The further evolution of the process described (using the clavicle exercise), in which the tissues guide the operator, requires a great deal of practice.

Hoover (1969a) explains:

> *The operator relaxes and becomes entirely passive as his sensory or listening hand detects any change in the clavicle and its surrounding tissues. A change in the clavicle and its surrounding tissues, if felt by the sensory/listening hand, sends information to the reflex centers which relay an order to the motor hand to move the arm in a manner so as to maintain the reciprocal balance, or neutral. If this is the proper move there will be a feeling of increasing ease of motion and improved tissue texture. This process continues through one or more motions until the state of maximum ease, or quiet, is obtained.*

4. Hoover's thoracic exercise

(Hoover 1969b)

Exercise 4(a) Suggested time for this part of the exercise is 4 minutes.

- Stand behind your seated partner, whose arms are folded across the chest.

- You should have previously assessed by palpation, observation and examination the thoracic or lumbar spine of your partner, and should now lightly place your listening hand on an area that appeared to be restricted, or in which the tissues are particularly hypertonic.
- Wait and do nothing as your hand 'tunes' in to the tissues.
- Make no assessments as to structural status.
- Wait for at least 15 seconds. Hoover says: 'The longer you wait the less structure you feel. The longer you keep the receiving fingers still, the more ready you are to pick up the first signals of segment response when you proceed to induce a movement demand'.
- With your other hand, and by voice, guide your partner/model into slight flexion and then extension.
- The motive hand should apply a very light touch, just a suggestion as to the direction towards which you want movement to take place.
- The listening hand does nothing but waits to feel the functional response of the tissues – ease and bind – as the spinal segments and tissues move into flexion and then extension.
- A wave-like movement should be noted as the segment/area being palpated is involved in the gross motion demanded of the spine.
- Changes in the tissue tension under palpation should be noted as the various phases of the movement are carried out.
- Practise the assessment at various segmental levels, and areas of the back, and try to feel the different status of the palpated tissues during the phases of the process, as bind starts, becomes more intense, eases somewhat and then becomes very easy, before a hint of bind reappears and then becomes intense again.
- Decide where the *maximum bind* is felt and where *maximum ease* occurs. These are the key pieces of information required for functional technique as you assiduously avoid bind and focus on ease.
- Try also to distinguish between the bind that is a normal physiological response to an area coming towards the end of its normal range of movement, and the bind that is a response to dysfunctional restriction.

Exercise 4(b) Suggested time for this part of the exercise is 3 minutes.

- Return to the starting position as in 4(a) and, while palpating an area of restriction or hypertonicity, induce pure side-bending to one side, and then the other while assessing for ease and bind in exactly the same way as in 4(a) (where flexion and extension were the directions used).

Exercise 4(c) Suggested time for this part of the exercise is 3 minutes.

- Return to the starting position as in 4(a) and 4(b) and, while palpating an area of restriction, or hypertonicity, induce rotation to one side and then the other while assessing for ease and bind in exactly the same way as in 4(a) and 4(b).

Different responses

Hoover describes variations in what you might feel, as a response from the tissues being palpated, during these various positional demands.

1. **Dynamic neutral:** This response to motion is an indication of normal physiological activity. There is minimal signalling during a wide range of motions in all directions. Hoover states it in the following way:

   This is the pure and unadulterated un-lesioned (i.e. not dysfunctional) segment, exhibiting a wide range of easy motion demand–response transactions.

2. **Borderline response:** This is an area or segment which gives some signals of a degree of bind fairly early in a few of the normal motion demands. The degree of bind will be minimal and much of the time ease, or dynamic neutral, will be noted. Hoover states that 'most segments act a bit like this'; they are neither fully 'well' nor 'sick'.
3. **The lesion response:** This is where bind is noted almost at the outset of almost all motion demands, with little indication of dynamic neutral.

   Note: Terminology has changed and what was called a 'lesion' in Hoover's day is now known as *somatic dysfunction*.

   Hoover suggests that you should:

   Try all directions of motion carefully. Try as hard as you can to find a motion demand that doesn't increase bind, but on the contrary, actually decreases bind and introduces a little ease … This is an important characteristic of the lesion (dysfunction).

Indeed, he states that the more severe the restriction the easier it will be to find one or more slight motion demands that produce a sense of ease or dynamic neutral, because the contrast between ease and bind will be so obvious.

Hoover's summary

Practice is suggested with dysfunctional joints and segments in order to become proficient.

Three major ingredients are required for doing this successfully (Hoover 1969b):

1. A focussed attention to the process of motion demand and motion response, while whatever is

being noted is categorized, as 'normal', 'slightly dysfunctional', 'frankly or severely dysfunctional' and so on.

2. A constant evaluation of the changes in the palpated response to motion in terms of *ease* and *bind*, with awareness that these represent increased and decreased levels of signalling and tissue response.

3. An awareness that in order to thoroughly evaluate tissue responses, all possible variations in motion demand are required, which calls for a structured sequence of movement demands.

Hoover suggests that these be verbalized (silently):

Mentally, set up a goal of finding ease, induce tentative motion demands until the response of ease and increasing ease is felt, verbalize the motion-demand which gives the response of ease in terms of flexion, extension, side-bending and rotation. Practice this experiment until real skills are developed. You are learning to find the particular ease-response to which the dysfunction is limited.

In addition, depending upon the region being evaluated, directions such as abduction, adduction, translation forwards, translation backwards, translation laterally and medially, translation superiorly and inferiorly, compression and distraction, etc. may need to be factored into this approach.

Greenman's functional exercise, below, introduces some of these elements.

Bowles describes the goal

Bowles (1964) summarizes succinctly what is being sought during such processes of assessment:

The activity used to test the segment (or joint) is largely endogenous, the observing instrument is highly non-perturbational, and the information gathered is about how well or how poorly our segment of structure is solving its problems. Should we find a sense of easy and non-distorted following of the structures, we diagnose the segment as normal. If we find a sense of binding, tenseness, tissue distortion, a feeling of lagging and complaining in any direction of the action, then we know the segment is having difficulty properly solving its problems.

The diagnosis would be of dysfunction.

5. Greenman's (1989) spinal 'stacking' exercise

The recommended time for this exercise is 10 minutes.

In previous exercises, individual directions and some simple combinations of movement have been used to assess the response of the palpated tissues in terms of ease and bind.

In this exercise, pairs of motion demands are made (e.g. flexion and extension). However, each of these assessments, after the first one, should commence from the point of ease discovered in relation to the previous motion demand assessed.

In this way, the ultimate position of maximal ease, of dynamic neutral, is equal to the sum of all the previously achieved positions of ease so that one position of ease is literally 'stacked' onto another.

*   Stand behind the individual/patient, whose arms are crossed on their chest, with hands on shoulders.
*   Place your listening hand on an upper thoracic segment and take your other arm across and in front of the person's folded arms, to engage their opposite shoulder or lateral chest wall.
*   Motion demands are made by verbal instruction as well as by slight encouragement from the motive hand.
*   A series of assessments is made for ease (Fig. 5.2) in each of the following pairs of direction:
    *   Flexion and extension
    *   Side-bending left and right
    *   Rotation left and right
    *   Translation anteriorly and posteriorly
    *   Lateral translation left and right
    *   Translation cephalad and caudad (traction and compression)
    *   Full inhalation and full exhalation.
*   The first element of the investigation should *always* be flexion and extension.
*   The final element of the investigation evaluates the influence on *ease* of the different phases of breathing, full inhalation and full exhalation.
*   However, apart from these two requirements, the sequence in which the other movements are performed is irrelevant, as long as they are all introduced so that each subsequent motion demand commences from the position of combined-ease, previously discovered.
*   The final respiratory demand indicates in which phase of breathing the most ease in the tissues is noted, and once this has been established that phase is 'stacked' onto the combined positions of ease previously identified.
*   This is held for approximately 90 seconds, after which the position of neutral is slowly readopted before the entire stacking sequence is performed again to evaluate changes.

6. Exercise in cervical translation palpation

Note: This is a modification of Greenman's (1989) exercise, in which he suggested the use of a muscle energy

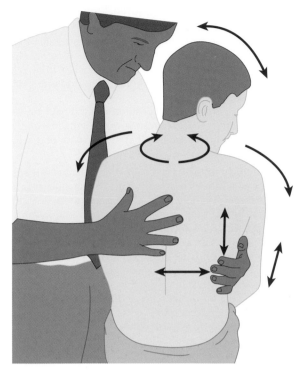

Figure 5.2 Functional palpation (or treatment) of a spinal region/segment, during which all possible directions of motion are assessed for their influence on the sense of 'ease and bind' in the palpated tissues. After the first position of ease is identified (sequence is irrelevant), each subsequent assessment commences from the position of ease (or combined positions of ease) identified by the previous assessment(s) in a process known as 'stacking'.

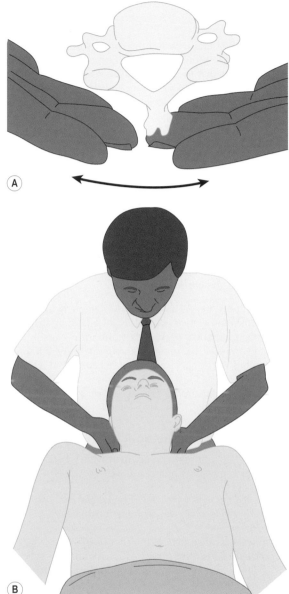

Figure 5.3 (A,B) Functional assessment and/or treatment of the cervical area involving translation/rotation restrictions.

technique to treat whatever restrictions are identified, when testing translation restrictions. In this variation, positional release (functional) techniques are suggested instead; however, the basic design of the exercise is as described by Greenman.

To easily palpate for side-flexion and rotation, a side-to-side *translation* ('shunt') movement is used, with the neck in one of three positions: neutral, moderate flexion and extension.

As segments below C2 are translated to one side, it automatically creates side-flexion and, because of the anatomical and physiological rules governing it, *rotation to the same side occurs* (Mimura et al. 1989).

This spinal coupling feature appears to be a predictable universal event in most of the cervical spine (i.e. side-flexion and rotation to the same side between C2 and C6); however, coupling in the remainder of the spine, while universal, is less predictable (Gibbons & Tehan 1998).

In order to evaluate cervical function using this effect, Greenman suggests that the practitioner should place the fingers as follows, on each side of the spine (Fig. 5.3):

- The supine patient's occiput rests on the practitioner's thenar eminences.
- The index finger pads rest on the articular pillars of C6, just above the transverse processes of C7, which can be palpated just anterior to the upper trapezius.

- The middle finger pads will be on C6, and the ring fingers on C5, with the little finger pads on C3.

Then:

- With these contacts, it is possible to examine for sensitivity, fibrosis and hypertonicity, as well as to apply lateral translation to cervical segments with the head in neutral, flexion or extension.
- In order to do this effectively, it is helpful to stabilize the superior segment to the one being examined.
- The heel of the hand helps to control movement of the head.
- With the head/neck in relative neutral (no flexion and no extension), translation to the right and then left is introduced (any segment) to assess freedom of movement (and by implication, side-flexion and rotation) in each direction.
- Say C5 is being stabilized with the finger pads, as translation to the left is introduced, the ability of C5 to freely side-flex and rotate on C6 is being evaluated when the neck is in neutral.
- If the joint – and/or associated soft tissues – are normal, this translation will cause a gapping of the left facet and a 'closing' of the right facet as left translation is performed, and vice versa.
- There will be a soft end-feel to the movement, without harsh or sudden braking.
- If, however, translation of the segment towards the right from the left produces a sense of resistance/bind, then the segment is restricted in its ability to side-flex left and (by implication) to rotate left.
- If translation right is restricted, then (comparatively) translation left will be more 'free'.
- If such a restriction is noted, the translation should be repeated, but this time with the head in extension instead of neutral.
- This is achieved by lifting the contact fingers on C5 (in this example) slightly towards the ceiling before reassessing the side-to-side translation.
- The head and neck should also be taken into slight flexion, and left-to-right translation should again be assessed.
- The objective is to ascertain which position (neutral, flexion, extension) creates the greatest degrees of *ease* and *bind* as any particular translation occurs.
- By implication, if translation left (whether in neutral, extension of flexion) is the most free, then translation in the opposite direction would be more restricted.
- Because of spinal coupling rules, this indicates that rotation is also likely to be more restricted in the direction opposite that in which translation was most free (i.e. greater freedom of translation left suggests greater restriction of rotation right).
- The question the assessment is asking is whether (at the segment being assessed) there is more freedom of translation movement in one direction or the other, in neutral, extension or flexion.
- If this freedom of movement is greater with the head extended, or neutral, or flexed, then that is the position to be used in treating any dysfunction or imbalance (as indicated by greater restriction in translation in the opposite direction) at that segment.
- Hold the translation position in the most obvious position of ease for 90 seconds and then re-evaluate the symmetry of translation movement.
- Movement should be more balanced.
- All segments up to C2 should be assessed and/or treated following the same guidelines.

Functional treatment of the knee – a case study

Johnston (1964) describes the way in which an acute knee restriction might be handled using a functional approach.

He stresses that the description given is unique to the particular pattern of dysfunction under consideration, and that quite different patterns of dysfunction and therapeutic input would be noted in each and every acute knee problem treated. We need to consider, in each case, 'this particular patient with this particular problem'.

A young male patient is described who had a painful left knee, of 3 months' duration, which could not fully straighten following a period of extensive kneeling.

On examination, the left leg remained slightly flexed at the knee, with tissues in the region somewhat warmer and more congested than in the normal right knee. Extension of the knee was painful and provided a rigid resistance as well as pain.

- Standing on the left of the patient the practitioner placed his right hand so that the palm was in contact with the patella, the thumb encircled the knee to contact the lateral aspect of the joint interspace while the second finger was in contact with the medial joint interspace.
- This *listening hand* maintained a contact light enough to appreciate subtle changes in tissue status (the sense of tension and rigidity in the tissues – described as bind) while also being able to assist in subsequent motion introduced by the other hand.
- The left hand firmly held the patient's left ankle (Fig. 5.4A).
- Initially, the extreme sense of bind was assessed by taking the joint into an extension direction – straightening the leg a little.
- As the knee was then returned to its position of slight flexion a sense of ease was noted in the palpated tissues.
- Various directions of motion were then explored and evaluated for the responses of ease and bind.

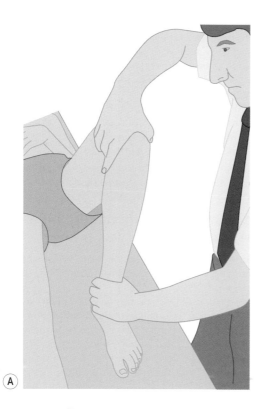

(A)

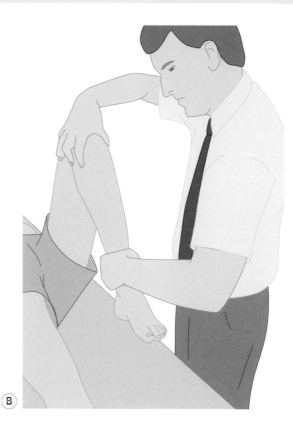

(B)

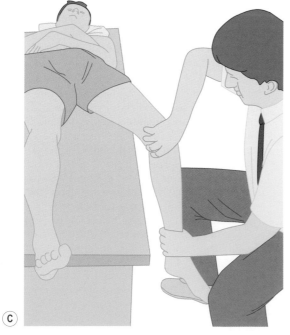

(C)

Figure 5.4 (A) Johnston's (1964) exercise for 'mapping out an enlarging pattern for the response of decreasing bind' in a knee joint. (B) Commonly a position of ease for the knee will be found in which introduction of hip and knee flexion is followed by the lower leg being internally rotated and abducted, while tissue status is monitored in the knee area. (C) An alternative position of ease for the strained knee may be found in which the hip is slightly extended and abducted while the lower limb is taken into flexion, abduction and/or internal rotation.

- The purpose of this was to map 'an enlarging pattern for the response of decreasing bind'.
- The knee was then moved into greater degrees of flexion, both elevated from the table and with the upper leg hanging below the edge of the table (Fig. 5.4B,C).
- Various motions were assessed, including abduction and adduction of the lower limb, internal and external rotation of the lower leg.
- The greatest degree of palpated ease was noted by the listening hand when the hip was flexed, the knee was markedly flexed and the lower leg was internally rotated and abducted.

Painless approach

Johnston highlights the value of such an approach in a painful condition:

> *Even when this testing involved the potentially painful ranges of motion, the increasing binding response at the fingertips is so immediate and is so dramatic a signal, to the operator, that these ranges need barely be engaged.*

- Treatment was carried out, following this evaluation sequence, with the supine patient's leg supported as described in the assessment process.
- The limb was raised to clear the table and taken into semi-flexion, as a torsion arc of internal rotation and abduction was introduced by the operator's left hand (holding the ankle), while the right hand monitored the response of the tissues around the knee, as well as supporting the knee in its flexed position.
- Alternative ranges and motions were occasionally tested during the procedure in order to 'remind' the operator's right hand to the sense of immediately increasing bind.
- With the knee markedly flexed, the thigh slightly abducted, and the lower leg held in its 'ease' position of internal rotation and abduction, a 'sudden change' in tissue tension was noted, which allowed a sense of freedom as the leg was returned to its resting position.
- It remained slightly flexed but with objectively less rigidity, an assessed improvement of around 15% in terms of its degree of acuteness.

Repetition of the whole process

Precisely the same sequence of assessment and treatment was then repeated once more. This repetition is not a precise repositioning of the knee in the previous position of ease, but rather a further evaluation during which a new ideal position of 'balanced neutral' is determined by the process of palpation and motion.

Johnston informs us that the subsequent evaluation of the position of maximal ease for the dysfunctional knee differed slightly from the previous one, as did the therapeutic holding position.

After these two functional treatments, the degree of dysfunction in terms of restriction and pain was reduced by approximately 40%.

At subsequent visits the process was carried further towards normalization so that: 'After five office visits during four weeks of continued improvement in use, the leg was able to be rested comfortably straight and the binding was no longer discernible at the knee' (Johnston 1964).

It is the experience of those using functional technique that a less chronic, less 'organized' degree of dysfunction would respond more rapidly than one, such as the case described, in which soft tissue changes in response to the strained tissues had become established for several months.

This functional diagnostic and treatment process takes longer to describe than to accomplish, for once the listening hand learns to evaluate ease and bind, and the operator learns to assess the variable positions open to motion, in any given setting, the whole process can take a matter of a very few minutes.

Functional treatment of the atlanto-occipital joint

This final purely functional 'exercise' is offered as a means of introducing functional technique methodology into clinical practice. It is almost universally applicable, has no contraindications, and builds on the basic exercises in functional methodology described in this chapter.

The only situations in which it would be difficult or impossible to apply this method would be if the patient were unable to relax and allow the procedure to be completed, over a period of several minutes.

- The patient is supine.
- The practitioner sits at the head of the table, slightly to one side facing the corner of the table.
- One hand (caudal hand) cradles the occiput with opposed index finger and thumb palpating the soft tissues adjacent to the atlas.
- The other hand is placed on the patient's forehead or the crown of the head.
- The caudal hand searches for feelings of 'ease' or 'comfort' or 'release' in the tissues surrounding the atlas, as the hand on the head directs it into a compound series of motions, one at a time.
- As each motion is 'tested' a position is identified where the tissues being palpated feel at their most relaxed or easy.
- This position of the head is used as the starting point for the next element in the sequence of assessments.

- In no particular order (apart from the first movements into flexion and extension), the following directions of motion are tested, seeking always the position of the head and neck which elicits the greatest degree of ease in the tissues around the atlas, to 'stack' onto the previously identified positions of ease (Fig. 5.5).

Note: Each motion assessment starts from the combined 'stacked' position of ease established by the previous assessments:

- Flexion/extension (suggested as the first directions of the sequence: Fig. 5.5A,B)
- Side-bending left and right (Fig. 5.5C)
- Rotation left and right (Fig. 5.5D)
- Antero-posterior translation (shunt, shift) (Fig. 5.5E)
- Side-to-side translation (Fig. 5.5F)
- Compression/traction (Fig. 5.5G)
- Inhalation/exhalation.

- Once '3-dimensional equilibrium' has been ascertained (known as dynamic neutral), in which a compound series of ease positions have been 'stacked', the patient is asked to inhale and exhale fully – to identify which stage of the breathing cycle enhances the sense of palpated 'ease' – and the patient is asked to hold the breath in that phase of the cycle for 10 seconds or so.
- The final combined position of ease is held for 90 seconds before *slowly* returning to neutral.

Note: After commencing with flexion and extension, and finishing with inhalation and exhalation – the sequence in which directions of movements are assessed is not relevant – provided as many variables as possible are employed in seeking the combined position of ease.

The effect of this held position of ease is to allow neural resetting to occur, reducing muscular tension, and also to encourage improved circulation and drainage through previously tense and possibly ischaemic or congested tissues.

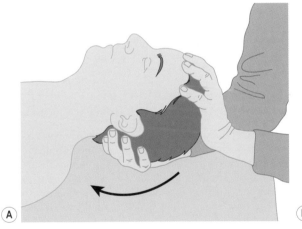

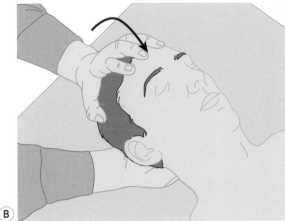

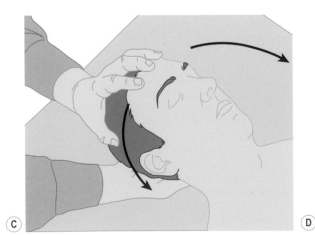

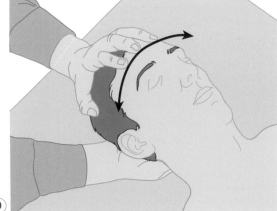

Figure 5.5 (A–G) Functional atlanto-occipital joint release.

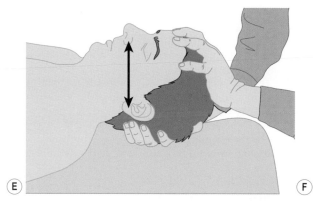

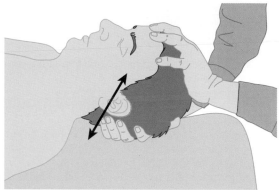

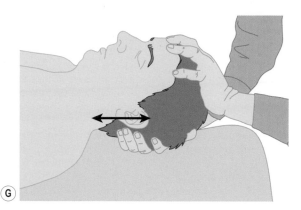

Figure 5.5, continued

Timing issues

The next section of this chapter looks at *Facilitated Positional Release* (FPR) that builds on the functional approach described above.

Clinical experience suggests that functional technique methods require holding for a minimum of 90 seconds in an 'ease' position, for beneficial changes to manifest. In contrast, facilitated positional release, as described below, reduces this to under 5 seconds by means of the addition to the procedures of facilitating features.

FACILITATED POSITIONAL RELEASE (FPR)

The nature of FPR

(DiGiovanna et al. 2004; Schiowitz 1990, 1991)

Schiowitz has described the method known as *facilitated positional release* (FPR), which incorporates elements of both SCS and functional technique, and appears to produce an accelerated resolution of hypertonicity and dysfunction.

He explains that FPR is in-line with other indirect methods which adopt positional placement towards a direction of freedom of motion, and away from restriction barriers.

1. What is 'special' about this approach is that FPR adds to this absolute requirement (movement away from the barrier of restriction), the need for a prior modification of the sagittal posture – so that, for example in a spinal area, a balance would first be achieved between flexion and extension. In spinal terms, the placing of regions into a neutral state, somewhere between extension and flexion, has the effect of releasing facet engagement.

2. FPR then adds to this the 'facilitating' elements, which might involve either compression or torsion, or a combination of both, inducing an initial soft-tissue release, relating to hypertonicity or restriction of motion.

3. Where muscles are being treated using FPR, a shortening process is called for. Specifically, Schiowitz recommends that 'larger superficial (easily palpable) muscles on the posterior aspect of the body should be placed into extension with ipsilateral

135

lateral flexion, while anteriorly situated muscles require flexion'. This is held for under 5 seconds before returning to a neutral position. If a muscle has a rotational function it needs to be placed in a shortened position, before a facilitating additional load is applied.

4. Extremity muscles require that associated articulations are 'in neutral' – freely movable with relaxed ligaments. Compression should be applied towards the articulation (long-axis compression) to shorten the affected muscles, after which abduction and/or external rotation *or* adduction and/or internal rotation are added, as the tissues being treated are palpated for maximal 'ease'. Once achieved, this is held for approximately 5 seconds.

The neurophysiology that Schiowitz describes (in DiGiovanna et al. 2004) in order to explain what happens during the application of FPR is based on the work of Korr (1975, 1976) and Bailey (1976) and correlates with facilitation and sensitization mechanisms suggested in earlier chapters of this book, in relation to the onset of somatic dysfunction. FPR appears to modify increased gamma motor neuron activity that may be affecting muscle spindle behaviour. 'This (reduction in gamma motor neuron activity) allows the extrafusal muscle fibers to lengthen to their normal relaxed state' (Carew 1985).

The placement of involved tissues or joints into a position of ease involves the practitioner *fine-tuning* the neurological feedback process, ensuring that the relaxation response is specific to the muscle fibres involved in the problem.

The 19th century origins of these methods: the Still technique

Van Buskirk (1996) has described methods taught by Andrew Taylor Still, the founder of osteopathic medicine, in the late 19th century, that mirror very closely – but not exactly – those described by Bowles, Johnston, Schiowitz and other pioneers of functional approaches. These methods were recorded by Hazzard (1905), and have been resurrected by Van Buskirk (2000).

Having identified the nature of a somatic dysfunction (see Chapter 1), the Still technique follows these steps:

1. The patient is passive throughout all procedures.
2. The diagnosis of the joint and the position at which surrounding tissue is least taut, are determined.
3. The joint and tissue are moved into the direction of ease in all planes.
4. The position is slightly exaggerated so as to increase the relaxation of the affected myofascial elements.
5. A force that is vectored parallel to the part of the body that is being used as a lever (i.e. head and neck, arm, leg, trunk) is applied in order to further relax the involved tissues. Traction or compression

are the most common forces applied for a few seconds.
6. While maintaining the vector force, the region and dysfunction are brought back towards the barrier directions and then back through the restrictions.
7. The force and motion will commonly mobilize the joint and release the tissue to the point that there may be a sudden release as reflected by a 'pop', 'click' or other such noise.
8. The forces are released and the region is brought back to neutral for reassessment of the dysfunction.

Example of Still technique for elevated first rib on the right

1. The practitioner stands on the supine patient's right side and locates the superior surface of the right first rib articulation, with his left thumb, to monitor tissue tension.
2. The patient's flexed elbow is held and is compressed and adducted to create a decoupling of the rib from its articulation. (*Note*: this reproduces the position of strain, see Chapter 1.)
3. Optionally, an isometric contraction may be added to the sequence by having the patient lightly push his elbow against the resistance of the patient's hand for a few seconds.
4. On release, compression is increased as the elbow is adducted further, then taken sweepingly superiorly in an arc towards abduction, and a return to the starting position (see video).
5. This exaggeration of the dysfunction should release the rib.

DO MUSCLES CAUSE JOINT PROBLEMS OR VICE VERSA?

Janda (1988) stated that it is not known whether dysfunction of muscles causes joint dysfunction or vice versa. However, he pointed to the undoubted fact that they massively influence each other, and that it is possible that a major element in the benefits noted following joint manipulation derives from the effects that such methods (high-velocity thrust, mobilization, etc.) have on associated soft tissues.

Steiner (1994) has specifically discussed the role of muscles in disc and facet syndromes and describes a possible sequence of events as follows:

• A strain involving body torsion, rapid stretch, loss of balance, etc. produces a myotatic stretch reflex response in, for example, a part of the erector spinae muscle group.

- The muscles contract to protect excessive joint movement, and spasm may result if there is an exaggerated response, and the tissues fail to assume normal tone following the strain.
- This limits free movement of the attached vertebrae, approximates them and causes compression and, possibly, bulging of the intervertebral discs and/or a forcing together of the articular facets.
- Bulging discs might encroach on a nerve root, producing disc-syndrome symptoms.
- Articular facets, when forced together, produce pressure on the intra-articular fluid, pushing it against the confining facet capsule, which becomes stretched and irritated.
- The sinuvertebral capsular nerves may therefore become irritated, provoking muscular guarding, initiating a self-perpetuating process of pain–spasm–pain.

Steiner continues:

From a physiological standpoint, correction or cure of the disc or facet syndromes should be the reversal of the process that produced them, eliminating muscle spasm and restoring normal motion.

He argues that before discectomy or facet rhizotomy is attempted, with the all-too-frequent 'failed disc-syndrome surgery' outcome, attention to the soft tissues and articular separation to reduce the spasm should be tried, to allow the bulging disc to recede and/or the facets to resume normal relationships (see Chapter 10 on the McKenzie approach, for another possible alternative to surgery.)

Clearly, osseous manipulation often has a place in achieving this objective. However, the evidence of clinical experience indicates that a soft-tissue approach may also be employed in order to allow restoration of functional integrity.

If, for example, joint restriction were the result of muscle hypertonicity, then complete or total release of this heightened tone would ensure a greater freedom of movement for the joint.

If, however, other intra-articular factors were causing the joint restriction then, although improvement of soft-tissue status, produced by a reduction in hypertonicity, would ease the situation somewhat, the basic restriction would remain unresolved.

FOCUS ON SOFT-TISSUE OR JOINT RESTRICTION USING FPR

Schiowitz (1991) suggests that FPR can either be directed towards local, palpable soft-tissue changes, or be used as a means of modifying the deeper muscles that might be involved in joint restriction:

It is sometimes difficult to make a clear diagnostic distinction as to which is the primary somatic dysfunction, changes in tissue texture or motion restriction. If in doubt, it is recommended that the palpable tissue changes be treated first. If motion restriction persists, then a technique designed to normalize deep muscles involved in the specific joint motion restriction should be applied.

In order to appreciate the way in which FPR is used, examples of its application are described below.

FPR treatment of soft-tissue changes in the spinal region

Schiowitz (1991) follows Jones's guidelines, which state that soft-tissue changes on the posterior aspect of the body should be treated in the first instance by taking them into extension, while those on the anterior aspect of the body require a degree of flexion to assist in their normalization, when using FPR.

However, he also reminds us that some muscles have contralateral side-bending functions, or a rotary component, or both. These muscles must be placed in their individual shortened positions. Schiowitz suggests that careful localization of the component motions of compression, forward- or backward-bending, and side-bending/rotation to the area of altered tissue texture, allows a more rapid and accurate outcome.

1. FPR for soft-tissue changes affecting spinal joints

1. After placing the patient into a relaxed neutral position, the first requirement is that the sagittal posture should be modified to create a flattening of the antero-posterior spinal curve in whichever spinal region needs treating; 'thus a mild reduction of the normal cervical and lumbar lordosis or the thoracic kyphosis is established', inducing a softening and shortening of the affected muscle(s).
2. Following this, additional elements of fine-tuning might involve compression and/or torsion (Fig. 5.6) in order to place dysfunctional tissue (or the articulation) in such a manner that 'it moves freely or is pain-free, or both'.
3. The position of ease achieved by this fine-tuning is then held for 3–4 seconds, before being released so that the area can be re-evaluated.

Note: The component elements that comprise the various facilitating forces, i.e. crowding or torsion, can be performed in any order.

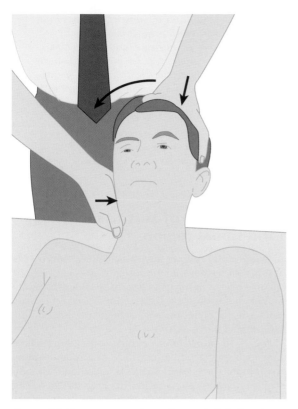

Figure 5.6 FPR treatment of anterior cervical dysfunction involves introduction of a reduced cervical curve followed by compression, side-bending and some slight torsion to achieve a sense of ease in palpated tissues.

2. Cervical restriction – FPR treatment method

When dealing with restrictions and dysfunctional states of the intervertebral (soft-tissue) structures, Schiowitz suggests that the associated vertebrae be placed into 'planes of freedom' of motion.

For this to be successful, the directions of 'ease' and 'bind' of a given segment need first to be evaluated.

If, for example, there is a restriction of a cervical vertebra in which it is found that, in relation to the vertebrae below, it cannot easily extend, side-bend right and rotate right, it would be logical, in order to establish a position of ease, to take it into flexion, side-bending left and rotation left, in relation to the vertebrae below, as a first stage of application of FPR.

If, in such an example, there were obvious discomfort/pain, or tissue changes palpable posterior to the articular facet of the third cervical vertebra, the following procedure (which needs to involve extension because the tissues are on the posterior aspect of the body) might be suggested.

1. The patient would be supine on the table, the practitioner either standing, or seated at the head of the table with a cushion on his lap.
2. The patient would have previously moved to a position in which the head was clear of the end of the table.
3. Contact would be made with the area of tissue texture alteration (right articular facet, third cervical vertebra in this case) by the practitioner's left index fingerpad, while at the same time, the head (occipital region) is being well supported by the right hand of the practitioner (Fig. 5.7A).
4. It is via the activity of this right hand that further positioning would mainly be achieved.
5. As noted previously, the first priority in FPR is to reduce the sagittal curve and this would be achieved by means of a slight flexion movement, introduced by the left hand.
6. The second component, compression, would then be introduced by application of light pressure through the long axis of the spine towards the feet (Fig. 5.7A).
7. The changes in tissue tone thus induced should be easily palpable by the contact finger ('listening finger') as a reduction in the sense of 'bind'.
8. No more than 0.5 kg (1 lb) of force should be involved in this compressive effort.
9. The next component of FPR, in this instance, would be the introduction of rotation/torsion, and this could be achieved by slight extension and side-bending to the right over the practitioner's contact that rests on the dysfunctional tissue, the right index finger.
10. Cervical spinal mechanics dictate that side-bending is impossible without some degree of rotation taking place towards the same side.
11. Therefore, rotation to the right would automatically occur as the neck was being side-flexed over the finger, so further easing and softening the tissues being treated (Fig. 5.7B).
12. This final position would be held for 3–4 seconds, before slowly returning the neck and head to neutral for reassessment of the degree of tissue change/release achieved by the procedure.

Note: If the crowding/long-axis compression caused discomfort, then traction or a slight torsional force should be used instead.

Note: It is important to recall that in regard to the atlanto-occipital joint, flexion should require a slight degree of movement only, and that atlanto-occipital mechanics involves contralateral directions of motion, i.e. side-flexion and rotation of the atlas are in opposite directions, unlike the rest of the cervical spine where side-flexion and rotation are towards the same side.

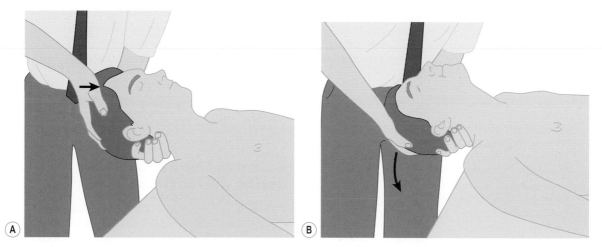

Figure 5.7 (A) FPR treatment of posterior cervical dysfunction involves introduction of a reduced cervical curve followed by compression, as palpating hand monitors tissues for a sense of ease. (B) Additional fine-tuning involves introduction of extension side-bending and some slight rotation until a sense of ease in palpated tissues is noted and held for 4–5 seconds.

Spinal joint – FPR treatment

The only difference between treating a soft-tissue change that may be affecting a spinal joint, and treating the spinal joint itself using FPR, is the degree of precision required in the positioning process.

Where the individual mechanics of restriction have been identified, the joint needs to be placed in 'all three planes of freedom of motion', into the directions of 'ease', using 'careful localization of the component motions'; in other words, in flexion, side-bending and rotation, having taken care to start from a position in which the normal sagittal curves have been somewhat reduced or neutralized.

3. FPR treatment of thoracic region dysfunction

1. The patient should be seated for treatment of thoracic soft-tissue dysfunction.
2. The example described here relates to tissue tension in the area of the sixth thoracic vertebral transverse process, on the right.
3. The practitioner stands behind and to the right, having placed a contact, palpating or 'listening' (left index) finger on the area to be treated (Fig. 5.8).
4. The practitioner places the right hand across the front of the patient's shoulders so that the practitioner's right hand rests on the patient's left shoulder and the practitioner's right axilla stabilizes the patient's right shoulder.
5. In order to reduce the antero-posterior curves, the patient is then asked to sit up straight.

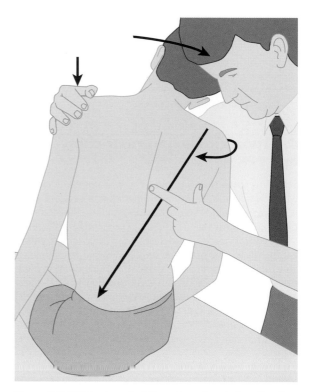

Figure 5.8 FPR treatment of thoracic region dysfunction (in this example 'tissue tension' to the right of the sixth thoracic vertebrae). One hand monitors tissue status as the patient is asked to 'sit straight' and to then slightly extend the spine. The practitioner then introduces compression from the right shoulder towards the left hip, which automatically produces right side-flexion at T6, and probably rotation to the left. Whatever the precise positional changes are, if ease is noted in the palpated tissues, the position is held for 4–5 seconds.

6. In a controlled manner, the patient is then told to 'lift the sternum towards the ceiling', so introducing a slight extension motion that is monitored by the contact (left index) finger in order to assess changes in tension/bind.

7. This extension movement is slightly assisted, but not forced, by the practitioner's right hand/arm.

8. When some ease is noted, the practitioner uses compressive effort through the right shoulder (via his own right axilla). The suggestion given by Schiowitz is that, 'this compressive motion should be applied as close to the patient's neck as possible, and directed downwards towards the patient's left hip'.

9. Once again, there is a monitoring, at the site of soft-tissue tension, of the effects of this compressive effort.

10. In spinal structures other than the cervical spine, side-flexion is commonly (but not always) accompanied by contralateral rotation.

11. In this case, compressive force applied through the right shoulder, towards the left hip, would introduce both right side-flexion and left rotation at the area being palpated.

12. If this produces a significant palpable softening, or 'ease', of the previously tense tissues, the position would be held for 3–4 seconds before returning to a neutral position for reassessment.

4. Thoracic flexion restriction and FPR

Schiowitz gives the example of a sixth thoracic vertebra which is free in its motions on the seventh vertebra when it moves easily into extension, side-bending right and rotation to the right.

The directions of restriction, therefore, which would engage the barrier would be into flexion, side-bending left and rotation left, and it is these directions of movement that would be utilized were a direct method (such as high-velocity thrust) being used to overcome that barrier, possibly involving the right articular facet joint.

However, since FPR is an indirect method, it is towards the directions of ease that we need to travel in order to achieve release.

1. The starting positions (patient seated, practitioner's palpating digit at the right sixth articular facet, shoulder contacts) should be precisely as described in the previous example (above) for tissue release.

2. This time, however, the compressive force would be applied straight downwards (inferiorly) from the shoulder towards the monitoring finger.

3. No increase in movement into extension is suggested, as this would reduce the chances of facet release.

4. When some ease was noted at this contact point from the compressive effort, a torsional side-bending and rotation movement to the right would be introduced until the freedom of motion was noted in the facet contact.

5. This would be held for 3–4 seconds, then released.

6. After repositioning into neutral, the range of motion which was previously restricted should be reassessed.

5. Prone FPR treatment for thoracic flexion dysfunction

1. For the same restriction (difficulty in moving into flexion and side-bending rotation to the left) the patient could be lying prone with the practitioner standing beside the table on the side opposite the dysfunctional vertebral restriction (Fig. 5.9).

2. The prone position would tend to introduce a mild degree of extension which can be enhanced by placement of a thin cushion under the patient's head/neck area.

3. In this example, standing on the left of the patient, the practitioner's left (monitoring) index finger would be placed on the right articular joint between the sixth and seventh thoracic vertebrae.

4. The practitioner's right hand would cup the area over the acromion process, easing this towards the patient's feet, parallel to the table, until a desirable 'softening' of the tissues was noted by the palpating digit. To compare this functional method with the counterstrain equivalent, see Figure 4.42A.

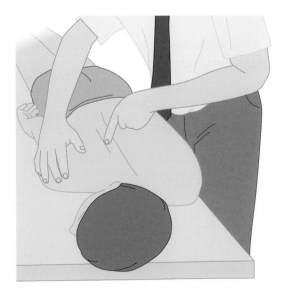

Figure 5.9 FPR treatment of thoracic flexion dysfunction.

5. This effort should be maintained as the practitioner leans backwards, in order to initiate a slight backward movement (towards the ceiling) of the patient's right shoulder, so adding a further degree of extension, together with side-flexion and rotation of the thoracic spine, up to the palpating finger, all the while maintaining the compression effort (light but firm).

6. A sense of increased ease should be noted in the palpated region, at which time the various positions and directions of pull and pressure may be fine-tuned in order to enhance ease to an optimal degree.

7. After holding the final position for 3–4 seconds, a return to neutral is allowed before reassessment of the dysfunctional area.

6. Thoracic extension restriction treatment

In the previous example, there was difficulty moving into flexion, and therefore part of the treatment protocol involved increasing extension.

If we change this to an example of someone with difficulty moving into extension (but with freedom moving into flexion), the same sequence would be used:

1. Reduction of antero-posterior curves
2. Slight increase of flexion, into 'ease'
3. Followed by the other components of side-flexion and rotation to induce and increase ease in the palpated tissue
4. All other elements remain the same.

7. FPR for third rib motion restriction

In this example, the third rib on the right is restricted and is prominent anteriorly – an inhalation restriction, producing an 'elevated' rib anteriorly.

1. The patient is seated and the practitioner stands in front with forearms placed as close to the neck as is comfortably possible.
2. The practitioner palpates the angle of the third rib with the left middle finger ('listening hand').
3. With the right forearm (resting on the patient's left shoulder area) lightly ease that shoulder posteriorly, causing the right side (and the affected rib) to rotate anteriorly exaggerating its anteriority on that side. The palpating digit should feel a slight slackening of tension.
4. The practitioners left forearm (resting on the patient's right shoulder area) applies slight downward pressure (to the floor), so introducing right side-bending *to the level of the affected* (and

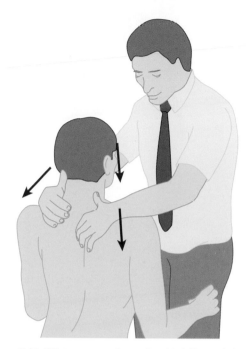

Figure 5.10 FPR treatment of anterior third rib restriction (inhalation restriction). The posterior articulation of that rib is palpated while the patient is taken into side flexion right and rotation left (exaggerating the distortion) together with a compressive crowding of the palpated tissues, before release and return to neutral.

palpated) *rib*. The palpating digit should feel a further slackening of tension.

5. A very slight increase in downward pressure (towards the floor) should be introduced by both forearms, reducing tension in the palpated area further.

6. The patient's upper body will effectively now be slightly side-flexed to the right and rotated to the left (Fig. 5.10).

7. Maintaining the compression vector, the patient should then be taken into left side-flexion and rotation to the right in order to return to the neutral position, at which time compression should be released.

8. Reassessment of the rib restriction should demonstrate both positional and functional improvement.

8. FPR treatment for lumbar restrictions and tissue change

This example is of an area of exaggerated tissue tension located on the right transverse process of the fourth lumbar vertebra.

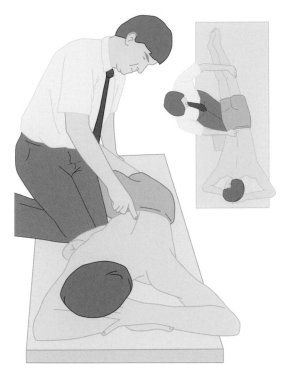

Figure 5.11 FPR treatment for lumbar restriction and tissue changes. Note that a pillow is used to reduce the antero-posterior curve of the lumbar spine while the practitioner introduces fine-tuning by positioning the legs to produce extension, side-flexion and rotation, until the palpating hand indicates that ease has been achieved. This is held for 3–4 seconds.

1. The patient lies prone with a pillow under the abdominal area, the purpose of which is to reduce the anterior lumbar curve.
2. The practitioner stands to the right of the table, having marked the area of tissue tension with the right index finger.
3. The practitioner places one or both knees on the table, at the level of the right hip joint, in order to offer a fulcrum over which the patient can be side-bent to the right (Fig. 5.11).
4. The practitioner's left hand draws the patient's legs towards the right side of the table, which effectively side-flexes the patient to the right.
5. This motion is continued slowly until tissue change (softening) is monitored by the index finger.
6. At this time, the practitioner changes the position of the left hand so that it grasps the anterior of the thigh, in order to be able to raise it into extension, at the same time introducing external rotation, until greater 'ease' is noted at the palpated monitoring point.

7. This is held for 3–4 seconds before a return to neutral is allowed, followed by reassessment.

Variations

Depending upon the nature of specific spinal restrictions, the same general rules would be applied. The basic requirements involve:

1. A reduction in the antero-posterior curve
2. A degree of crowding (or sometimes distraction)
3. Plus the spinal (or other) joint being taken to a combined position of freedoms of motion, away from the direction(s) of bind and into ease.

The examples given for thoracic and cervical normalization using FPR should make the general principles clear.

MUSCULAR CORRECTIONS USING FPR: PIRIFORMIS AS AN EXAMPLE

Schiowitz has described FPR application in treatment of piriformis and gluteal dysfunctions.

1. The distinctive FPR feature is introduced first –the patient is prone with a cushion under the abdomen to neutralize the lumbar curve.
2. The practitioner is positioned (possibly seated) on the side of dysfunction (right side in this example) facing cephalad.
3. The practitioner's left hand monitors a key area of tissue dysfunction, or a tender point, as in SCS.
4. The patient's flexed right knee and thigh are taken over the edge of the table and allowed to hang down, supported at the knee by the practitioner's right hand.
5. Flexion is introduced at the hip and knee by the practitioner, until an ease is sensed in the palpated tissues, or pain reduces.
6. The patient's thigh is then either abducted or adducted towards the table until further ease is noted in the palpated tissues.
7. The patient's knee is used as a lever to introduce either internal or external rotation at the hip, whichever produces the greatest reduction in tension under the palpating hand/finger (Fig. 5.12A).
8. Once a maximal degree of ease has been achieved, or pain is reduced by 70%, light compression is introduced through the long axis of the thigh towards the monitoring hand, where a marked reduction in tissue tension may be noted. *Note*: Compression is not shown in the accompanying video demonstration.
9. This is held for 3–4 seconds if facilitation is used, or for up to 90 seconds, if not, before a return to neutral and reassessment (Fig. 5.12B).

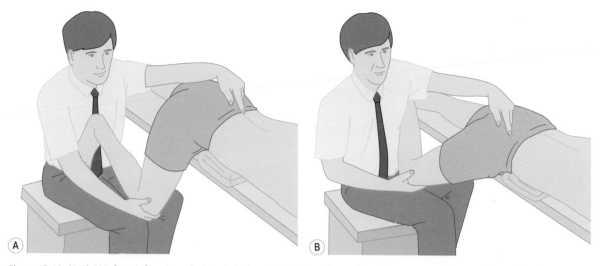

Figure 5.12 (A,B) FPR for piriformis and gluteal dysfunction involves the patient lying prone with a cushion under the abdomen. For right-sided dysfunction the right leg is flexed at both hip and knee, and abducted over the edge of the table while internal or external rotation of the thigh (whichever produces greater 'ease' in the palpated tissues) is used to fine-tune a position of ease. Light compression through the long axis of the femur may be applied to facilitate ease.

CLINICAL EVIDENCE OF FUNCTIONAL TECHNIQUE AND FPR EFFICACY

- Both counterstrain and FPR have been reported (Boyajian-O'Neill et al. 2008) to be effective in treatment of piriformis syndrome (DiGiovanna et al. 2004; Grant 1987).
- McSweeney et al. (2012) have demonstrated the immediate increase in pain thresholds in the lumbar spine, following functional technique applied to the sigmoid colon. 'This novel study provides new experimental evidence that visceral manual therapy can produce immediate hypoalgesia in somatic structures segmentally related to the organ being mobilised'.
- Kain et al. (2011) report that in a randomized clinical study, FPR (which they describe as 'triplanar indirect myofascial release') produced 'significant increases in range of motion … for flexion, extension and abduction' of the shoulder joint.

SIMILARITIES AND DIFFERENCES BETWEEN FPR AND SCS

The similarities and differences that exist when FPR (this chapter) and SCS (Chapters 2 and 3) are

Table 5.1 Similarities and differences between SCS and FPR

	SCS	FPR
Indirect approach	Yes	Yes
Monitoring contact	Pain point	Tissue tension
Find position of ease	Yes	Yes
Holding time	30–90 seconds	3–4 seconds
Uses facilitating crowding	Optional	Yes

compared, should by now be clear (see the summary in Table 5.1).

One major advantage of FPR seems to lie in its reduced (hence 'facilitated') time for holding the position of ease.

Another is of course the fact that no pain is induced in tender points, merely a palpation of ease (as in functional technique).

Note: There are no good reasons to avoid using facilitating compression in the application of SCS, and indeed the author strongly recommends that this be done, as long as (when using SCS) pain in the tender point reduces and no additional pain is caused.

143

CONTRAINDICATIONS

There are no contraindications to FPR, except that its value lies most profoundly in acute and sub-acute problems, with its ability to modify chronic tissue changes being limited to the same degree as other positional release methods.

POSITIONAL RELEASE AND CRANIAL MOBILITY

There is little, if any, debate regarding the pliability and plasticity of infant skulls. However, in order for cranial manipulation of adults, as currently taught and practised, to be taken seriously, it is necessary to establish whether or not there is evidence of verifiable motion between the cranial bones during and throughout adult life.

Sutherland (1939) suggested that there is demonstrable – if minute – motion at many of the cranial articulations. He also described the influence of the intracranial ligaments and fascia on cranial motion, which he suggested acted (at least in part for they certainly have other functions) to balance motion within the skull.

The reciprocal tension membranes (mainly the tentorium cerebelli and the falx cerebri), which are themselves extensions of the meninges, along with other contiguous and continuous dural structures, were described by Sutherland as taking part in a movement sequence which, because of their direct link (via the dura and the cord) between the occiput and the sacrum, produced a craniosacral movement sequence in which force was transmitted via the dura to the sacrum, producing an involuntary motion.

Five key elements of the cranial hypothesis that Sutherland (1939) proposed were:

1. An inherent motility of the brain and spinal cord
2. Fluctuating movement of the CSF
3. Motility of intracranial and spinal membranes
4. Mobility of the bones of the skull
5. Involuntary sacral motion between the ilia.

Do these propositions stand up to examination?

Evidence suggests that motility of the brain has been demonstrated (Frymann 1971). Cranial motion may contribute towards the composite of forces/pulses which it has been suggested go towards producing, what is known as, the cranial rhythmic impulse – CRI (Greenman 1989; McPartland & Mein 1997; Magoun 1976).

The CSF fluctuates, but its role remains unclear in terms of cranial motion. Whether it helps drive the observed motion of the brain or whether its motion is a by-product of cranial (and brain) motion remains uncertain.

The intracranial membranous structures (falx cerebri, etc.) attach to the internal skull and give shape to the venous sinuses. Any dysfunction involving the cranial bones would influence the status of these soft-tissue structures and vice versa. To what degree they influence sacral motion is questionable.

The bones of the skull appear to have minute motion potential at their sutures (Zanakis 1996). Whether this is simply plasticity that allows accommodation to intra- and extracranial forces or whether constant rhythmical motion, the CRI, drives a distinct cranial motion, is debatable.

The clinical implications of restrictions of the reported cranial articulations remain disputed as to precise implications.

There seems to be involuntary motion of the sacrum between the ilia, but the means whereby this occurs remains unclear (or at least unproven), as does the significance of this motion in terms of cranial mechanics.

In adults, most cranial treatments that attempt to normalize perceived restrictions or to influence function, involve indirect, positional release-type techniques.

Treatment of cranial structures

Upledger & Vredevoogd (1983) suggest that in order for cranial structures to be satisfactorily and safely treated, 'indirect' approaches are best.

By following any restricted structure to its easy unforced limit, in the direction towards which it moves most easily ('the direction towards which it exhibits the greatest range of inherent motion'), a sense may be noted in which the tissues seem to 'push back' from that extreme position, at which time the practitioner is advised to become 'immovable', not forcing the tissues against the resistance barrier, or trying to urge it towards greater 'ease', but simply refusing to allow movement.

It is not within the scope of this text to fully explore cranial concepts, some of which have been validated by animal and human research. However, a brief summary is needed in order for positional release applications to the cranial structures to be understood in the context of their clinical use (Chaitow 2005; Marmarou et al. 1975; Moskalenko 1961; Upledger & Vredevoogd 1983).

Greenman (1989) summarizes cranial flexibility as follows:

Craniosacral motion involves a combination of articular mobility and change in the tensions within the (intracranial) membranes. It is through the membranes' attachment that the synchronous movement of the cranium and the sacrum occurs.

During cranial motion, he explains:

The sutures appear to be organized to permit and guide certain types of movement between the cranial bones. These are intimately attached to the dura, and the sutures contain vascular and nervous system elements. The fibers within the sutures appear to be present in directions, which permit and yield to certain motions.

In one model of cranial theory, the movement of the cranial elements is said to be driven, at least in part, by a coiling and uncoiling process in which the cerebral hemispheres appear to swing upwards during what is known as cranial flexion, and then to descend again during the extension mode of the cranial cycle.

As the flexion phase occurs, the paired and unpaired bones of the head are thought to respond in symmetrical fashion, which is both palpable and capable of being assessed for restriction.

A variety of other theories exist to explain cranial motion (Chaitow 2005; Heisey & Adams 1993), ranging from biomechanical explanations, in which respiration and muscular activity are the prime movers, to circulatory models, in which venomotion and CSF fluctuations are responsible, and even compound 'entrainment' theories, in which the body's multiple oscillations and pulsations combine to form harmonic influences (McPartland & Mein 1997). The truth is that while an undoubted, if minute degree of motility (self-actuated movement) and mobility (movement induced by external features) can be demonstrated at the cranial sutures (Lewandoski et al. 1996), most explanations for the mechanisms involved are as yet hypothetical.

Motions noted at the sphenobasilar junction

It has been suggested by Upledger & Vredevoogd (1983), and others that the following movements take place simultaneously (it is important to realize that cranial motion is a plastic one rather than one involving gross movement):

- A reduction in the vertical diameter of the skull.
- A reduction in the antero-posterior diameter.
- An increase in the cranial transverse diameter.

These 'movements' are extremely small, in the region of 0.25 mm (250 microns) at the sagittal suture (Zanakis 1996).

Put simply, this means the skull gets 'flatter', narrower from front to back, and wider from side to side. It is proposed that this happens as the occiput eases forwards at its base, causing the sphenoid to rise at its synchondrosis (Fig. 5.13).

Because of its unique structure, this then causes the great wings of the sphenoid to rotate anteriorly, followed by the frontal and facial bones. The temporals and other cranial bones are then said to accommodate this motion by externally rotating.

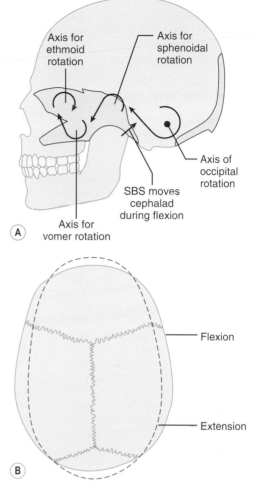

Figure 5.13 (A) Schematic representation of theorized cranial motion. During flexion, the occiput is thought to move antero-superior, which causes the sphenoid to rise at its synchondrosis. Simultaneous movement occurs in the frontal, facial and nasal bones as indicated. The extension phase of this motion involves a return to a neutral position. (B) The flexion phase of cranial motion ('inhalation phase') causes the skull as a whole to widen and flatten minutely.

Two cranial exercises

Two exercises are described below that should allow the reader to get a sense of the subtlety of cranial methodology and of the influence of positioning in order to effect a change.

Caution

D'Ambrogio & Roth (1997) caution that:

With any cranial treatment it is recommended that certain precautions be taken. Symptoms and signs of space-occupying lesions and acute head trauma are clear contraindications. A history of seizures or previous cerebrovascular accident should be approached with caution.

1. Exercise in sphenobasilar assessment and treatment

A useful exercise can be performed in which the model/patient is supine and the practitioner sits to the right or left near the head of the table.

1. The caudad hand rests on the table holding the occipital area so that the occipital squama closest to the practitioner rests on the hyperthenar eminence while the tips of the fingers support the opposite occipital angle (Fig. 5.14).
2. The cephalad hand rests over the frontal bone so that the thumb lies on one great wing of the sphenoid, with the tips of the fingers on the other great wing, with as little contact as possible on the frontal bone.
3. If the hand is small, the contacts can be made on the lateral angles of the frontal bone.
4. It is necessary to sit quietly in this position for some minutes in an attempt to palpate cranial motion.
5. As sphenobasilar flexion commences (as a sense of 'fullness' is noted in the palpating hand), apparent occipital movement may be noted in a caudad and anterior direction; simultaneously the great wings of the sphenoid may seem to rotate anteriorly and caudally around their transverse axis.

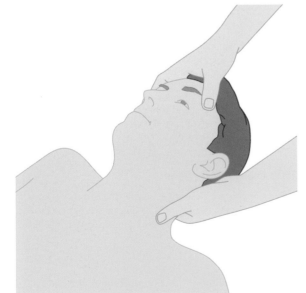

Figure 5.14 Sphenobasilar assessment: hand positions for palpation of the occiput and great wings of the sphenoid.

6. Encouragement of these motions can be introduced in order to assess any existing restriction.
7. This is achieved by using very light (grams rather than ounces) pressure in the appropriate directions to impede the movement described.
8. During sphenobasilar extension (as the sense of fullness in the palpating hand recedes), a return to neutral may be noted, as cranial motion appears to return to the starting position.
9. Whichever of these motions (flexion, extension) is assessed as being *least* restricted should then be encouraged.
10. As this is done, a very slight 'yielding' motion may be noted at the end of the range.
11. The tissues should be held in this direction of greatest ease until a sense occurs of the tissues 'pushing back' towards the neutral position.
12. A great deal of sensitivity is needed in order to achieve this successfully.

Note: It is worth emphasizing the author's belief that while the cranial movements described may be palpated and perceived by the sensitive individual, precisely what is moving, and what moves it, as well as clinical relevance, remains uncertain. The description of cranial motion given above expresses Upledger's (1984) suggestion as to what may be happening (a widely held view in craniosacral circles) but remains unsubstantiated (Chaitow 2005).

2. Temporal freedom of movement palpation exercise

(Fig. 5.15)

Sit at the head of the supine model/patient.

1. Interlock your fingers (or have the hands cupped, with one in the other) so that the head is cradled, your thumbs are on, and are parallel with, the anterior surfaces of the mastoid processes, while the thenar eminences support the mastoid portion of the bone (Fig. 5.15A).
2. Your index fingers should cross each other and be in direct contact.
3. Assess the freedom of flexion of one side and then the other.
4. This is achieved by focussing on the thumb contact on one side at a time.
5. As the temporal bones move into the flexion phase the mastoid appears to ease very slightly posteriorly and medially (Fig. 5.15B).
6. This is more a sense of 'give' or plasticity, than actual movement.
7. Assess one side and then the other several times, using a very small amount of contact pressure – no more than would be comfortable were this applied to your open eye.

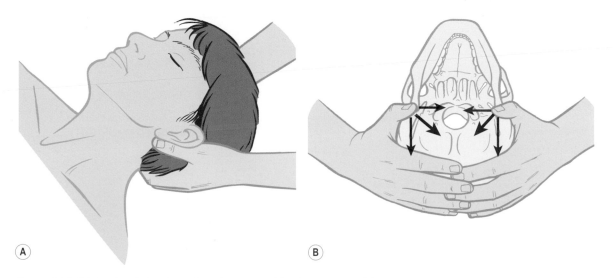

Figure 5.15 (A) Hand and thumb positions for temporal freedom exercise. (B) Directions of motion of the mastoid to encourage temporal flexion.

8. By pivoting the middle joints of your index fingers against each other in rhythm with cranial flexion and extension (a very slight sense of fullness in the palms of the hands equates with the flexion phase), this can be achieved without use of actual hand or thumb strength.

9. The amount of pressure introduced at the mastoid should be in grams only, and should only be attempting to evaluate whether there is symmetry of easy motion on each side.

10. Test slight variations in the directions of applied pressure (grams only!) as shown with Figure 5.15B.

11. If one side appears to 'move' more freely into flexion, to be more resilient, more plastic, have more give, this is the side of relative freedom of movement.

12. To evaluate whether this can be modified towards better balance (equal degree of freedom of movement bilaterally), ease the 'free' side towards its direction of free movement (posteromedially) and hold it there, while at the same time placing the thumb on the other side posterior to the mastoid in order to ease it anterolaterally.

13. Hold this for four or five cycles of inhalation/exhalation, or until a sense of pressure against your palpating thumbs is noted.

14. At that time, release the pressure (grams only!) and reassess to see whether the exercise has created a more balanced sense of motion or plasticity.

CLINICAL EVIDENCE OF CRANIAL TREATMENT EFFICACY

- Berkowitz (2014) reports as follows: 'This case involves a patient seen in the Osteopathic Manipulative Medicine Clinic with sudden, painless onset of loss of visual field five weeks following craniotomy for meningioma removal. … The patient's loss of visual field resolved completely immediately following the application of osteopathy in the cranial field. While the synchronicity may suggest that the two events are causally linked, further clinical evidence is required before such an effect can be attributed to osteopathic intervention'.

- Other reports have indicated the potential benefits of cranial treatment (functional) of visual dysfunction (Sandhouse et al 2010; Wolf 1991).

- Hayden & Mulligan (2009) report on the outcomes of an open, controlled trial in which 28 infants with colic were either treated with cranial methods – once weekly for 4 weeks, or received no treatment. Outcomes showed: 'overall decline in crying was 63% (treated) and 23% (not treated), respectively; improvement in sleeping was 11% and 2%, respectively. Treated infants also required less parental attention than the untreated group'.

THIS CHAPTER

This chapter has explored aspects of functional (including cranially applied) and facilitated positional release techniques – offering some of the theoretical underpinnings of these methods together with practical exercises, along with examples of research evidence as to their possible clinical usefulness.

NEXT CHAPTER

Additional evidence is offered in the next chapter that outlines the use of these – and counterstrain – methods, in particular clinical settings, including use for hospitalized/bed-bound patients, as well as in chronic pain situations.

REFERENCES

Bailey, H., 1976. Some problems in making osteopathic spinal manipulative therapy appropriate and specific. Journal of the American Osteopathic Association 75, 486–499.

Berkowitz, M.R., 2014. Application of osteopathy in the cranial field to treat left superior homonymous hemianopsia. International Journal of Osteopathic Medicine 17, 119–122.

Bowles, C., 1955. A Functional Orientation for Technic: Part 1. Academy of Applied Osteopathy Year Book, Colorado Springs.

Bowles, C., 1956. A Functional Orientation for Technic: Part 2. Academy of Applied Osteopathy Year Book, Colorado Springs.

Bowles, C., 1957. A Functional Orientation for Technic: Part 3. Academy of Applied Osteopathy Year Book, Colorado Springs.

Bowles, C., 1964. The Musculoskeletal Segment as a Problem-Solving Machine. Academy of Applied Osteopathy Yearbook, Colorado Springs.

Bowles, C., 1981. Functional technique – a modern perspective. Journal of the American Osteopathic Association 80, 326–331.

Boyajian-O'Neill, L.A., McClain, R.L., Coleman, M.K., et al., 2008. Diagnosis and management of piriformis syndrome: an osteopathic approach. Journal of the American Osteopathic Association 108, 657–664.

Carew, T., 1985. The control of reflex action. In: Kandel, E. (Ed.), Principles of Neural Science, second ed. Elsevier Science, New York.

Chaitow, L., 2005. Cranial Manipulation: Theory and Practice. Churchill Livingstone, Edinburgh.

D'Ambrogio, K., Roth, G., 1997. Positional Release Therapy. Mosby, St Louis, MO.

DiGiovanna, E., Schiowitz, S., Dowling, D., 2004. An Osteopathic Approach to Diagnosis and Treatment, third revised ed. Lippincott Williams and Wilkins, Philadelphia, PA.

Frymann, V., 1971. A study of the rhythmic motions of the living cranium. Journal of the American Osteopathic Association 70, 828–945.

Gibbons, P., Tehan, P., 1998. Muscle energy concepts and coupled motion of the spine. Manual Therapy 3, 95–101.

Grant, J.H., 1987. Leg length inequality in piriformis syndrome. Journal of the American Osteopathic Association 87, 456.

Greenman, P., 1989. Principles of Manual Medicine. Williams & Wilkins, Baltimore, MD.

Hayden, C., Mulligan, B., 2009. A preliminary assessment of the impact of cranial osteopathy for the relief of infantile colic. Complementary Therapies in Clinical Practice 15, 198–203.

Hazzard, C., 1905. The Practice and Applied Therapeutics of Osteopathy, third ed. Journal Printing Co, Kirksville, MO.

Heisey, S., Adams, T., 1993. Role of cranial bone mobility in cranial compliance. Neurosurgery 33, 869–877.

Hoover, H.V., 1957. Functional Technique. Academy of Applied Osteopathy Yearbook, Colorado Springs.

Hoover, H.V., 1969a. Collected Papers. Academy of Applied Osteopathy Yearbook, Colorado Springs.

Hoover, H.V., 1969b. A Method for Teaching Functional Technic. Academy of Applied Osteopathy Yearbook, Colorado Springs.

Janda, V., 1988. In: Grant, R. (Ed.), Physical Therapy of the Cervical and Thoracic Spine. Churchill Livingstone, New York.

Johnston, W., 1964. Strategy of a Functional Approach in Acute Knee Problems. Academy of Applied Osteopathy Yearbook, Colorado Springs.

Johnston, W.L., 1988a. Segmental definition: Part I. A focal point for diagnosis of somatic dysfunction. Journal of the American Osteopathic Association 88, 99–105.

Johnston, W.L., 1988b. Segmental definition: Part II. Application of an indirect method in osteopathic manipulative treatment. Journal of the American Osteopathic Association 88, 211–217.

Johnston, W., Robertson, A., Stiles, E., 1969. Finding a Common Denominator. Academy of Applied Osteopathy Yearbook, Colorado Springs.

Kain, J., Martorello, L., Swanson, E., et al., 2011. Comparison of an indirect tri-planar myofascial release (MFR) technique and a hot pack for increasing range of motion. Journal of Bodywork and Movement Therapies 15, 63–67.

Korr, I., 1947. The neural basis for the osteopathic lesion. Journal of the American Osteopathic Association 47, 191.

Korr, I., 1975. Proprioceptors and somatic dysfunction. Journal of the American Osteopathic Association 74, 638–650.

Korr, I., 1976. Spinal Cord as Organizer of the Disease Process. Academy of Applied Osteopathy Yearbook, Colorado Springs.

Lewandoski, M., Drasby, E., Morgan, M., et al., 1996. Kinematic system demonstrates cranial bone movement about the cranial sutures. Journal of the American Osteopathic Association 96, 551.

McPartland, J.M., Mein, J., 1997. Entrainment and the cranial rhythmic impulse. Alternative Therapies in Health and Medicine 3, 40–45.

McSweeney, T.P., Thomson, O.P., Johnston, R., 2012. The immediate effects of sigmoid colon manipulation on pressure pain thresholds in the lumbar spine. Journal of Bodywork and Movement Therapies 16, 416–423.

Magoun, H., 1976. Osteopathy in the Cranial Field. Journal Printing Co, Kirksville, MO.

Marmarou, A., Shulman, K., LaMorgese, J., 1975. Compartmental analysis of compliance and outflow resistance of CSF system. Journal of Neurosurgery 43, 523–534.

Mimura, M., Moriya, H., Watanabe, T., et al., 1989. Three-dimensional motion analysis of the cervical spine with special reference to the axial rotation. Spine 14, 1135–1139.

Moskalenko, Y., 1961. Cerebral pulsation in the closed cranial cavity. Izvestiia Academii Nauk Biologicheskaia 4, 620–629.

Sandhouse, M.E., Shechtman, D., Sorkin, R., et al., 2010. Effect of osteopathy in the cranial field on visual function – a pilot study. Journal of the American Osteopathic Association 110, 239–243.

Schiowitz, S., 1990. Facilitated positional release. Journal of the American Osteopathic Association 90, 145–156.

Schiowitz, S., 1991. Facilitated positional release. In: DiGiovanna, E. (Ed.), An Osteopathic Approach to Diagnosis and Treatment. Lippincott, Philadelphia, PA.

Steiner, C., 1994. Osteopathic manipulative treatment – what does it really do? Journal of the American Osteopathic Association 94, 85–87.

Sutherland, W., 1939. The Cranial Bowl. Privately published, Mankato, MN.

Upledger, J., 1984. Cranial Sacral Therapy. Eastland Press, Seattle.

Upledger, J., Vredevoogd, J., 1983. Craniosacral Therapy. Eastland Press, Seattle, WA.

Van Buskirk, R.L., 1996. A manipulative technique of Andrew Taylor Still as reported by Charles Hazzard, DO, in 1905. Journal of the American Osteopathic Association 96, 597–602.

Van Buskirk, R.L., 2000. The Still Technique Manual. Applications of a Rediscovered Technique of Andrew Taylor Still. American Academy of Osteopathy, Indianapolis, IN.

Wolf, A.H., 1997. Osteopathic manipulative procedure in disorders of the eye. Journal of the American Osteopathic Association 7, 31.

Zanakis, N., 1996. Studies of CRI in man using a tilt table. Journal of the American Osteopathic Association 96, 552.

Chapter | 6 |

Positional release methods in special situations

This chapter builds on methods described in earlier chapters, by describing approaches suitable for:

Specific conditions, situations:

- Myofascial pain (see Box 6.1)
- Fibromyalgia (see Box 6.1).

Particular settings:

- Bed-bound
- Postoperative situations.

Abbreviations:

- TrPs – myofascial trigger points (a feature of acute or chronic myofascial pain)
- TePs – tender points; specified areas used in diagnosis of fibromyalgia (see later in this chapter)
- CMP – chronic myofascial pain (previously known as 'myofascial pain syndrome', but no longer regarded as a syndrome)
- FM – fibromyalgia (previously known as 'fibromyalgia syndrome', but no longer regarded as a syndrome).

MYOFASCIAL PAIN, TRIGGER POINTS AND CENTRAL SENSITIZATION (CS)

Pain is the most frequent presenting symptom in medical practice in the industrialized world, and musculoskeletal pain forms a major element of that category of symptoms.

According to leading researchers into the topic, Wall & Melzack (1990), myofascial trigger points are a key element in all chronic pain, and are often the main factor maintaining it.

There appears to be a direct link between localized, e.g. myofascial pain and the evolution of chronic syndromes, such as fibromyalgia (FM) (Baldry 2010).

- Fernández-de-las-Peñas et al. (2005) have also reported on the distinct connection between myofascial trigger point activity and a wide range of pain problems and sympathetic nervous system aberrations.
- There is increasing evidence that trigger points contribute to the development of central sensitization, and as such may cause or contribute to various chronic pain syndromes (Cuadrado et al. 2008; Giamberardino et al. 2007).

Ge et al. (2009) note that: 'The local and referred pain patterns induced from active TrPs bilaterally, in the upper trapezius muscle are similar to ongoing pain patterns in the neck and shoulder region in FM. Active TrPs may serve as one of the sources of noxious input leading to the sensitization of spinal and supraspinal pain pathways in FM'.

Ge (2010) further reports that: 'Research highlights the importance of active TrPs in FM patients. Most of the tender point (TeP) sites in FM are TrPs. Active TrPs may serve as a peripheral generator of fibromyalgia pain and inactivation of active TrPs may thus be an alternative for the treatment of FM'.

- Niddam et al. (2008) found that individuals with chronic myofascial pain (CMP) had abnormal central processing with enhanced brain activity in the somatosensory and limbic regions, suppressed activity in the hippocampus, and hyperalgesia in response to electrical stimulation and compression of trigger points. Trigger point therapy appears to improve such abnormal pain processing (Dommerholt et al. 2006).

It is clearly of major importance that practitioners and therapists have available safe and effective methods for handling myofascial and other chronic pain conditions, such as the fibromyalgia (FM) (Wolfe et al. 1990).

Mense (1993, 2008) has reported:

Clinical examination reveals sites of excessive sensitivity to palpation of tender points (TeP), at which mild externally applied pressure causes pain. Many of these TePs are located at the myotendinous junction, rather than near the belly of the muscle, where trigger points are more likely to be found.

Trigger (and other non-referring pain) points commonly lie in muscles that have been stressed in a variety of ways, often as a result of:

- Postural imbalances (Harden 2007; Lewit 1999)
- Congenital factors – short leg problems or small hemipelvis (Simons et al. 1999)
- Occupational or leisure overuse patterns (Bron & Dommerholt 2012)
- Emotional states reflecting into the soft tissues (McNulty et al. 1994)
- Referred/reflex involvement of the viscera producing facilitated (neurologically hyper-reactive) segments paraspinally (Beal 1985; Hong 1994; Simons 1999)
- Hypermobility (Muller 2003)
- Trauma (see Chapter 2 for discussion on the evolution of dysfunction via adaptation) (Fig. 6.1).

Reducing central sensitization by deactivating myofascial trigger points

A study by Affaitati et al. (2011) involved 56 female patients with FM and CMP, and 56 female patients with FM joint pain. These were all randomly divided into active treatment (lidocaine injection ×2/hydrofor-electrophoresis ×2) or placebo groups.

In the active groups, the number and intensity of myofascial/joint episodes and pain medication consumption decreased, and pressure thresholds at trigger point/joint increased ($p < 0.001$). FM pain intensity decreased and all thresholds increased progressively ($p < 0.0001$). At a 3-week follow-up, FM pain reduction was maintained.

Conclusion

Localized muscle/joint pains impact significantly on FM, probably through increased central sensitization due to the peripheral input, and their systematic identification and treatment are recommended in fibromyalgia.

To summarize

Both local muscle, as well as joint pains, *directly* influence increased central sensitization (CS) and successful treatment of these, leads to reduced CS.

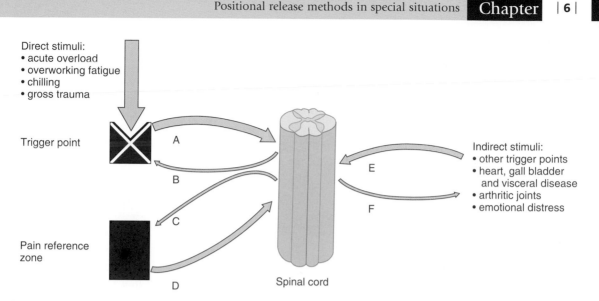

Figure 6.1 Direct stress influence can affect the hyper-reactive neural structure of a myofascial trigger point, leading to increased activity (A, B) as well as referring sensations (pain, paraesthesiae, increased sympathetic activity) to a target area (C, D) which feeds back into the cord to increase the background stress load. Other stimuli reach the cord from distant trigger points and additional dysfunctional areas (E, F).

Trigger point characteristics

- The leading researchers into trigger points (TrPs), Simons et al. (1999), define trigger points as: hyperirritable foci, lying within taut bands of muscle, which are painful on compression and which refer pain or other symptoms at a distant site ('target area').
- Embryonic TrPs tend to develop as 'satellites' of existing triggers in the target area, and in time, these produce their own satellites.
- According to Wall & Melzack (1990), nearly 80% of TrPs are in exactly the same positions as known acupuncture points, as used in traditional Chinese medicine.
- Painful points ('tender points') that do not refer symptoms to a distant site are often latent trigger points, that need only to experience additional degrees of stress in order to create greater facilitation, and so be transformed into active TrPs.
- The taut band in which TrPs lie will twitch if a finger is run across it, and is tight but not usually fibrosed, and it will commonly soften and relax if the appropriate treatment is applied – something fibrotic tissue cannot do (Hong 1994).
- Muscles that contain TrPs will often hurt when they are contracted (i.e. when they are working) and they will almost always be painful if stretched.
- TrPs are areas of lowered oxygen supply due to inadequate local circulation. Such muscles will therefore fatigue rapidly (Shah & Phillips 2003).

- The fact that muscles in which TrPs cannot reach a normal resting length – being held almost constantly in a shortened position – makes them an ideal target for the methods of positional release, since such muscles will happily be shortened further but will resist being lengthened.
- Simons et al. (1999) have established that until a muscle housing a TrP can reach its normal resting length, without pain or effort, attempts to deactivate a TrP will only achieve temporary relief, as it will reactivate after treatment.
- Stretching of the muscles housing a TrP, using either active or passive methods, is a useful way of treating the shortness as well as the TrP, since this can reduce the contraction (taut band) as well as increasing circulation to the area – something which positional release methods, such as SCS, can also achieve (Vernon & Schneider 2009).
- There are many variably successful ways of treating TrPs, including acupuncture, procaine injections, direct manual pressure (with the thumb, etc.), stretching the muscle, ice therapy, etc. Whatever is done, unless the muscle can be induced to reach its normal resting length, any such treatment will be of limited value.
- Some of these methods (pressure, acupuncture) cause the release in the body and the brain of natural pain-killing substances – endorphins and endocannabinoids – which explains one of the ways in which pain might be reduced (McPartland 2008).

- Pain is also relieved when one sensation (digital pressure, needle, etc.) is substituted for another (the original pain). In this way, pain messages are partially or totally blocked, or partially prevented from reaching or being registered by the brain.
- Methods that improve the circulatory imbalance will affect TrPs, which contain areas of ischaemic tissue, and in this way appear to deactivate them (Gerwin 2005; Hong 1994).
- The target area to which a TrP refers pain will be the same in everyone if the TrP is in the same position – but this pattern of pain distribution does not seem to relate to known nerve pathways.
- TrPs involve a self-perpetuating cycle (pain leading to increased tone leading to more pain) and may not deactivate unless adequately treated.
- The way in which a TrP influences pain in a distant site may involve neurological mechanisms, however just how TrPs influence their symptoms remains unclear.
- Remarkable research by Langevin & Yandow (2002) has shed much new light on the possibility that fascial structures are the means whereby sensation is transmitted.
- TrPs lie in parts of muscles most prone to mechanical stress, often close to origins and insertions, and also, very commonly, they are situated on fascial cleavage planes (Langevin & Yandow 2002).

What causes the trigger point to develop?

Simons et al. (1999) are the physicians who, above all others, have helped our understanding of trigger points. They have described the evolution of TrPs as follows:

> In the core of the trigger lies a muscle spindle which is in trouble for some reason. Visualise a spindle like a strand of yarn in a knitted sweater … a metabolic crisis takes place which increases the temperature locally in the trigger point, shortens a minute part of the muscle (sarcomere) – like a snag in a sweater – and reduces the supply of oxygen and nutrients into the trigger point. During this disturbed episode an influx of calcium occurs and the muscle spindle does not have enough energy to pump the calcium outside the cell where it belongs. Thus a vicious cycle is maintained and the muscle spindle can't seem to loosen up and the affected muscle can't relax.

Simons tested his concept and found that at the core of a trigger point, there is an oxygen deficit compared with the muscle tissue which surrounds it.

Travell & Simons (1992) confirmed that the following factors can all help to maintain and enhance trigger point activity:

- Nutritional deficiency, especially vitamin C, B-complex and iron
- Hormonal imbalances (low thyroid, menopausal or premenstrual situations, for example)
- Infections (bacteria, viruses or yeast)
- Allergies (wheat and dairy in particular)
- Low oxygenation of tissues (aggravated by tension, stress, inactivity, poor respiration).

Bron & Dommerholt (2012) simplify the aetiological features when they assert:

> There is general agreement that any kind of muscle overuse or direct trauma to the muscle can lead to the development of TrPs. Muscle overload is thought to be the result of sustained or repetitive low-level muscle contractions, eccentric muscle contractions, and maximal or submaximal concentric muscle contractions.

Muscle pain and breathing dysfunction

Trigger point activity is particularly prevalent in the muscles of the neck/shoulder region, which also act as accessory breathing muscles, particularly the scalenes (Gerwin 1991; Sachse 1995).

In situations of increased anxiety and chronic fatigue, the incidence of borderline or frank over-breathing is frequent, and may be associated with a wide range of secondary symptoms including headaches, neck, shoulder and arm pain, dizziness, palpitations, fainting, spinal and abdominal discomfort, digestive symptoms relating to diaphragmatic weakness and stress, as well as the anxiety-related phenomena of panic attacks and phobic behaviour (Bass & Gardner 1985; Njoo et al. 1995; Perri & Halford 2004).

Clinically, where upper chest breathing is a feature, the upper fixators of the shoulders and the intercostal, pectoral and paraspinal muscles of the thoracic region are likely to palpate as tense, often fibrotic, with active trigger points being common (Chaitow et al. 2014; Roll & Theorell 1987).

Successful breathing retraining and normalization of energy levels seems in such cases to be accelerated and enhanced following initial normalization of the functional integrity of the muscles involved in respiration, directly or indirectly (latissimus dorsi, psoas, quadratus lumborum) (Lum 1984).

Pelvic pain and myofascial trigger points

Slocumb (1984), Weiss (2001) and Fitzgerald et al. (2009) have all shown that in a large proportion of chronic pelvic pain problems in women, often destined for surgical intervention, the prime cause of the symptoms involves TrPs activity in muscles of the lower abdomen, perineum, inner thigh and even on the walls of the vagina.

They have also demonstrated that appropriate deactivation of these TrPs can remove or relieve symptoms of both interstitial cystitis and chronic pelvic pain.

Strain/counterstrain and trigger points

Simons et al. (1999) discuss strain/counterstrain in relation to the treatment of trigger points, and suggest that most of the TePs listed in Jones's original book (Jones 1981), and many of those described in subsequent PRT texts (D'Ambrogio & Roth 1997), are close to attachment trigger point sites.

This is, however, not universally true:

Of the 65 tender points (in Jones' original book), nine were identified at the attachment region of a named muscle. Forty-four points were located either at the region of a muscular attachment where one might find an attachment trigger point, or, occasionally, at the belly of a muscle where a central trigger point might be located.

If at least some, and possibly the majority, of Jones's TePs, appear to be the same phenomena as Simons & Travell's TrPs, logic suggests that a therapeutic approach that effectively deactivates one (the tender point) should beneficially affect the other (trigger point).

See Chapter 2, Box 2.4, for discussion on TrPs and TePs – similarities and differences.

Treatment of TrPs using positional release methods

Numerous studies confirm the value of positional release methods – either singly within combinations on its own (Dardzinski et al. 2000; Ibáñez-García et al. 2009; Meseguer et al. 2006) or a combination of methods, including counterstrain – described as *integrated neuromuscular inhibition technique* (INIT), which is explained below (Chaitow 1994; Nagrale et al. 2010).

Before describing positional release as part of the INIT trigger point treatment protocol, the methods for identifying TrPs are required.

PALPATION

Palpation tests for tender and trigger points

In 1992, a study was conducted by two leading figures in the study of myofascial pain, in order to evaluate the accuracy of TrP palpation, by experts responsible for diagnosis of fibromyalgia (FM) or chronic myofascial pain (CMP) (Wolfe et al. 1992).

- Volunteers from three groups were tested – some with FM, some with CMP and some with no pain or any other symptoms.
- The FM patients were easily identified – 38% of the FM patients were found to have active trigger points.
- Of the CMP patients, only 23.4% were identified as having trigger points, and of the normal volunteers, less than 2% had any.
- Most of the CMP patients had tender points in sites usually tested in FM, and would have qualified for this diagnosis as well.

Recommended trigger point palpation method

There are a variety of palpation methods by means of which trigger (or tender) points can rapidly be identified, among which the simplest and possibly the most effective is use of what is termed 'drag' palpation, as fully discussed in Chapter 2 (Chaitow 1991).

- A light passage of a single digit, finger or thumb, across the skin ('feather-light touch') elicits a sense of hesitation, or 'drag', when the skin has an increased water content compared with surrounding skin.
- This increased hydrosis (sweat) seems to correlate with increased sympathetic activity, which accompanies local tissue dysfunction in general and trigger point activity in particular (Lewit 1999).

Lewit (1999) additionally suggests that the skin overlying a trigger point will exhibit reduced elasticity when lightly stretched apart, as compared with surrounding skin.

Lewit terms such phenomena 'hyperalgesic skin zones' and identifies a further characteristic: a reduced degree of movement of the skin over the underlying fascia, palpable when attempting to slide or 'roll' the skin.

These three features of skin change offer simple and effective clues as to underlying dysfunction:

- Reduced sliding movement of skin on fascia
- Reduced local elasticity
- Increased hydrosis.

Systematic approaches to the charting of TrP locations (and their deactivation) are also offered by systems such as neuromuscular technique (NMT), in which a methodical sequence of palpatory searches are carried out, based on the trigger point 'maps', as described by Simons et al. (1999).

When attempting to palpate for TrPs at depth, not simply using skin signs, a particularly useful phrase to keep in mind is that used by Stanley Lief DC, co-developer of NMT (Chaitow 1996):

> *To discover local changes (such as TrPs) it is necessary to constantly vary palpation pressure, to 'meet and match' tissue tensions.*

D'Ambrogio & Roth (1997), put it differently:

> *Tissue must be entered gently, and only necessary pressure must be used to palpate through the layers of tissue.*

Note: Counterstrain – as detailed in Chapter 4 – may be used on its own as an effective TrP treatment, however treatment has been found to produce more effective and lasting effects when combined with other modalities.

Integrated neuromuscular inhibition technique (INIT)

(Chaitow 1994)

Counterstrain may be used in combination with other modalities such as is used in integrated neuromuscular inhibition technique (INIT). The method of INIT is explained below:

- Pyszora et al. (2010) reported that a combination of INIT and kinesio-taping proved effective in palliative care of severely ill individuals: *minimizing the complications and effects of disease and optimizing patients' condition.*
- Abha et al. (2010) demonstrated that INIT was: *highly effective in the treatment of trigger point pain in the upper trapezius muscle.*
- A similar outcome was reported by Nagrale et al. (2010) in relation to neck pain resulting from myofascial trigger points.
- A study was conducted (Nayak 2013) at Rajiv Gandhi University of Health Sciences, Bangalore, to establish the efficacy of INIT combined with therapeutic ultrasound (US), compared with INIT with placebo ultrasound in the treatment of acute neck pain, associated with myofascial trigger points in the upper trapezius muscles. The study concluded that INIT used with US, and INIT used with placebo US, are both effective

in decreasing pain, decreasing neck disability and improving range of motion. However, those receiving INIT + therapeutic US showed significantly more improvement than those receiving INIT plus placebo.

INIT method

1. It is reasonable to assume, and palpation confirms, that when a TrP is being palpated by direct finger or thumb pressure, and when the very tissues in which the trigger point lies are positioned in such a way as to take away the pain (entirely or at least to a great extent), the most (dis)stressed fibres in which the trigger point is housed are in a position of relative ease (Fig. 6.2, INIT methodology is outlined in the caption for this figure).
2. At this time, the TrP would be under direct inhibitory pressure (mild or perhaps intermittent) and would have been positioned so that the tissues housing it are relaxed (relatively or completely).
3. Following a period of 20–30 seconds of this position of ease and inhibitory pressure, the patient is asked to introduce an isometric contraction into the tissues and to hold this for 7–10 seconds – involving the precise fibres which had been repositioned to obtain the strain/counterstrain release.
4. The effect of this isometric contraction would be to produce (following the contraction) a degree of reduction in tone in these tissues (as a result of post-isometric relaxation).
5. The hypertonic or contracted tissues could then be gently stretched for up to 30 seconds, as in any muscle energy procedure, with the strong likelihood that the specifically targeted fibres would be stretched.
6. Following this, a whole muscle isometric contraction, followed by a whole muscle stretch (also for up to 30 seconds) is then carried out.

Clinical relevance

As detailed above, there exists a great deal of agreement that much of the pain, and the peripheral stimulus that leads to, or helps maintain, central sensitization, involves local myofascial (TrP) pain.

With this in mind, it can be seen that non-invasive, and effective, methods – such as counterstrain and other positional release methods – offer a useful combination of modalities for clinical use in management of chronic pain syndromes, such as FM.

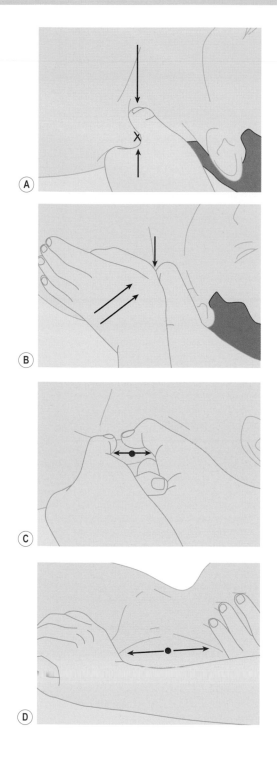

Figure 6.2 (A) First stage of INIT in which a tender/pain/trigger point in upper trapezius is located and ischaemically compressed, either intermittently or persistently. (B) The pain is removed from the tender/pain/trigger point by finding a position of ease, which is held for at least 20 seconds, following which an isometric contraction is achieved involving the local tissues housing the point. (C) Following the holding of the isometric contraction for 5–7 seconds, the local muscle tissues in which the point lies are stretched. (D) The whole muscle is stretched after a further whole muscle isometric contraction. This completes the INIT sequence.

FIBROMYALGIA SYNDROME (FM)

FM is defined by *Mosby's Medical Dictionary* as:

> *A form of nonarticular rheumatism characterized by musculo-skeletal pain, spasms, stiffness, fatigue, and severe sleep disturbance. Common sites of pain or stiffness include the lower back, neck, shoulder region, arms, hands, knees, hips, thighs, legs, and feet. These sites are known as trigger points. Physical therapy, non-steroidal anti-inflammatory drugs, and muscle relaxants provide temporary relief. Also called fibrositis, soft tissue rheumatism. (See Boxes 6.1, 6.2.)*

Counterstrain and fibromyalgia

Osteopathic physicians using strain/counterstrain (SCS) and muscle energy techniques (MET), as well as other osteopathic methods, have conducted numerous studies involving patients with a firm diagnosis of FM.

Among the studies in which (SCS) was a major form of treatment of FM are the following:

1. Doctors at the Chicago College of Osteopathic Medicine measured the effects of osteopathic manipulative therapy (OMT – which included both SCS and MET) on the intensity of pain in tender points involving 18 patients who met all the criteria for FM. Each had six visits/treatments and it was found, over a 1-year period, that 12 of the patients responded well, in that their tender points became less sensitive (14% reduction against a 34% increase in the six patients who did not respond well). Most of the patients – the responders and the non-responders who had received SCS and MET – showed (using thermographic imaging) that their tender points were more symmetrically spread after the course than before. Activities of daily living were significantly improved and general pain symptoms decreased (Stoltz 1993).

1.   History of widespread pain

Pain is considered widespread when all of the following are present:

- Pain in the left side of the body
- Pain in the right side of the body
- Pain above the waist
- Pain below the waist.

In addition, the patient should complain of pain in the spine or the neck or front of the chest, or thoracic spine or low back.

2.   Pain in 11 of 18 palpated sites

There should be pain on pressure (around 4 kg of pressure maximum) on not less than 11 of the following sites:

- Either side of the base of the skull where the suboccipital muscles insert
- Either side of the side of the neck between the fifth and seventh cervical vertebrae (technically described as between the 'anterior aspects of intertransverse spaces')
- Either side of the body on the midpoint of the muscle, which runs from the neck to the shoulder (upper trapezius)
- Either side of the body on the origin of the supraspinatus muscle which runs along the upper border of the shoulder blade
- Either side, on the upper surface of the rib, where the second rib meets the breast bone, in the pectoral muscle
- On the outer aspect of either elbow just below the prominence (epicondyle)
- In the large buttock muscles, either side, on the upper outer aspect in the fold in front of the muscle (gluteus medius)
- Just behind the large prominence of either hip joint in the muscular insertion of piriformis muscle
- On either knee in the fatty pad just above the inner aspect of the joint.

Box 6.2 **Similarities and differences between fibromyalgia (FM) and chronic myofascial pain (CMP)**

FM and CMP are *similar*, in that both:

- Are affected by cold weather
- May involve increased sympathetic nerve activity and may involve conditions such as Raynaud's phenomenon
- Have tension headaches and paraesthesia as a major associated symptom
- Are unaffected by anti-inflammatory, pain-killing medication whether of the cortisone type or standard formulations.

FM and CMP are *different*, in that:

- CMP affects males and females equally; fibromyalgia affects mainly females.
- CMP is usually local to an area such as the neck and shoulders, or low back and legs, although it can affect a number of parts of the body at the same time while fibromyalgia is a generalized problem, often involving all four 'corners' of the body at the same time.
- Muscles which contain areas that feel 'like a tight rubber band' are found in the muscles of around 30% of people with CMP and more than 60% of people with FM.
- People with FM have poorer muscular endurance than do people with CMP.
- CMP can sometimes be severe enough to cause disturbed sleep; in fibromyalgia the sleep disturbance has a more causative role, and is a pronounced feature of the condition.
- Patients with CMP usually do not suffer from morning stiffness, whereas those with fibromyalgia do.
- Fatigue is not usually associated with CMP, while it is common in fibromyalgia.
- CMP can sometimes lead to depression (reactive) and anxiety, whereas in a small percentage of fibromyalgia cases (some leading researchers believe), these conditions can be causative.
- Conditions, such as irritable bowel syndrome, dysmenorrhoea and a subjective feeling of 'swollen joints' are noted in fibromyalgia, but seldom in CMP.
- Low-dosage tricyclic antidepressant drugs are helpful in dealing with the sleep problems associated with FM, and many of the symptoms of fibromyalgia – but not those of CMP.
- Exercise programmes (cardiovascular fitness) can help some fibromyalgia patients, according to experts; but this is not a useful approach in CMP.

2. Osteopathic physicians at Kirksville College of Osteopathic Medicine treated 19 patients classified as having fibromyalgia, using SCS and MET approaches, for 4 weeks, one treatment each week. Some 84.2% of the patients showed improved sleep patterns and 94.7% reported a significant reduction in pain after this short course of treatment (Lo et al. 1992).

3. Doctors at Texas College of Osteopathic Medicine selected three groups of FM patients, one of which

received OMT including SCS, another had OMT plus self-teaching (study of the condition and self-help measures) and a third group received only moist-heat treatment. The group with the lowest level of reported pain after 6 months of care was that receiving OMT, although benefits were also noted in the self-teaching group (Gamber et al. 1993).

4. Another group of doctors from Texas, in a study involving 37 patients with FM (Rubin et al. 1990), tested the differences resulting from using: drugs only (ibuprofen, alprazolam); osteopathic treatment (including SCS) plus medication; osteopathic treatment plus a dummy medication (placebo); a placebo only. The results showed that:

   ▪ Drug therapy alone resulted in significantly less tenderness being reported than did drugs and osteopathy, or the use of placebo and osteopathic treatment or placebo alone.

   ▪ Patients receiving placebo plus osteopathic manipulation reported significantly less fatigue than the other groups.

   ▪ The group receiving medication and (mainly) osteopathic soft tissue attention, showed the greatest improvement in their quality of life.

5. Gamber et al. (2002) assessed the relative benefits of osteopathic methods, including SCS – with and without patient education regarding the condition, moist heat and standard medical care. Significant findings between the four treatment groups on measures of pain threshold, perceived pain, attitude toward treatment, activities of daily living, and perceived functional ability were found. All of these findings favoured use of osteopathic (SCS) methods. This study found osteopathic care, combined with standard medical care, was more efficacious in treating FM than standard care alone.

The main conditions that predispose to, or which accompany, fibromyalgia are summarized in Box 6.3.

Attention to underlying causes

Common-sense, as well as clinical experience, dictates that the management of FM and CMP should involve re-education (postural, breathing, relaxation, etc.), as well as the elimination of factors that may have contributed to the evolution, maintenance and/or aggravation of these conditions. This might well involve ergonomic evaluation of home and workplace, as well as the introduction and dedicated application of postural, exercise and/or breathing pattern re-education methods.

Unless soft tissue and other changes are accurately identified and addressed, no therapeutic method will do more than produce short-term relief.

> **Box 6.3 Main associated conditions which predispose towards and accompany fibromyalgia**
>
> These include the following (Block 1993; Duna & Wilke 1993; Fishbain 1989; Goldenberg 1993; Jacobsen 1992; Kalik 1989; Rothschild 1991):
>
> - Of people with FM, 100% have muscular pain, aching and/or stiffness (especially in the morning)
> - Almost all suffer fatigue and badly disturbed sleep with consequent reduction in production of growth hormone
> - Symptoms are almost always worse in cold or humid weather
> - The majority of people with FM have a history of injury – sometimes serious but often only minor – within the year before the symptoms started
> - 70–100% (different studies show variable numbers) are found to have depression (though this is more likely to be a result of the muscular pain rather than part of the cause)
> - 34–73% have irritable bowel syndrome
> - 44–56% have severe headaches
> - 30–50% have Raynaud's phenomenon
> - 24% suffer from anxiety
> - 18% have dry eyes and/or mouth (sicca syndrome)
> - 12% have osteoarthritis
> - 7% have rheumatoid arthritis
> - An as yet unidentified number of people with FM have had silicone breast implants and a newly identified silicone breast implant syndrome (SBIS) is now being defined
> - Between 3% and 6% are found to have substance (drugs/alcohol) abuse problems.

In order for restrictions, imbalances and malcoordination in the musculoskeletal system to be satisfactorily addressed, and where possible reversed, the individual needs to be appropriately treated as well as taught improved patterns of use.

In order for appropriate treatment to be offered, assessment methods are needed that lead to identification and modification of:

- Patterns of misuse, overuse, etc.
- Postural imbalances
- Chronically shortened postural muscles
- Chronically weakened muscles
- Patterns of functional malcoordination and imbalance
- Local changes within muscles (such as trigger points) and other soft tissues (e.g. fascia)
- Joint restrictions
- Functional imbalances in gait, respiration, etc.

HOSPITALIZED PATIENTS

Problems of manual treatment delivery in hospital

Acutely ill patients have very special problems and needs when being considered for manual treatment. These relate to their inability to be moved more than a little, their difficulty in cooperating in a manual treatment, possibly because of 'multiple intravenous and subclavian taps, monitors or various types of catheters', as well as their current particular state of vulnerability, either due to illness or to their being pre- or post-surgical (Schwartz 1986).

Edward Stiles (1976), then director of osteopathic medicine at Waterville Osteopathic Hospital in Maine, evaluated the usefulness of osteopathic attention to patients in hospital settings (Stiles 1976). He found that general osteopathic attention is of value in treating pre- and postoperative patients, especially with regard to excursion of the rib cage in order to establish maximum ventilating ability:

> *This is particularly important for patients undergoing upper gastrointestinal or thoracic surgery, since a decrease in excursion of the rib cage can increase the patient's susceptibility to splinting of the thoracic cage and impede ventilating ability.*

Stiles found that few methods achieved this end more effectively than the application of variants of positional release methods, which are particularly relevant in the context of pain, restriction – and limitation of the ability to change the patient's position, as described regarding bed-bound patients, later in this chapter.

Box 6.4 lists examples of major benefits resulting from use of positional release methods in hospitalized patients.

Postoperative situations

Postoperative uses of positional release

Dickey (1989) focussed attention on the particular needs of the many thousands of people undergoing surgery each year, via median sternotomy, in which the rib cage is opened anteriorly to allow access to the heart and other thoracic structures. More than 250 000 patients undergo coronary bypass graft surgery annually (in the USA alone). This surgery is accomplished via a median sternotomy incision, an approach that has been gaining widespread acceptance.

- In this form of surgery, an incision is made from the suprasternal notch to below the xiphoid process.

Box 6.4 Three examples of the efficacy of indirect methods (including SCS) in hospital settings

1. Reduced duration of postoperative hospital stay

Osteopathic manipulative treatment (including SCS and functional techniques) are seen to be easily implemented and cost-effective in terms of shortening hospital stays, resulting from effective relief of acute pain. Patients who receive morphine preoperatively and osteopathic attention postoperatively tend to have less postoperative pain and require less intravenously administered morphine. In addition, those receiving osteopathic attention demonstrate early ambulation and body movement, as well as decreased postoperative morbidity and mortality and increased patient satisfaction (Noll et al. 2000).

2. Shorter hospital stay for patients with pancreatitis

In an outcomes research study, Radjieski et al. (1998) randomly assigned six patients with pancreatitis to receive standard care plus daily osteopathic manipulative treatment (comprising myofascial release, soft tissue and strain/counterstrain techniques) for the duration of their hospitalization or to receive only standard care (eight patients). Osteopathic treatment involved 10–20 minutes daily of a standardized protocol, with attending physicians blinded as to group assignment. Results indicated that patients who received osteopathic attention averaged significantly fewer days in the hospital before discharge (mean reduction, 3.5 days) than control subjects, although there were no significant differences in time to food intake or in use of pain medications.

3. Shorter hospitalization and duration of intravenous antibiotics for elderly pneumonia patients

Elderly patients hospitalized with acute pneumonia were recruited and randomly placed into two groups: 28 in the treatment group and 30 in the control group. The treatment group received a standardized osteopathic attention protocol (including SCS and functional methods), while the control group received a light touch protocol. There was no statistical difference between groups for age, sex or simplified acute physiology scores. The treatment group had a significantly shorter duration of intravenous antibiotic treatment and a shorter hospital stay (Noll et al. 2000).

- The soft tissues below the skin are treated with diathermy to stem bleeding and the sternum is divided by an electric bone saw, the exposed edges being covered with bone wax.
- The sternum is then retracted with the upper level being placed at the level of the second rib.
- Following whatever surgical intervention is involved, the sternal margins are brought together and held by stainless steel sutures.
- There are often drainage tubes exiting from below the xiphoid following surgery.

The degree of stress and injury endured by all the tissues of the region is clearly major, especially considering that the open-chest situation may have been maintained for many hours. The sequels to this trauma are many and varied, as Dickey (1989) explains, and include:

Dehiscence, substernal and pericardial infection, nonunion of the sternum, pericardial constriction, phrenic nerve injuries, rib fractures and brachial plexus injuries.

Fully 23.5% of patients undergoing these procedures develop brachial plexus injuries.

Dickey reports on this surgical procedure being carried out experimentally on 10 cadavers, of which seven sustained first rib fractures with the fractured ends often impaling the lower trunks of the brachial plexus. While such negative effects are usually noted immediately postoperatively, many problems do not emerge until later and these might include structural and functional changes in chest mechanics that do not become evident for weeks or months, particularly restrictions affecting thoracic vertebrae and the rib cage, as well as fascial and diaphragmatic changes.

Dickey (1989) has outlined a number of appropriate manual methods for helping in recovery, including positional release methods. He stresses the importance of structural evaluation and treatment, both before and after surgery, with the manual therapeutic methods being of various types. However, it is specifically those positional release approaches that he advocates that are discussed in the context of this book.

Because of the wide retraction involved, the upper ribs (because of their firmer attachments) sustain the greatest degree of strain. Interosseous contraction, fascial strain and diaphragmatic dysfunction may all be palpable and to an intent, if implicable.

It is as well to be reminded that patients undergoing this form of surgery are likely to be past middle age, commonly with a range of existing musculoskeletal restrictions and dysfunctions and therefore with a limited prospect of normal function being completely restored (Nicholas & Oleski 2002; O-Yurvati 2005).

Functional treatment of surgically traumatized tissues

This is a part of functional technique methodology in which, rather than using a 'tender point' monitor, the tissues being treated are evaluated for their directions of freedom of movement (ease), and are held in those directions until a spontaneous change takes place (Fig. 6.3).

- The patient should be supine.
- The practitioner places one hand between the scapulae with the other hand resting on the surface of the midline of the sternum (Fig. 6.3).
- Each hand, independently, tests tissue preference in both a clockwise and then an anticlockwise direction, allowing assessment of the 'tissue preference pattern' relating to the skin and superficial fascia.
- In other words, the hands on the tissues are asking, 'in which direction do these tissues move most easily?', as the anterior and posterior assessments are made.
- Once assessed and identified, the tissues (anterior and posterior simultaneously), are taken in their respective directions of motion, towards the

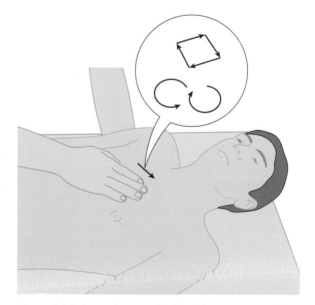

Figure 6.3 Release of traumatized fascial structures. In this figure, the practitioner's left hand lies between the patient's scapulae, while the right hand lies on the sternum. The hands independently assess the 'tissue preference patterns' (Dickey 1989). These 'positions of ease' are held for up to 90 seconds, in order to allow distorted fascial patterns to modify or normalize.

directions of preferred movement that they currently exhibit.

- Whichever direction of rotation is most 'easy' should be held – simultaneously front and back (90 seconds minimum), each in their preferred direction – until tension eases.
- This will commonly release recently acquired stress patterns in the fascia, possibly revealing older patterns which can then be addressed.
- This approach should be applied at least weekly until distorted fascial patterns are resolved or cease to alter, possibly indicating an intractably fixed state.

Normal, unstressed tissues should exhibit an equal excursion in both directions of rotation, although this is seldom found in adults, even if surgical trauma has not been a factor (Lewit 1999; Zink & Lawson 1979). Compare this method with the seated version described in Chapter 1, Functional technique variation: integrated neuromuscular release.

Research validation

In order to determine the effects on cardiac haemodynamics of this method, O-Yurvati et al. (2005) documented the effects of functional positional release (FuPR), applied to traumatized thoracic tissues – as part of a broader osteopathic intervention – following coronary artery bypass graft (CABG).

- Ten subjects undergoing CABG were compared, pre-treatment, versus post-treatment, involving measurements of thoracic impedance, mixed venous oxygen saturation and cardiac index.
- Immediately following CABG surgery, FuPR was provided to *anaesthetized and pharmacologically paralysed patients* to alleviate anatomical dysfunction of the rib cage, caused by median sternotomy, and to improve respiratory function.

This approach involved the practitioner placing one hand under the supine patient, to rest/palpate tissues between the scapulae. Simultaneously, the other hand was placed anteriorly, directly over the surgically traumatized tissues. Just sufficient pressure was exerted to allow the superficial skin and fascia to be moved in the directions being tested (Fig. 6.3).

- Each hand, independently, evaluated tissue preference directions – superior/inferior?
- Lateral to the left/lateral to the right?
- Clockwise/anticlockwise?
- Each evaluation commenced from the 'ease' position of the previous evaluation(s).

Once the final ease position was identified, by each hand independently, the tissues were maintained in those positions for 90 seconds before a slow return to the starting position.

Results: Improved peripheral circulation and increased mixed venous oxygen saturation was evident after the treatment – accompanied by a significant improvement in cardiac index.

See also Chapter 1 notes on Integrated neuromuscular release and Figure 1.3.

Functional release of the diaphragm attachment area

- The patient is supine and the practitioner stands at waist level facing cephalad, and places his hands over the middle and lower thoracic structures, fingers along the rib shafts (Fig. 6.4).
- Treating the structure being palpated as a cylinder, the hands test the preference that this cylinder has to rotate around its central axis, one way and then the other: does the lower thorax rotate with more ease to the right or to the left?
- Once the direction of greatest rotational ease has been established, and with the lower thorax rotated into this 'preferred' direction, side-bending one way and then the other is evaluated: when rotation has been made toward ease, does the lower thorax side-flex with more ease to the right or to the left?
- Once these two pieces of information have been established, the combined positions of ease, are 'stacked' onto each other, i.e. the lower thorax is

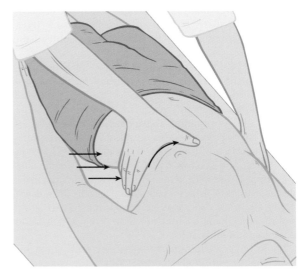

Figure 6.4 In this functional approach, the lower thoracic cage is taken into its preferred directions of rotation and side flexion, where it is held for up to 90 seconds, in order to relax the diaphragmatic attachment areas. See also Figure 1.2 and the functional exercise described in that chapter.

rotated towards its easiest direction, and then side-flexion is introduced, also towards the easiest direction.

- These positions are held for up to 90 seconds followed by a slow release.
- At this time, the diaphragm should be found to function more normally, accompanied by a relaxation of associated soft tissues, and a more symmetrical rotation and side-flexion potential of the previously restricted tissues.

Indirect rib treatment

See also SCS rib treatment description in Chapter 5.

Dickey suggests that following the nonspecific fascial release method described above (Fig. 6.3), standard rib function tests should be performed in order to identify ribs that are not symmetrical in their range of movement during the respiratory cycle, so that treatment can be introduced in order to assist in normalizing what has become restricted.

In the early postoperative phase, a classical osteopathic positional release approach is suggested (Kimberly 1980).

Method

- The patient sits on one side of a treatment table and the practitioner sits facing the opposite way, on the other side.
- In this way, by half-turning towards the patient, there is easy access to the lateral chest wall.
- Having previously identified ribs that are restricted in their range of motion, using standard assessment procedures (as described in Chapter 3), the practitioner places his hands so that the index and middle fingers of one hand contact the restricted rib to be treated, facing forwards along the anterior aspect of the rib, while the other index and middle finger contact the same rib, facing backwards along the posterior aspect (Fig. 6.5).
- The thumbs rest touching each other, tip-to-tip, at the mid-axillary line.
- The patient is asked to sit erect and to lean gently towards the practitioner, so that the ribs and the fingers make good contact.
- In this way, no force is exerted by the practitioner towards the ribs, and the patient controls the degree

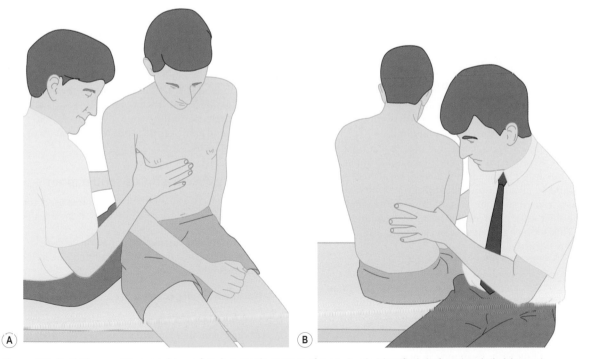

(A) (B)

Figure 6.5 (A,B) The practitioner achieves firm but gentle contact of a previously identified dysfunctional rib (elevated, depressed, restricted). The patient controls the degree of hand pressure by leaning towards the practitioner and then slightly turning towards the side opposite that being treated, which releases the demifacets. The patient then inhales and exhales as the practitioner assesses the phase at which the rib is most at ease. The patient holds this phase for as long as is comfortable, one or more times, until improved function is noted (Dickey 1989). The patient may need to repeat the breathing phase several times in order to achieve freedom of motion for a restricted rib at any treatment session.

of pressure being applied, which should be just enough to maintain firm contact.

- At this point, the patient is asked to *slightly* and *slowly* rotate the trunk away from the side being treated, which effectively eases the rib away from its demifacets.
- When the practitioner senses that this has been achieved, the patient is instructed to partially inhale and to then exhale in order for an evaluation to be made as to which phase of the cycle induces the greatest sense of *palpable ease*; freedom from tension.
- This evaluation is communicated to the patient, who is asked to hold the breath in the phase that induces maximum ease, for as long as is comfortable.
- The practitioner should be maintaining contact on the rib in order to achieve the maximal degree of ease.
- Any sense that tension, 'bind', is returning calls for a slight modification (fine-tuning) in the direction in which the rib is being held.

The patient may need to repeat the breathing phase several times in order to achieve freedom of motion for a restricted rib at any treatment session, which should be repeated not less than weekly until the ribs have all been released to the degree that is possible.

SCS techniques for rib dysfunction correction, as outlined in Chapter 4, can also be employed in order to support this method.

Improving lymphatic drainage

In patients who have undergone surgery, there may well be lymphatic stasis, as evidenced by swelling/oedema in the region of the posterior axillary fold.

Dickey (1989) suggests that the practitioner should: 'Assess the tissue preference patterns of the upper arm and the forearm, independently'. Once established, both sites should be taken towards the direction of the tissue preference, 'with slight compression through the elbow and the shoulder until he or she perceives the tension relaxing'.

This approach is repeated at each visit until tissue drainage is normal.

It is not difficult to see the similarities between the postoperative methods suggested by Dickey and the concepts of SCS and functional technique, as described elsewhere in the book. See in particular the various aspects of the Spencer sequence as described in Chapter 4, and also Hoover's clavicle and thoracic exercises in Chapter 5.

The commonality is the sensing of *directions of ease* in tissues, along with a supportive, non-invasive holding of the tissues in that state, until resolution occurs, whether the structures being treated are osseous (ribs, shoulder joint, clavicle) or soft (fascia, muscle).

Unlike SCS, these methods do not involve the use of pain-monitoring points, with the position of maximal ease being achieved entirely by means of palpation assessment.

SCS methods in bed-bound hospital patients

Schwartz (1986) notes that SCS, which is one of the primary manipulative methods routinely used in osteopathic hospitals, is of particular value in mobilization of the mechanical aspects of respiration, including, 'clavicle, ribs, sternum and anterior and posterior vertebral segments, as well as the diaphragm'.

Patients due for surgery are routinely treated in order to normalize respiratory function, as well as being treated for postoperative ileus.

The potential value and importance of methods that are non-invasive and easily adapted to bed-bound patients or those in considerable pain or distress, speaks for itself.

The methods described involve patients in medical and surgical, obstetric and paediatric wards, including pre- and post-surgical patients, some of whom have undergone cystotomy, gastrotomy and other major surgery.

Schwartz (1986) confirms Jones's assertion that all counterstrain positions are capable of being modified and successfully applied to bed-bound patients, saying that, 'without exception, this observation has been found to be valid'. (See Chapters 3 and 4 for more detail of SCS usage.)

Note: The descriptions in this chapter by Schwartz (1986) were based on the original Jones's formulaic model of SCS.

It may not be possible when treating bed-bound, hospitalized individuals to fully employ the Goodheart approach, as described in Chapter 4, in which the individual describes painful or restricted movements, which are then used to guide the therapist to the location of ideal 'tender point' sites.

Schwartz's description of tender points

Schwartz (1986) described the tender points used as monitors in SCS application as being:

> *Pea-sized bundles or swellings of fascia, muscle tendrils, connective tissue and nerve fibers as well as some vascular elements.*

Interestingly, unlike many other authors, he notes that:

> *Generally, but not always, pressure on the tender point will cause pain at a site distant to the point itself.*

This description of course defines such a point as a trigger point, as well as a tender point.

He also acknowledges that:

> *Tender points resemble both Chapman's neurolymphatic reflexes, and Travell's*

myofascial trigger points (Owens 1982; Travell & Simons 1983).

Schwartz highlights the difference between SCS and other methods that use such points in treatment by saying:

Other methods invade the point itself, for example by needle in acupuncture, injection of lidocaine into the point, or the use of pressure or ultrasound to destroy the tender point.

Note: See earlier in this chapter for a description of an integrated trigger-point deactivation sequence (Integrated neuromuscular inhibition technique, INIT).

Palpating change

Schwartz suggests that when using SCS, if a position of ease is achieved and tenderness vanishes from the palpated point, one of a number of sensations may become apparent to the practitioner/therapist, a 'sudden release', or a 'wobble', or a 'give' or a 'melting away' – all of which may indicate a change in the tissues in response to the positional changes, which has been brought about by the practitioner/therapist.

Two phases of the positioning process are emphasized, the first being 'gross' movement, which takes the area or the patient to the approximate position of ease, and 'fine-tuning', which further reduces pain from the palpated tender point.

Guidelines for use of counterstrain in bed-bound patients

In the summaries of suggestions for bed-bound patients that follow, only the particular modifications necessary in such a setting are emphasized. For more detailed descriptions, see Chapter 4.

Remember that:

- Unusually sensitive local areas ('tender points') represent aspects of a local dysfunction
- Tender points will usually be found in hypertonic, shortened soft tissues
- Active contraction of those tissues, or movements that stretch them, are likely to feel restricted or uncomfortable, or frankly painful, to the individual
- Positioning the tissues in ways that increase their 'shortness', while palpating a reduction in tone, combined with reduced 'tenderness scores', guides you to the position of ease that may allow spontaneous release to occur.

Note: Many of the illustrations of these 'bed-bound' methods are to be found in earlier chapters (see Chapters 3 and 4 particularly).

1. Anterior cervical dysfunction in bed-bound individuals

- Anterior cervical tender points located around the tips of the transverse processes are easily accessible in a bed-bound patient, as are the positions of ease (see Fig. 4.12A), which almost all require a degree of flexion, together with side-bending towards, and rotation away from, the side of the tender point.

2. Posterior cervical dysfunction in bed-bound individuals

- The posterior cervical points lie on or around the tips of the spinous processes and require extension of the head on the neck, and/or the neck as a whole (see Fig. 4.16A), which is more easily achieved in bed-bound patients if they are side-lying, with – it is suggested – the painful side uppermost, since (according to Schwartz's guidelines) the main side-bending and rotation into 'ease' needs to be towards the pain side, which would be difficult were the patient lying on the painful side.
- The C3 posterior point may require extension *or* flexion to create ease, and both directions should be gently attempted until the greatest reduction in sensitivity is achieved.

3. Posterior thoracic spinal dysfunction in bed-bound individuals

- Posterior thoracic and lumbar spinal tender points lie close to the spinous processes in the upper thoracic area, becoming increasingly lateral, lying on or around the transverse processes in the lower thoracic and lumbar vertebrae.
- The upper four thoracic segments are best treated with the patient side-lying with the arms resting, if possible, at the level of the shoulders (see Fig. 4.42) and with the upper arm supported by a pillow in order to avoid the introduction of rotation.
- The patient's upper spine should be extended to the level of the tender point in order to reduce or remove the palpated tenderness
- For the middle thoracic vertebrae, posterior points are also treated with the patient side-lying, but this time the arms are held above the head as the patient moves into extension.
- The lower four thoracic vertebrae are treated for posterior tender points (extension strains) with the patient supine and the practitioner/therapist standing on the dysfunctional side, with one hand under the patient to palpate the point.

- The patient's hand on the side opposite the pain is held, and the arm drawn across the chest towards the practitioner, so that the shoulder on that side lifts 30–45° from the bed, at which time fine-tuning should remove residual pain.
- If the patient's condition means that turning onto the side is not possible, then the method suggested for the lower thoracic vertebrae can be substituted for the side-lying posture described above.

4. Posterior lumbar dysfunction in bed-bound individuals

- Posterior lumbar tender points, which are described and illustrated in this chapter, and which are usually treated with the patient prone, can also be efficiently dealt with in the side-lying position.
- L1, L2, L3 and L4 involve the side-lying patient, dysfunction side uppermost.
- L1 and L2 (see Fig. 4.44B) require the upper leg being taken into straight extension and then either abduction or adduction, and/or rotation (of the leg) one way or the other, whichever combination provides the greater ease.
- In treatment of L3 and L4, as well as upper-pole L5 (lying between the fifth lumbar spinous process and the first sacral spinous process, see Fig. 4.4B) and the lower-pole L5 point (located midway on the body of the sacrum, see Fig. 4.4B), abduction and extension of the leg is introduced, and fine-tuning is achieved by variations in the degree of extension, as well as by the introduction of rotation internally or externally of the foot.
- For treatment of what is known as the middle-pole L5 tender point (in the superior sulcus of the sacrum), the side-lying patient's upper leg (dysfunction side) is flexed at hip and knee and this rests on the practitioner/therapist's thigh.
- This is fine-tuned by movement of the leg into greater or lesser degrees of hip flexion (see Fig. 4.44C) and by the degree of abduction or abduction needed to produce ease.
- The patient's ipsilateral arm may then be used in fine-tuning by having it hang forward and down over the edge of the bed.

5. Anterior thoracic dysfunction in bed-bound individuals

Anterior thoracic tender points lie on the anterior or surface of the thorax, the first six on the midline and the lower ones slightly lateral to it, bilaterally at approximately 1–2 cm (half to 1 inch) intervals, so that from T8 onwards the tender points lie in the abdominal musculature.

- These points relate directly to respiratory dysfunction and respond dramatically quickly to SCS methodology.
- The improvement in breathing function is commonly immediately apparent to the patient.
- In bed-bound patients, the patient is supine and there is usually a need for pillows or bolsters to assist in supporting them as flexion is introduced (see Fig 4.40A).
- For the first six anterior thoracic tender points (lying on the sternum) the patient's arms are allowed to rest slightly away from the body, and the knees and hips are flexed, feet resting on the bed. The only movement usually needed to ease tenderness is flexion of the head and neck towards the chest (the lower the point the greater the degree of flexion).
- Fine-tuning involves movement of the head slightly towards or away from the palpated pain site.
- For tender point treatment from T7 onwards, the patient's buttocks are rested on a pillow, so that the segment involved is unsupported, allowing it to fall into flexion.
- Alternatively, the practitioner/therapist can support the flexed knees and bring them towards the head, so flexing the lumbar and thoracic spine (see Fig. 4.41B).
- Fine-tuning may involve crossing the patient's ankles or side-bending to or away from the side of palpated tenderness, whichever combination reduces sensitivity more.

6. Anterior lumbar dysfunction in bed-bound individuals

Anterior lumbar (see Fig. 4.4A) tender points require a similar positioning to that called for by the thoracic points.

Rib dysfunction and interspace dysfunction. The appropriate treatment for rib dysfunction and interspace dysfunction are described in this chapter and can be applied to bed-bound patients without any modification.

Schwartz (1986) reports that:

> Interspace dysfunctions are implicated in costochondritis, the persistent chest pain of the patient who has suffered acute myocardial infarction, 'atypical' angina and anterior chest wall syndrome. They are strongly implicated along with depressed and elevated ribs in restricted motion of ribs … and thus contribute to the etiology and morbidity of many respiratory illnesses.

THIS CHAPTER

This chapter has provided detail in the use of positional release methods in particular clinical settings, including for hospitalized/bed-bound patients, as well as in chronic pain situations, such as fibromyalgia.

NEXT CHAPTER

The next chapter summarizes particular aspects of the use of positional release methods relative to fascial dysfunction.

REFERENCES

Abha, S., Angusamy, R., Sumit, K., et al., 2010. Efficacy of post-isometric relaxation versus integrated neuromuscular ischaemic technique in the treatment of upper trapezius trigger points. Indian Journal of Physiotherapy and Occupational Therapy 4, 1–5.

Affaitati, G., Costantini, R., Fabrizio, A., et al., 2011. Effects of treatment of peripheral pain generators in fibromyalgia patients. European Journal of Pain 15, 61–69.

Baldry, P., 2010. Myofascial Pain and Fibromyalgia Syndromes. Churchill Livingstone, Edinburgh.

Bass, C., Gardner, W., 1985. Respiratory abnormalities in chronic symptomatic hyperventilation. British Medical Journal 290, 1387–1390.

Beal, M., 1985. Viscerosomatic reflexes review. Journal of the American Osteopathic Association 85, 786–800.

Block, S., 1993. Fibromyalgia and the rheumatisms. Controversies in Rheumatology 19, 61–78.

Bron, C., Dommerholt, J., 2012. Etiology of myofascial trigger points. Current Pain and Headache Reports 16, 439–444.

Chaitow, L., 1991. Palpatory Literacy. HarperCollins, London.

Chaitow, L., 1994. INIT in treatment of pain and trigger points. British Journal of Osteopathy XIII, 17–21.

Chaitow, L., 1996. Modern Neuromuscular Techniques. Churchill Livingstone, Edinburgh.

Chaitow, L., Bradley, D., Gilbert, C., 2014. Recognizing and Treating Breathing Disorders: A Multidisciplinary Approach, second ed. Churchill Livingstone, Edinburgh.

Cuadrado, M., Young, W.B., Fernández-de-las-Peñas, C., et al., 2008. Migrainous colpalgia: body pain and allodynia associated with migraine attacks. Cephalalgia: An International Journal of Headache 28, 87–91.

D'Ambrogio, K., Roth, G., 1997. Positional Release Therapy. Mosby, St. Louis, MO.

Dardzinski, J.A., Ostrov, B.E., Hamann, L.S., 2000. Myofascial pain unresponsive to standard treatment. Successful use of a strain and counterstrain technique with physical therapy. Journal of Clinical Rheumatology 6, 169–174.

Dickey, J., 1989. Postoperative osteopathic manipulative management of median sternotomy patients. Journal of the American Osteopathic Association 89, 1309–1322.

Dommerholt, J., Bron, C., Franssen, J., et al., 2006. Myofascial trigger points; an evidence-informed review. Journal of Manual and Manipulative Therapy 14, 203–221.

Duna, G., Wilke, W., 1993. Diagnosis, etiology and therapy of fibromyalgia. Comprehensive Therapy 19, 60–63.

Fernández-de-las-Peñas, C., Sohrbeck Campo, M., Fernandez Carnero, J., et al., 2005. Manual therapies in myofascial trigger point treatment: a systematic review. Journal of Bodywork and Movement Therapies 9, 27–34.

Fishbain, D., 1989. Diagnosis of patients with myofascial pain syndrome. Archives of Physical and Medical Rehabilitation 70, 433–438.

Fitzgerald, M.P., Anderson, R.U., Potts, J., et al., 2009. Randomized multicenter feasibility trial of myofascial physical therapy for the treatment of urological chronic pelvic pain syndromes. Journal of Urology 182, 570–580.

Gamber, R.G., Rubin, B.R., Jiminez, C.A., 1993. Treatment of fibromyalgia with OMT and self-learned techniques [abstract]. Journal of the American Osteopathic Association 93, 870.

Gamber, R.G., Shores, J.H., Russo, D.P., et al., 2002. Osteopathic manipulative treatment in conjunction with medication relieves pain associated with fibromyalgia syndrome: results of a randomized clinical pilot project. Journal of the American Osteopathic Association 102, 321–325.

Ge, H.-Y., Nie, H., Madeleine, P., et al., 2009. Contribution of the local and referred pain from active myofascial trigger points in fibromyalgia syndrome. Pain 147, 233–240.

Ge, H.-Y., Wang, Y., Danneskiold-Samsøe, B., et al., 2010. Predetermined sites of examination for tender points in fibromyalgia syndrome are frequently associated with myofascial trigger points. Journal of Pain 11, 644–651.

Gerwin, R., 1991. Neurobiology of the myofascial trigger point. Bailliere's Clinical Rheumatology 88, 747–762.

Gerwin, R.D., 2005. A review of myofascial pain and fibromyalgia – factors that promote their persistence. Acupuncture in Medicine 23, 121–134.

Giamberardino, M., Tafuri, E., Savini, A., et al., 2007. Contribution of myofascial trigger points to migraine symptoms. Journal of Pain 8, 869–878.

Goldenberg, D.L., 1993. Fibromyalgia, chronic fatigue syndrome, and myofascial pain syndrome. Current

Opinion in Rheumatology 5, 199–208.

Harden, R., 2007. Muscle pain syndromes. American Journal of Physical Medicine and Rehabilitation 86, S47–S58.

Hong, C.Z., 1994. Lidocaine injection versus dry needling to myofascial trigger point. The importance of the local twitch response. American Journal of Physical Medicine and Rehabilitation 73, 256–263.

Ibáñez-García, J., Alburquerque-Sendín, F., Rodríguez-Blanco, C., et al., 2009. Changes in masseter muscle trigger points following strain-counterstrain or neuro-muscular technique. Journal of Bodywork and Movement Therapies 13, 2–10.

Jacobsen, S., 1992. Dynamic muscular endurance in primary fibromyalgia compared with chronic myofascial pain syndrome. Archives of Physical and Medical Rehabilitation 73, 170–173.

Jones, L., 1981. Strain/Counterstrain. Academy of Applied Osteopathy, Colorado Springs.

Kalik, J., 1989. Fibromyalgia: diagnosis and treatment of an important rheumatologic condition. Journal of Osteopathic Medicine 90, 10–19.

Kimberly, P. (Ed.), 1980. Outline of Osteopathic Manipulative Procedures. Kirksville College of Osteopathic Medicine, Kirksville, MO.

Langevin, H., Yandow, J., 2002. Relationship of acupuncture points and meridians to connective tissue planes. Anatomical Record (New Anat.) 269, 257–265.

Lewit, K., 1999. Manipulative Therapy in Rehabilitation of the Locomotor System. Butterworths, London.

Lo, K., Kuchera, M.L., Preston, S.C., et al., 1992. Osteopathic manipulative treatment in fibromyalgia syndrome. Journal of the American Osteopathic Association 92, 1177.

Lum, L., 1984. Editorial: Hyperventilation and anxiety state. Journal of the Royal Society of Medicine Jan, 1–4.

McNulty, W., Gervirtz, R., Hubbard, D., et al., 1994. Needle electromyographic evaluation of trigger point response to a psychological stressor. Psychophysiology 31, 313–316.

McPartland, J.M., 2008. Expression of the endocannabinoid system in fibroblasts and myofascial tissues. Journal of Bodywork and Movement Therapies 12, 169–182.

Mense, S., 1993. Nociception from skeletal muscle in relation to clinical muscle pain. Pain 54, 241–290.

Mense, S., 2008. Muscle pain: mechanisms and clinical significance. Deutsches Ärzteblatt International 105, 214–219.

Meseguer, A., Fernández-de-las-Peñas, C., Navarro-Poza, J.L., et al., 2006. Immediate effects of the strain/counterstrain technique in local pain evoked by tender points in the upper trapezius muscle. Clinical Chiropractic 9, 112–118.

Mosby's Medical Dictionary. 2009. eighth ed. Elsevier, St. Louis, Missouri.

Muller, K., Kreutzfeldt, A., Schwesig, R., et al., 2003. Hypermobility and chronic back pain. Manuelle Medizin 41, 105–109.

Nagrale, A., 2010. The efficacy of an integrated neuromuscular inhibition technique on upper trapezius trigger points in subjects with non-specific neck pain: a randomized controlled trial. Journal of Manual and Manipulative Therapy 18, 3743.

Nayak, P.P., 2013. A Study to Establish the Efficacy of INIT Combined with Therapeutic Ultrasound, Compared with INIT with Placebo Ultrasound in the Treatment of Acute Myofascial Trigger Point in Upper Trapezius. Dissertation. The Oxford College of Physiotherapy, Hongasandra, Bangalore.

Nicholas, A., Oleski, S., 2002. Osteopathic manipulative treatment for postoperative pain. Journal of the American Osteopathic Association 102, S5–S8.

Niddam, D.M., Chan, R.C., Lee, S.H., et al., 2008. Central representation of hyperalgesia from myofascial trigger point. Neuroimage 39, 1299–1306.

Njoo, K.H., Van der Does, E., 1995. The occurrence and inter-rater reliability of myofascial trigger points on quadratus lumborum and gluteus medius. Pain 61, 159.

Noll, D., Shores, J., Gamber, R., 2000. Benefits of osteopathic manipulative

treatment for hospitalized elderly patients with pneumonia. Journal of the American Osteopathic Association 100, 776–782.

Owens, C., 1982. An Endocrine Interpretation of Chapman's Reflexes. Academy of Applied Osteopathy, Colorado Springs.

O-Yurvati, A.H., Carnes, M.S., Clearfield, M.B., et al., 2005. Hemodynamic effects of osteopathic manipulative treatment immediately after coronary artery bypass graft surgery. Journal of the American Osteopathic Association 105, 475–481.

Perri, M., Halford, E., 2004. Pain and faulty breathing – a pilot study. Journal of Bodywork and Movement Therapies 8, 237–312.

Pyszora, A., Wójcik, A., Krajnik, M., 2010. Are soft tissue therapies and Kinesio Taping useful for symptom management in palliative care? Advances in Palliative Medicine 9, 87–92.

Radjieski, J.M., Lumley, M.A., Cantieri, M.S., 1998. Effect of osteopathic manipulative treatment of length of stay for pancreatitis: a randomized pilot study. Journal of the American Osteopathic Association 98, 264–272.

Roll, M., Theorell, T., 1987. Acute chest pain without obvious cause before age 40 – personality and recent life events. Journal of Psychosomatic Research 31, 215–221.

Rothschild, B., 1991. Fibromyalgia: an explanation for the aches and pains of the nineties. Comprehensive Therapy 17, 9–14.

Rubin, B.R., Gamber, R.G., Cortez, C.A., et al., 1990. Treatment options in fibromyalgia syndrome. Journal of the American Osteopathic Association 90, 844–845.

Sachse, J., 1995. The thoracic region region's pathogenetic relations and increased muscle tension. Manuelle Medizin 33, 163–172.

Schwartz, H., 1986. The use of counterstrain in an acutely ill in-hospital population. Journal of the American Osteopathic Association 86, 433–442.

Shah, J., Phillips, T., 2003. A novel microanalytical technique for assaying soft tissue demonstrates significant quantitative biomechanical differences in 3 clinically distinct groups: normal, latent and active. Archives of Physical Medicine and Rehabilitation 84, A4.

Simons, D., Travell, J., Simons, L., 1999. Myofascial Pain and Dysfunction – the Trigger Point Manual. Williams & Wilkins, Baltimore, MD.

Slocumb, J., 1984. Neurological factors in chronic pelvic pain trigger points and abdominal pelvic pain. American Journal of Obstetrics and Gynecology 49, 536.

Stiles, E.G., 1976. Osteopathic manipulation in a hospital environment. Journal of the American Osteopathic Association 76, 243–258.

Stoltz, A., 1993. Effects of OMT on the tender points of FM. Journal of the

American Osteopathic Association 93, 866.

Travell, J., Simons, D., 1983. Myofascial Pain and Dysfunction, vol. 1. Williams & Wilkins, Baltimore, MD.

Travell, J., Simons, D., 1992. Trigger Point Manual. Williams & Wilkins, Baltimore, MD.

Vernon, H., Schneider, M., 2009. Chiropractic management of myofascial trigger points and myofascial pain syndrome: a systematic review of the literature. Journal of Manipulative and Physiological Therapeutics 32, 14–24.

Wall, P., Melzack, R., 1990. The Textbook of Pain. Churchill Livingstone, Edinburgh.

Weiss, J., 2001. Pelvic floor myofascial trigger points: manual therapy for

interstitial cystitis and the urgency-frequency syndrome. Journal of Urology 166, 2226–2231.

Wolfe, F., Simons, D., Fricton, J., et al., 1992. The fibromyalgia and myofascial pain syndromes: a preliminary study of tender points and trigger points in persons with fibromyalgia, myofascial pain syndrome and no disease. Journal of Rheumatology 19, 944–951.

Wolfe, F., Smythe, H., Yunus, M., et al., 1990. American College of Rheumatology. 1990. Criteria for classification of fibromyalgia. Arthritis and Rheumatism 33, 160–172.

Zink, G., Lawson, W., 1979. Osteopathic structural examination and functional interpretation of the soma. Osteopathic Annals 7, 433–440.

Chapter | 7 |

Positional release and fascia

This short chapter provides background information as to the potential for use of positional release techniques (PRT) in management of specifically fascia-related conditions. In addition, research in which fascial function – for example mechanotransduction – offers insights into clinical effects is described.

Some of this information has been included in earlier chapters, however it is hoped that, by drawing fascia-related information together, readers may be helped to reflect on potential applications of PRT methods, in particular clinical situations.

CONNECTIVE TISSUE AND FASCIAL CONCEPTS

Fascia offers a unifying medium, a structure that literally 'ties everything together', from the soles of the feet, to the meninges surrounding the brain.

This ubiquitous material offers support, separation and structure to all other soft tissues and because of this, produces distant effects whenever dysfunction occurs in it (Schleip et al. 2012; Swanson 2013).

Levin (1986) has described fascia as comprising innumerable building blocks, shaped as icosahedrons (20-sided structures) that produce, in effect, kinetic chains in which tensions are transmitted to-and-from every part of the body, partly by hydrostatic pressure (Fig. 7.1).

Some years earlier Deane Juhan (1998) reflected on fascia's tensegrity feature:

> *Besides this hydrostatic pressure (which is exerted by every fascial compartment, not just the outer wrapping), the connective tissue framework – in conjunction with active muscles – provides another kind of tensional force that is crucial to the upright structure of the skeleton. We are not made up of stacks of building blocks resting securely upon one another, but rather of poles and guy-wires, whose stability relies not upon flat-stacked surfaces but upon proper angles of the poles and balanced tensions on the wires. Buckminster Fuller coined the term 'tensegrity' to describe this principle of structure, and his inventive experiments with it have clarified it as one of nature's favorite devices for achieving a maximum of stability with a minimum of materials.*

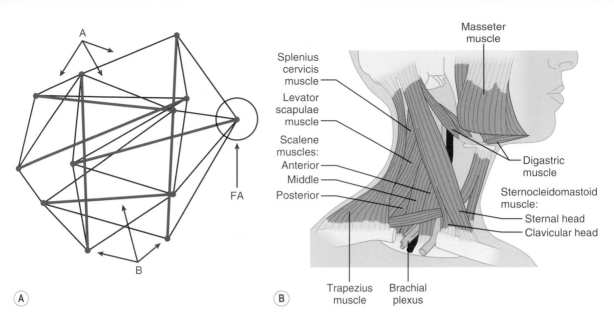

Figure 7.1 (A) Biotensegrity model (after Swanson 2013). A: Tensional elements of the biotensegrity structure, including: microfilaments, muscles, tendons, ligaments, etc. B: Compression elements of a biotensegrity structure, including DNA helix, microtubules, ribs, bones, fascia. FA: Focal adhesion complex within cells that connects the cytoskeleton and the extracellular matrix. (B) Cervical muscles and ligaments, illustrating a macro-tensegrity-like pattern to be found throughout the body.

Juhan continues:

This principle of tensegrity describes precisely the relationship between the connective tissues, the muscles, and the skeleton. There is not a single horizontal surface anywhere in the skeleton that provides a stable base for anything to be stacked upon it. Our design was not conceived by a stonemason. Weight applied to any bone would cause it to slide right off its joints if it were not for the tensional balances that hold it in place and control its pivoting. Like the beams in a simple tensegrity structure, our bones act more as spacers than as compressional members; more weight is actually borne by the connective system of cables than by the bony beams.

With these models in mind, of stacked and packed icosahedrons, as well as tensegrity structures which easily comply with compressive and tension forces, and the unique plastic and elastic properties of connective tissue, we have the possibility of visualizing a structure capable of absorbing and accommodating to a variety of forces and adaptations. The beneficial effects of holding tissues at ease when stressed also emerges.

As D'Ambrogio & Roth (1997) explain:

A perceived condition in one area of the body may have its origin in another area and therapeutic action at the source will
have an immediate effect on all secondary areas, including the site of symptom manifestation. It may also account for some of the physiologic effects that produce the [spontaneous] release phenomenon.

FASCIAL 'MERIDIANS'

Langevin & Yandow (2002) have suggested (Box 7.1) that fascial structures provide a medium for the transmission of sensations including pain. This goes a long way to offering an explanation for a variety of apparently unconnected elements, such as:

- The similarity between acupuncture points and trigger points
- The means whereby patterns of pain relate to such points
- How distant effects may be achieved by stimulation of such points (needling or manual)
- The nature of acupuncture meridians
- How positioning of tissues can modify the behaviour of what appear to be pain-generating 'points'.

Chains, trains and positional release

Myers (1997) has described a number of clinically useful sets of myofascial chains – the connections between

One of the important features of acupuncture theory is that needling of appropriately selected acupuncture points has predictable effects remote from the site of needle insertion, and that these effects are mediated by means of the acupuncture meridian system.

Langevin & Yandow (2002) note that: '*To date, physiological models attempting to explain these remote effects have invoked systemic mechanisms involving the nervous system*' (Pomeranz 2001).

Langevin & Yandow go on to report that their research shows that signal transduction appears to occur through connective tissue, probably involving sensory mechanoreceptors.

They hypothesize that the network of acupuncture points and meridians can be viewed as a representation of the network formed by interstitial connective tissue.

This hypothesis is supported by ultrasound images showing connective tissue cleavage planes at most traditional acupuncture points in humans.

They found that fully 80% of charted acupuncture points lie close to intermuscular or intramuscular connective tissue planes.

They see acupuncture points as representing a convergence of connective tissue planes and being involved in the 'sum of all body energetic phenomena (e.g. metabolism, movement, signalling, information exchange)'.

Implications

The implications of these concepts in relation to positional release methods seems clear – that normalization, or improved function, of connective tissue dysfunction may potentially modify this 'signalling' mechanism, and might well explain how and why positional release effects its results.

The idea that pain perceived in sensitive and distressed tissues by applied manual pressure (as in counterstrain methodology), can be relieved by positioning, suggests that the 'ease' position is one in which disturbed signalling may be able to normalize?

The superficial front line (Fig. 7.2A):

- The anterior compartment and the periosteum of the tibia, link the dorsal surface of the toes to the tibial tuberosity.
- Rectus femoris, links the tibial tuberosity to the anterior inferior iliac spine and pubic tubercle.
- Rectus abdominis, as well as the pectoralis and sternalis fascia, link the pubic tubercle and the anterior inferior iliac spine with the manubrium, with sternocleidomastoid, linking the manubrium with the mastoid process of the temporal bone.

The back-of-the-arm lines (Fig. 7.2B):

- The broad sweep of trapezius links the occipital ridge and the cervical spinous processes to the spine of the scapula and the clavicle.
- The deltoid, together with the lateral intermuscular septum, connects the scapula and clavicle with the lateral epicondyle.
- The lateral epicondyle is joined to the hand and fingers by the common extensor tendon.
- Another track on the back of the arm can arise from the rhomboids, which link the thoracic transverse processes to the medial border of the scapula.
- The scapula in turn is linked to the olecranon of the ulna by infraspinatus and the triceps.
- The olecranon of the ulna connects to the small finger by means of the periosteum of the ulna.
- A 'stabilization' feature in the back of the arm involves latissimus dorsi and the thoracolumbar fascia, with its attachments to the lower limb.

The front-of-the-arm lines (Fig. 7.2C):

- Latissimus dorsi, teres major and pectoralis major attach to the humerus, close to the medial intramuscular septum (MIS), connecting it to the back of the trunk.
- The MIS connects the humerus to the medial epicondyle, which connects with the palmar hand and fingers by means of the common flexor tendon.
- An additional line on the front of the arm involves pectoralis minor, the costocoracoid ligament, the brachial neurovascular bundle and the fascia clavi-pectoralis, which attach to the coracoid process.
- The coracoid process also provides the attachment for biceps brachii (or brachialis) linking this to the radius and the thumb, by means of the flexor compartment of the forearm.
- A 'stabilization' line on the front of the arm involves pectoralis major attaching to the ribs, as do the external obliques, which then run to the pubic tubercle, where a connection is made to the contralateral adductor longus, gracilis, pes anserinus, and the tibial periosteum.

different structures ('long functional continuities'), which he terms 'anatomy trains'.

These are not distinct from tensegrity features, but are more specific linkages that may be seen to be connected when some positional release methods are performed. In particular, SCS methods for normalizing rib restrictions can involve some bizarre positioning of the entire body, with remarkable effects (see Chapter 4, pp. 98, 99).

These figures are examples of Myers' fascial 'trains' (and there are a number of others – for details see Myers (2013) *Anatomy Trains*).

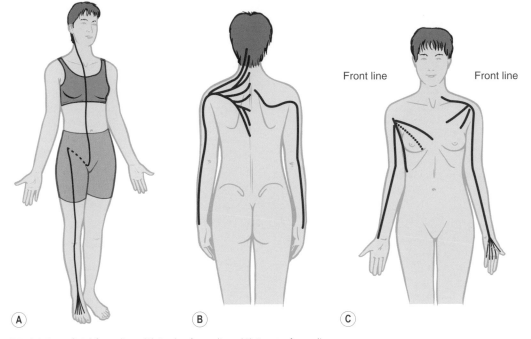

Figure 7.2 (A) Superficial front line. (B) Back-of-arm line. (C) Front-of-arm line.

It seems possible – indeed probable that in taking a distressed, strained (chronic or acute) muscle or joint painlessly into a position that allows for a reduction in tone in the tissues involved, some modification takes place of neural reporting, as well as local circulation being improved (see Chapter 2 for research discussion). Any changes in tone are then likely to be reflected in the chains to which the strained tissues belong.

D'Ambrogio & Roth (1997) summarize what is thought to happen to the fascia during PRT as follows:

> *It is hypothesized that PRT, by reducing the tension on the myofascial system, also engages the fascial components of dysfunction. The reduction in tension on the collagenous cross-linkages appears to induce a disengagement of the electrochemical bonds and a conversion back [from the gel-like] to the sol [solate] state.*

COMMON COMPENSATORY – FASCIAL – PATTERNS

In Chapter 2, the 'common compensatory pattern' was discussed and illustrated (see Box 2.2, and Fig. 2.1). According to the studies of Zink & Lawson (1979) and

Pope (2003), the modified fascial status of most individuals appears to provide a well-compensated pattern.

Where the pattern is found to be poorly-compensated (see Chapter 2), individuals appear to experience less than optimal health, and may demonstrate unpredictable reactions to stress, including the inevitable adaptive demands of manual treatment.

It is suggested that roughly 20% of individuals, are ideal candidates for the non-invasive, indirect, positional release approaches as outlined in previous chapters.

This is not meant to suggest that the remaining 80% (roughly) who are 'well-compensated' would not also benefit from positional release methods, should this be indicated.

CELLULAR FASCIAL RESEARCH AND COUNTERSTRAIN

A number of laboratory studies have suggested that when 'stressed', fibroblast cells (the principal active cells of connective tissue) modify their genetic behaviour and excrete inflammatory materials.

These changes – involving a process known as mechano-transduction – are capable of being reversed by altering the load applications to the cells – mimicking either counterstrain, or myofascial release.

The architectural shape of a cell matters – and as this changes due to altered levels of load, so do its functions. Of particular relevance to this book is the importance in that change in cell shape, of *reduced load*, such as occurs in positional release.

Also relevant, and as noted later in this chapter, these observations are reflected in clinical studies, for example involving plantar fasciitis (Urse 2012), or soft-tissue density (Barnes et al. 2013).

Studies

- Dodd et al. (2006) report that: '*Human fibroblasts respond to strain by secreting inflammatory cytokines, undergoing hyperplasia, and altering cell shape and alignment … and that biophysical [tissue changes] – whether resulting from injury, somatic dysfunction, or [soft tissue manipulation, such as SCS] – affects range of motion, pain, and local inflammation*'.

- In 2007 Standley & Meltzer observed that: '*Data from [this] study suggest that fibroblast proliferation and expression/secretion of pro-inflammatory and anti-inflammatory interleukins may contribute to the clinical efficacy of indirect osteopathic manipulative techniques*'.

- Standley & Meltzer (2008) reported on various clinically applied fascial strains (counterstrain, as well as myofascial release) used to treat somatic dysfunctions. These methods produced positive clinical outcomes, such as reduced pain, reduced analgesic use and improved range of motion. They note that '*it is clear that strain direction, frequency and duration, impact important fibroblast physiological functions known to mediate pain, inflammation and range of motion*'.

- Meltzer et al. (2010) note that traumatized fascia disrupts normal biomechanics of the body, increasing tension exerted on the system and causing myofascial pain and reduced range of motion. They found that resulting inflammatory responses by fibroblast cells can be reversed by changes in load on the tissues, delivered by either counterstrain or myofascial release, and that such changes may take only 60 seconds to manifest.

Analgesic and anti-inflammatory effects of counterstrain

Building on the laboratory evidence listed above, a number of studies and reports have indicated clinical benefits that include pain reduction and anti-inflammatory effects:

- Counterstrain has been shown to beneficially influence *plantar fasciitis*, '*Clinical improvement occurs in subjects with plantar fasciitis in response to counterstrain treatment [SCS]. The clinical response is accompanied by mechanical, but not electrical, changes in the reflex responses of the calf muscles*' (Wynne et al. 2006).

- Urse (2012) has described the counterstrain method for treatment of *plantar fasciitis* as follows: '*The supine patient's ipsilateral knee is flexed, and a plantar tender point [an area of local hypersensitivity] is identified where the fascia inserts onto the calcaneus. One thumb is used to monitor the tender point … [while] … the opposite hand plantar flexes the toes and ankle curving around the tender point. Additional adjustment to the tension may be accomplished by supination or pronation of the foot, until there is symptomatic relief of the tenderness underlying the monitoring thumb*'. This *position-of-ease* is maintained for up to 90 seconds, before a slow return to neutral and reassessment.

- In treatment of *Achilles tendonitis*, Howel (2006) noted changes in reported pain, following treatment involving counterstrain: '*subjects indicated significant clinical improvement in soreness, stiffness, and swelling, … Because subjects' soreness ratings also declined immediately after treatment, decreased nociceptor activity may play an additional role in somatic dysfunction, perhaps by altering stretch reflex amplitude*'.

- Dardzinski et al. (2000) reported: '*SCS techniques should be considered … as adjunctive therapy for patients previously unresponsive to standard treatment for myofascial pain syndrome*'. '*Symptoms of a 30-year-old distance runner with iliotibial band friction syndrome (ITBFS) were reduced with the help of OMT, specifically SCS. This technique allows for relief of pain at a tender point by moving the affected body part into its position of greatest comfort, aiding in the reduction of proprioceptor activity. The tender point was located from ≈2 cm proximal to the lateral femoral epicondyle. There is no prior documentation of the osteopathic manipulation of this specific tender point. Thus, this case report reflects an initial identification of a distal iliotibial band tender point, and a new therapeutic modality for ITBFS*' (Pedowitz 2005).

Counterstrain, balanced ligamentous tension and fascial stiffness

Specific therapeutic effects of both counterstrain (see Chapters 3 and 4) and balanced ligamentous tension (Chapter 8), on both symptoms, as well as 'tissue stiffness' changes, emerge from a study by Barnes et al. (2013).

Changes in 'tissue stiffness' measured before and after manual treatment is one way of evaluating the effects of the methods used. Change – whether an increase or a reduction in stiffness in tissues, is known as *hysteresis*. A 2013 study, conducted by Barnes et al., measured altered degrees of stiffness in fascia (i.e. hysteresis) after different manual methods.

The protocol was as follows:

1. Cervical articular somatic dysfunctions were identified in 240 individuals, using carefully controlled palpation assessment methods.
2. Once dysfunction (e.g. restriction or pain) had been identified, and before treatment (or sham treatment) was applied, the degree of stiffness in the dysfunctional tissues was measured, using an instrument designed for that purpose – a durometer.
3. The durometer measured the density/stiffness of the myofascial tissues overlying each cervical segment, using a single consistent piezoelectric impulse. This allowed four different tissue characteristics to be identified – fixation, mobility, frequency and motoricity (described as 'the overall degree of change of a segment') – including 'resistance' and range of motion. Put simply, the measurement identified relative degrees of mobility and stiffness.
4. Four different techniques were used: *Balanced ligamentous tension*, as described in Chapter 8; *Muscle energy technique* (not discussed in this book apart from being an element of INIT, see Chapter 6.); *High velocity manipulation* (also not discussed); and *Counterstrain*, see Chapters 3, 4 and 9. A single application of these four methods, as well as a sham technique, were randomly applied to the most severe areas of the dysfunctional cervical tissues of all participants.
5. At 10 minutes after the single treatment, the changes in tissue 'stiffness' (i.e. hysteresis) were again measured, using a durometer.
6. When the degree of restriction/stiffness present, before and after the single use of one of the four (or sham) methods above, the results showed that counterstrain (see Chapters 3 and 4) produced the greatest changes, compared with the other methods or sham treatment.

The results of this study suggest that the behaviour of soft tissues associated with restricted joints – (neck in this case) can be rapidly modified (becoming 'less stiff') using *any of the four methods* tested – *with the greatest effect observed following counterstrain*.

Of possible interest are some of the concluding remarks of the researchers in this study:

- 'It became apparent that in many instances, treating a single identified key dysfunction sometimes modified other underlying or adjacent somatic dysfunctions'.

- The results 'seemed to suggest that different cervical levels responded better to specific treatments'.
- Classification of the dysfunctions as 'acute' (ostensibly containing more fluid in the tissues) or 'chronic' (ostensibly stiffer tissues) might also lead to sub-analysis and better interpretation of the … changes.

What emerges from the laboratory studies of fibroblast behaviour when stressed and 'de-stressed' (e.g. by modelled counterstrain), and the studies of fasciitis and the experimental study of 'stiffness' by Barnes and colleagues – is that fascial structures appear to respond well to methods that 'de-stress' them, as in the unloading approaches of counterstrain and balanced ligamentous tension (see Chapter 8).

THE EFFECTS OF ALTERED LOAD ON LIGAMENTOUS REFLEXES

Goodheart's modified counterstrain methods (as described in Chapter 4) involve additional compressive or distraction load applied following identification of a 'position of ease'.

Schiowitz's facilitated positional release (FPR) (as described in Chapter 5) also involves an additional 'facilitating' force, applied to a functionally achieved position of ease.

One possible explanation for the effects of the 'loading' facilitating force is offered by Solomonow (2009), a leading researcher into ligament function. He notes that ligaments are sensory organs and have significant input to reflexive/synergistic activation of muscles. For example, muscular activity associated with the reflex from the anterior cruciate ligament acts to prevent distraction of the joint, while simultaneously reducing the strain in the ligament.

There is also evidence that *ligamentomuscular reflexes* have inhibitory effects on muscles associated with the related joint, inhibiting muscles that destabilize the joint, or increasing antagonist coactivation, to help stabilize the joint. One potential therapeutic use of this ligamentous function is found in any positional release method that includes crowding (compaction) of joints as part of the protocol.

The 'crowding' of ligaments

Solomonow spent many years researching the functions of ligaments, and in doing so, identified their sensory potential and many of the major ligamentomuscular reflexes that have inhibitory effects on associated muscles.

If you apply only 60–90 seconds of relaxing compression on a joint … an hour plus of relaxation of muscles may result. This may come not only from ligaments, but also from capsules and tendons.

Personal communication 8 January, 2009

Such effects would be temporary (20–30 minutes) but this would be sufficient to allow enhanced ability to mobilize or exercise previously restricted structures.

Wong (2012) summarizes current thinking regarding ligamentomuscular reflexes and SCS:

Ligamentous strain inhibits muscle contractions that increase strain, or stimulates muscles that reduce strain, to protect the ligament (Krogsgaard et al., 2002). For instance, anterior cruciate ligament strain inhibits quadriceps and stimulates hamstring contractions to reduce anterior tibial distraction (Dyhre-Poulsen and Krogsgaard, 2000).

Ligamentous reflex activation also elicits regional muscle responses that indirectly influence joints (Solomonow and Lewis, 2002). Research is needed to explore whether Counterstrain may alter the protective ligamento-muscular reflex and thus reduce dysfunction by shortening joint ligaments or synergistic muscles (Chaitow, 2009).

Hydraulic effects

Coincidently, crowding (compression) of soft tissues would have an effect on the water content of fascia, leading to temporary (also 20–30 minutes) of reduced stiffness of fascial structures – with similar enhanced mobility during that period.

THIS CHAPTER

This chapter has provided information and evidence of various fascial relationships with positional release approaches, including cellular research that suggest anti-inflammatory effects, possible 'signalling' features, the influence of 'muscle-chains', possible reflexive factors, as well as changes in stiffness/density following counterstrain – possibly involving hydraulic effects.

NEXT CHAPTER

The next chapter, by Raymond J. Hruby, DO, provides a detailed overview of balanced ligamentous tension techniques.

REFERENCES

Barnes, P., Laboy, F., Noto-Bell, L., et al., 2013. A comparative study of cervical hysteresis characteristics after various osteopathic manipulative treatment (OMT) modalities. Journal of Bodywork and Movement Therapies 17, 89–94.

D'Ambrogio, K., Roth, G., 1997. Positional Release Therapy. Mosby, St Louis.

Dardzinski, J.A., Ostrov, B.E., Hamann, L.S., 2000. Myofascial pain unresponsive to standard, treatment: successful use of a strain/counterstrain technique with physical therapy. Journal of Clinical Rheumatology 6, 169–174.

Dodd, J.G., Good, M.M., Nguyen, T.L., et al., 2006. In-vitro biophysical strain model for understanding mechanisms of osteopathic manipulative treatment. Journal of the American Osteopathic Association 106, 157–166.

Howell, J.N., Cabell, K.S., Chila, A.G., et al., 2006. Stretch reflex and

Hoffmann reflex responses to osteopathic manipulative treatment in subjects with Achilles tendinitis. Journal of the American Osteopathic Association 106, 537–545.

Juhan, D., 1998. Job's Body, second ed. Station Hill Press, Barrytown, NY.

Langevin, H., Yandow, J., 2002. Relationship of acupuncture points and meridians to connective tissue planes. The Anatomical Record (New Anat.) 269, 257–265.

Levin, S., 1986. The Icosahedron as the Three-Dimensional Finite Element in Biomechanical Support. Proceedings of the Society of General Systems Research on Mental Images, Values and Reality, May. Society of Systems Research, Philadelphia, PA.

Meltzer, K.R., Cao, T.V., Schad, J.F., et al., 2010. In vitro modeling of repetitive motion injury and myofascial release. Journal of Bodywork and Movement Therapies 14, 162.

Myers, T., 1997. Anatomy trains. Journal of Bodywork and Movement Therapies 1, 91–101.

Myers, T., 2013. Anatomy Trains: Myofascial Meridians for Manual and Movement Therapists, third ed. Churchill Livingstone, Edinburgh.

Pedowitz, R., 2005. Use of osteopathic manipulative treatment for iliotibial band friction syndrome. Journal of the American Osteopathic Association 105, 563–567.

Pomeranz, B., 2001. Acupuncture analgesia basic research. In: Stux, G., Hammerschlag, R. (Eds.), Clinical Acupuncture Scientific Basis. Springer-Verlag, Berlin.

Pope, R.E., 2003. The common compensatory pattern: its origin and relationship to the postural model. American Academy of Osteopathy Journal 14, 19–40.

Schleip, R., Findley, T., Chaitow, L., et al., 2012. Fascia: The Tensional Network of the Human Body.

Elsevier Churchill Livingstone, Edinburgh.

Standley, P., Meltzer, K., 2007. Modeled repetitive motion strain and indirect osteopathic manipulative techniques in regulation of human fibroblast proliferation and interleukin secretion. Journal of the American Osteopathic Association 107, 527–536.

Standley, P., Meltzer, K., 2008. In vitro modeling of repetitive motion strain and manual medicine treatments: potential roles for pro- and anti-inflammatory cytokines. Journal

of Bodywork and Movement Therapies 12, 201–203.

Solomonow, M., 2009. Ligaments: a source of musculoskeletal disorders. Journal of Bodywork and Movement Therapies 13, 136–154.

Swanson, R.L., 2013. Biotensegrity: a unifying theory of biological architecture. Journal of the American Osteopathic Association 113, 34–52.

Urse, G.N., 2012. Plantar fasciitis: a review. Osteopathic Family Physician 4, 68–71.

Wong, C.K., 2012. Strain counterstrain: current concepts and clinical

evidence. Manual Therapy 17, 2–8.

Wynne, M.M., Burns, J.M., Eland, D.C., et al., 2006. Effect of counterstrain on stretch reflexes, Hoffmann reflexes, and clinical outcomes in subjects with plantar fasciitis. Journal of the American Osteopathic Association 106, 547–556.

Zink, G., Lawson, W., 1979. Osteopathic structural examination and functional interpretation of the soma. Osteopathic Annals 7, 433–440.

Chapter | 8 |

Balanced ligamentous tension techniques

Raymond J. Hruby

BACKGROUND

The concepts of balanced ligamentous tension (BLT), balanced membranous tension (BMT) and the associated osteopathic manipulative treatment techniques were first described by William G. Sutherland, DO (DiGiovanna et al. 2005; Magoun 1976; Speece & Crow 2001). Sutherland was a graduate of the American School of Osteopathy and a student of Andrew Taylor Still, MD, DO, the founder of the osteopathic profession. Dr Sutherland is well known as the discoverer and developer of osteopathy in the cranial field. Although commonly referred to as 'cranial techniques', Sutherland rejected this terminology, as he felt that it implied that his techniques were separate from osteopathy as applied to the rest of the human body. Sutherland firmly believed, and always stated, that he was merely applying Still's original principles to the head. To prove his point, Sutherland taught a course to his followers in 1947, wherein he neither discussed nor demonstrated any procedures for the cranium; rather, he spent the entire time teaching his students how to apply his approach throughout the body. The concepts and techniques taught by Sutherland in this course were documented by one of his students, Howard A. Lippincott, DO, and published under the title *The Osteopathic Technique of Wm. G. Sutherland, D.O.*, in the 1949 Yearbook of the American Academy of Osteopathy (Lippincott 1949).

BASIC CONCEPTS

The principles of BLT are formulated around an understanding of ligamentous articular mechanisms. Ligaments regulate and guide the movement in all the articulatory mechanisms of the body. In most joints, they act as checks to the voluntary actions of muscles. The placement of the ligaments around a joint creates various fulcrums and checks within which the complex movements of the bones occur. Sutherland described this as a ligamentous articular mechanism. A further concept to be aware of is that, while bony position may change, the overall tensions on the ligaments remain in a symmetrical arrangement. In other words, as long as a joint is moved within its physiological range of motion, the tensions within the associated ligaments will remain in balance. Sutherland called this a 'balanced ligamentous articular mechanism'. In his model, the joints in the body are viewed as balanced ligamentous articular mechanisms. The ligaments provide proprioceptive information to guide the muscle response to joint position, and the ligaments guide the motion of the articular components.

To further elucidate this concept of balanced tensions in ligamentous structures, Sutherland introduced the terms 'reciprocal tension ligaments' and 'reciprocal tension mechanism' as additional descriptors of the ligamentous articular mechanism (Magoun 1976). A key concept is that, within the physiological range of motion of a joint, the ligamentous tension remains constant. The ligaments are neither stretched nor lax. The mechanical motion of the joint comes about as a result of a change in the shape of the joint space, rather than from any overall changes in ligamentous tension around the joint (Carriero 2003).

DEFINITIONS

In light of the above concepts, Sutherland (Magoun 1976) introduced the following terms as part of his treatment model:

1. **Balanced ligamentous tension (BLT)**: the concept that, in a normal, physiologically moving joint, the overall tension of the associated ligaments is symmetrical or balanced.
2. **Ligamentous articular strain (LAS)**: the type of somatic dysfunction characterized by abnormal tensions (strain) in some or all of a joint's ligamentous structures, as a result of trauma, inflammation or other abnormal conditions.

The reader should note that, in Sutherland's model of osteopathy in the cranial field, the dura is considered the ligamentous articular mechanism for the cranium. Accordingly, the terms 'balanced membranous tension' and 'membranous articular strain' were used by Sutherland to describe these principles as applied to the cranium. Further discussion of these cranial applications is beyond the scope of this chapter.

LIGAMENTOUS ARTICULAR STRAIN

As mentioned, ligamentous articular strain (LAS) is the name given to the specific type of somatic dysfunction associated with BLT technique. What is the nature of this type of somatic dysfunction (see Chapter 2) and how does it occur? A simple definition of LAS is that it is any somatic dysfunction resulting in abnormal ligamentous tension or strain. Lippincott (1949) explained Sutherland's original concept as follows:

Osteopathic lesions are strains of the tissues of the body. When they involve joints it is the ligaments that are primarily affected so the term 'ligamentous articular strain' is the one preferred by Dr. Sutherland. The ligaments of a joint are normally on a balanced, reciprocal tension and seldom if ever are they completely relaxed throughout the normal range of movement. When the motion is carried beyond that range the tension is unbalanced and the elements of the ligamentous structure which limit motion in that direction are strained and weakened. The lesion is maintained by the overbalance of the reciprocal tension by the elements, which have not been strained. This locks the articular mechanism or prevents its free and normal movement. The unbalanced tension causes the bones to assume a position that is nearer that in which the strain was produced than would be the case if the tension were normal, and the weakened part of the ligaments permits motion in the direction of the lesion in excess of normal. The range of movement in the opposite direction is limited by the more firm and unopposed tension of the elements which had not been strained.

LAS may also be understood by first examining the characteristics associated with physiological joint motion, and then reasoning what happens to alter this motion when certain adverse conditions are put into place. Carriero (2003) offers this view:

The type of motion which may occur at any given articulation is determined by the shape of the joint surfaces, the position of the ligaments, and the forces of the muscles acting upon the joint. Ligaments do not stretch and contract as muscles do; consequently, the tension in a ligament has very little variation. The tension distributed throughout the ligaments of any given joint is balanced. In normal movements, as the joint changes position, the relationships between the joint's ligaments also change, but the total tension within the ligamentous articular mechanism does not. The distribution of tension between the ligaments is altered, however, when the joint is affected by injury, inflammation, and/or mechanical forces. This is what happens in somatic dysfunction. The distribution and vector of tension within any given ligament will change according to the position of strain in the joint. However, the shared tension within the ligamentous articular mechanism of any given joint remains constant as long as the ligament is not damaged. This has been called a reciprocal tension mechanism. Of course, the balance within the ligamentous articular mechanism can be strained if the joint is inappropriately moved beyond its physiologic range of motion. In the former case, it is the balance of tension, which is distorted. In the latter case, the fibers of the ligament are subjected to microscopic tears and stretch. While this (the latter case) will most assuredly result in a strain to the balance of the articular ligaments, the ligaments do not need to be disrupted for the balance to be distorted. The distortion in balance is a mechanical strain, which may or may not involve an anatomical one. In any somatic dysfunction, there is always a strain in the balanced ligamentous articular mechanism.

PROPOSED MECHANISM OF ACTION OF BLT

Applying the principles of BLT involves establishing fulcrums and levers that are used to direct changes to the ligamentous articular strains. The general principle involves the introduction of a fulcrum by the practitioner and then having the patient provide an activating force. The activating forces can include respiration, postural changes and induced changes in fluid pressures, for example. The practitioner balances all the forces within the ligamentous structures of the joint being treated so that a fulcrum is established. The activating forces can then be used to correct the somatic dysfunction (Carriero 2003; Crow 2011; Speece et al. 2001).

The precise mechanism of action by which physiological motion is restored using BLT is not known. A commonly held theory is that positioning the affected joint in such a way as to minimize the ligamentous tensions around it (that is, achieve a point of balanced ligamentous tension) results in a reduction in afferent input from the affected joint structures to the central nervous system. This allows for the central nervous system to respond by re-establishing a more physiological state of motor control of the joint. Activating forces, such as patient positioning, postural adjustments, and respiration appear to facilitate the reestablishment of normal motor control, and enhance the success of the treatment process (Van Buskirk 1990).

BLT AND OTHER POSITIONAL RELEASE TECHNIQUES

BLT is one of a number of manual treatment modalities that may be classified as a type of positional release technique. In general, positional release techniques all utilize a similar therapeutic principle: the involved joint or tissue is placed in a more neutral position, which is typically perceived by the practitioner as the position where there is palpable relaxation of the involved tissues, such as

muscles, fascia, ligaments and tendons. The patient is maintained in this position until the involved tissues have become completely relaxed (Seffinger & Hruby 2007). Clinically, the patient perceives the neutral position as one where there is marked reduction or elimination of pain or discomfort, which persists when the treatment is completed. In order to appreciate similarities and contrasts among some commonly known positional release techniques, the reader is referred to Table 8.1, which includes definitions and brief descriptions of these techniques. (See also the discussion on positional release variations in Chapter 1.)

PRINCIPLES OF DIAGNOSIS

A specific diagnostic evaluation method for BLT has not been described. A diagnosis of LAS is arrived at by first performing an osteopathic structural examination and determining the presence of any specific joint somatic dysfunction(s). If a somatic dysfunction is found, the practitioner can use palpation in conjunction with the patient's respiratory cooperation efforts to test the dysfunctional joint in all of its planes of motion until the position of maximum ease is found. The practitioner also notes how the tissue feels at the end of range of motion testing, otherwise known as 'end feel'. The quality of the end feel indicates the most likely type of motion restriction present: articular, muscular, fascial, oedema-based or ligamentous. The end feel associated with LAS has been described as hard, abrupt and with near total loss of tissue elasticity. Such a finding thus makes BLT an excellent technique choice to treat the LAS associated with the joint in question (Ehrenfeuchter 2011).

PRINCIPLES OF TREATMENT

The first (and most critical) step in treatment using BLT is for the practitioner to place the strained articular mechanism in a position where all the tensions on the ligaments are at their minimum. This position is referred to as the point of balanced ligamentous tension (Carriero 2003). Once achieved, the practitioner can then utilize one or more of the activating forces previously described to treat the LAS in the involved joint structure. The treatment principles of BLT were first described by Lippincott (1949), as follows:

Since it is the ligaments that are primarily involved in the maintenance of the lesion it is they, not muscular leverage, that are used as the main agency for reduction. The articulation is carried in the direction of the lesion, exaggerating the lesion

Table 8.1 Some representative positional release techniques

Technique	Definition	Description
Counterstrain	A system of diagnosis and treatment that considers the dysfunction to be a continuing, inappropriate strain reflex, which is inhibited by applying a position of mild strain in the direction exactly opposite to that of the reflex; this is accomplished by specific directed positioning about the point of tenderness to achieve the desired therapeutic response.	The practitioner locates a specific counterstrain point, called a 'tender point', usually thought to be associated with musculotendinous or fascial tissues, and associated with somatic dysfunction(s) present in joint structures. While monitoring the tender point, the practitioner positions the patient until the tenderness to palpation at the counterstrain point is minimized. The practitioner holds the patient in this position for 90 seconds and then slowly and passively returns the patient to a neutral position. The tender point is reassessed to determine success of the treatment.
Facilitated positional release	A system of indirect myofascial release treatment. The component region of the body is placed into a neutral position, diminishing tissue and joint tension in all planes, and an activating force (compression or torsion) is added.	The involved joint or region placed into its neutral position in order to unload the tissue tensions that are present. An activating force, such as compression and/or torsion is applied and maintained, followed by further positioning of the somatic dysfunction into all three planes of relative freedom. The entire process up to this point only takes a few seconds. The dysfunction is then reassessed.
Functional	An indirect treatment approach that involves finding the dynamic balance point and one of the following: applying an indirect guiding force, holding the position or adding compression to exaggerate position and allowing for spontaneous readjustment. The osteopathic practitioner guides the manipulative procedure while the dysfunctional area is being palpated in order to obtain a continuous feedback of the physiological response to induced motion. The osteopathic practitioner guides the dysfunctional part so as to create a decreasing sense of tissue resistance (increased compliance).	The practitioner places the dysfunction in the position of greatest ease and maintains this position. One hand monitors the dysfunction (sensory hand) and the other hand (motor hand) positions the patient. As the sensory hand feels the tissues begin to release, the motor hand moves the body in that direction and keeps the affected area from returning to the previous position. The practitioner continues this process until the dysfunction is resolved.
Myofascial release (MFR)	A system of diagnosis and treatment first described by Andrew Taylor Still and his early students, which engages continual palpatory feedback to achieve release of myofascial tissues. With direct MFR, a myofascial tissue restrictive barrier is engaged for the myofascial tissues and the tissue is loaded with a constant force until tissue release occurs. With indirect MFR, the dysfunctional tissues are guided along the path of least resistance until free movement is achieved.	The direct form of MFR engages the restrictive barrier of the affected myofascial tissue. A constant force on the tissues is maintained until a release occurs. Direct MFR attempts to effect changes in the myofascial structures by stretching or elongation of fascia. The practitioner applies slow movements through the various layers of the fascia until the deep layers are reached. The indirect method involves applying a gentle stretch and allowing the fascia to spontaneously release, sometimes referred to as 'unwinding'. The restricted tissues are guided into the position of ease until free movement results.

Table 8.1 Continued

Technique	Definition	Description
Osteopathy in the cranial field	A system of diagnosis and treatment by an osteopathic practitioner using the primary respiratory mechanism and balanced membranous tension.	This technique involves the application of BLT principles to the cranial and/or sacral region. The dural membrane is considered the 'ligamentous' structure that is strained, and the term 'balanced membranous tension' is used to refer to the strain mechanism and the technique that is applied in this paradigm.
Visceral	A system of diagnosis and treatment directed to the viscera to improve physiological function.	Using the myofascial release principles described above, the affected organ is moved toward its position of ease, in order to minimize tensions on its associated fascial attachments. When a release occurs, the practitioner notes the presence of normal physiological motion in the fascial structures and/or a restoration of the normal inherent motion of the affected organ.

Source: Chila A G (Executive Ed.). 2011. Glossary of osteopathic terminology. In: Foundations of Osteopathic Medicine, 2nd edn. Lippincott Williams & Wilkins, Philadelphia, PA.

position as far as is necessary to cause the tension of the weakened elements of the ligamentous structure to be equal to or slightly in excess of the tension of those that were not strained. This is the point of balanced tension. Forcing the joint to move beyond that point adds to the strain which is already present. Forcing the articulation back and away from the direction of lesion strains the ligaments that are normal and unopposed, and if it is done with thrusts or jerks there is definite possibility of separating fibers of the ligaments from their bony attachments. When the tension is properly balanced the respiratory or muscular cooperation of the patient is employed to overcome the resistance of the defense mechanism of the body to the release of the lesion. If the patient holds the breath in or out as long as possible there is a period during his involuntary efforts to resume breathing when the release takes place. In appendicular lesions the patient holds the articulation in the position of exaggeration and the release occurs through the agency of the ligaments when or just before the muscles are relaxed.

More recent osteopathic authors have elaborated on these principles, based on clinical experience. For example, Speece & Crow (2001) give the following explanation of the principles of BLT:

Once an area of dysfunction has been located, compress or decompress the joint or fascial plane to disengage the injury so that the displaced bone can be moved. [This is similar to pushing in the clutch on

a car to shift gears.] Then carry the injured part in the direction of least resistance, returning it to the original position to which it was forced during the injury. Carrying the injury the way it wants to go is an indirect method of treatment and is also one that follows the direction of the somatic dysfunction. Remember that just after the initial injury, the injured part sprang back toward a normal position but was caught in limbo – part way between the position of the injury and the normal functional position. So, when correcting the injury, you must carry the injured part back to the exact position of injury and maintain that position until the body rebalances all the connective tissue surrounding the dysfunction, and draws the part back to its normal functional physiologic position. This can be done using a direct technique, and indirect technique, or a combination of direct and indirect methods.

Practitioners of BLT (Crow 2011; DiGiovanna et al. 2005; Speece & Crow 2001) agree that there are three primary components to the application of the technique: disengagement, exaggeration and balance.

1. *Disengagement*: The practitioner applies gentle compression or traction to the dysfunctional joint or fascial plane, to obtain the maximum amount of motion available without resistance.
2. *Exaggeration*: The practitioner moves the area of dysfunction toward its position of ease or, in other words, back to the original position of injury, until the point of balanced ligamentous tension is achieved.

3. *Balance*: The practitioner maintains this position of 'ease' and may recruit the assistance of the previously discussed activating forces until a release occurs. The practitioner continuously monitors the dysfunctional joint, and may need to shift the positioning periodically in order to maintain the point of balanced ligamentous tension throughout the treatment process. The joint will move gently in the direction of exaggeration, and then back to the point of balanced ligamentous tension. When the release occurs, the affected joint will slowly move back to its normal physiological position.

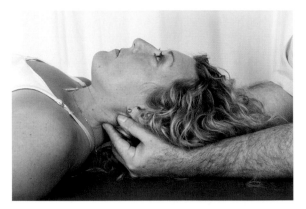

Figure 8.1 Treatment position for lower cervical spine.

INDICATIONS AND CONTRAINDICATIONS

Specific indications (Nicholas & Nicholas 2012) for the use of BLT are:

1. Acute or chronic somatic dysfunction of articular structures
2. Ligamentous sprains or strains
3. Somatic dysfunction of myofascial structures
4. Areas of lymphatic congestion or local oedema.

There are few contraindications to BLT, and most authors consider them to be relative contraindications. They are as follows:

1. Fracture, dislocation or gross instability of the region to be addressed
2. Malignancy, infection or severe osteoporosis at the site of treatment.

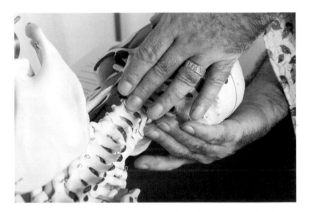

Figure 8.2 Skeleton view showing hand placement for lower cervical spine treatment.

SAFETY AND EFFICACY

Practitioners of BLT (Nicholas & Nicholas 2012; Seffinger & Hruby 2007) consider the technique to be safe and effective. There are no known or reported injuries, side-effects or serious complications resulting from the use of BLT for the treatment of LAS.

REPRESENTATIVE TECHNIQUES

Cervical spine

Lower cervical spine (C3–C7)

(Figs 8.1, 8.2)

1. The patient is supine.
2. The practitioner is seated at the head of the treatment table.

3. The practitioner cradles the patient's occiput with both hands, with the thenar and hypothenar eminences contacting the superior nuchal line, and the pads of the middle fingers contacting the articular pillars of the cervical segment to be treated.
4. The practitioner then slides the pads of the middle fingers inferiorly to a point just below the restricted segment.
5. The practitioner then applies an anterior and superior movement with the middle finger pads, drawing the fingers toward the thenar and hypothenar eminences until the point of BLT is achieved.
6. The practitioner maintains the point of BLT by monitoring the tissue tension between the two hands.
7. The practitioner may add an activating force by having the patient hold his or her breath in either inhalation or exhalation, whichever phase facilitates the maintenance of the point of BLT.

8. Release of the ligamentous tension will be felt either prior to, or at the point when the patient can no longer hold his or her breathing.

Atlantoaxial (AA) joint

(Figs 8.1, 8.2)

1. The AA joint may be treated using the same hand position as for the lower cervical spine, while contacting the appropriate articular pillars.

Occipitoatlantal joint

(Figs 8.3, 8.4)

1. The patient is supine.
2. The practitioner is seated at the head of the treatment table.
3. The practitioner cradles the patient's occiput in one hand, with the thenar and hypothenar eminences

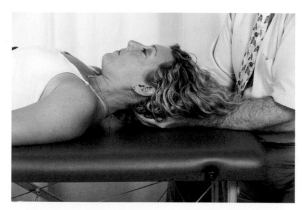

Figure 8.3 Treatment position for the occipitoatlantal joint.

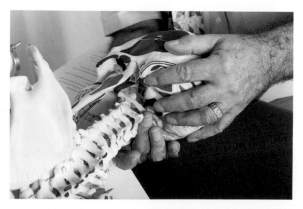

Figure 8.4 Skeletal view showing hand placement for treatment of the occipitoatlantal joint.

contacting the superior nuchal line, and the middle finger in the midline and pointing toward the opisthion (the median point of the posterior border of the foramen magnum).

4. The index and ring fingers are lateral to the midline and approximately in the plane of the occipital condyles.
5. The practitioner's other hand is placed under the upper cervical spinal region, with the pad of the middle finger resting in the midline just superior to the C2 spinous process.
6. The patient is asked to dorsiflex the feet.
7. While the head rests comfortably in the practitioner's hands, the patient is then instructed to slowly tuck the chin toward the chest until the point of BLT is achieved.
8. At this point, the practitioner will feel the finger pad on C2 move superiorly and contact the tubercle of C1.
9. The practitioner maintains the point of BLT between C1 and the occiput by monitoring the tissue tension between the two hands.
10. The practitioner may add an activating force by having the patient hold his or her breath in either inhalation or exhalation, whichever phase facilitates the maintenance of the point of BLT.
11. Release of the ligamentous tension will be felt either prior to, or at the point when the patient can no longer hold his or her breathing.

Thoracic and lumbar spine

Lower thoracic and lumbar spine

(Figs 8.5–8.7)

1. The patient is supine.
2. The practitioner sits at the side of the table.

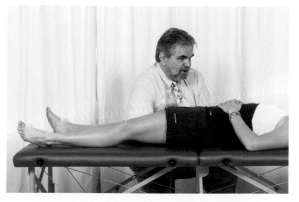

Figure 8.5 Physician and patient position for treatment of the lower thoracic or lumber spine.

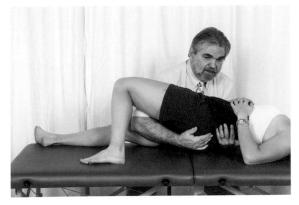

Figure 8.6 Hand position for lower thoracic or lumbar spine treatment.

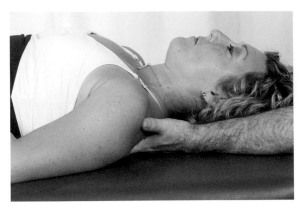

Figure 8.8 Treatment position for the upper thoracic spine.

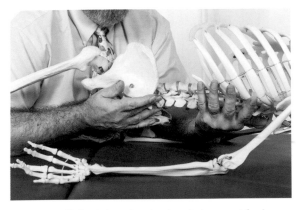

Figure 8.7 Skeletal view showing hand placement for lower thoracic or lumbar spine treatment.

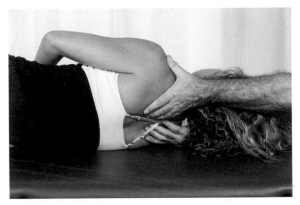

Figure 8.9 Lateral view showing hand position for upper thoracic spine treatment.

3. The practitioner places one hand on the sacrum, with the fingertips at the lumbosacral junction and the sacrum resting comfortably in the palm of the hand.

4. The practitioner's other hand is placed transversely over the vertebra to be treated, with the spinous process in the palm of the hand, the finger pads in contact with the paravertebral muscles farthest from the practitioner, and the thenar and hypothenar eminences in contact with the paravertebral muscles nearest the practitioner.

5. While maintaining the sacrum in position, the practitioner moves the affected vertebral segment in an anterior and superior direction until the point of BLT is achieved.

6. The practitioner may add an activating force by having the patient hold his or her breath in either inhalation or exhalation, whichever phase facilitates the maintenance of the point of BLT.

7. Release of the ligamentous tension will be felt either prior to, or at the point when the patient can no longer hold his or her breathing.

Upper thoracic spine

(Figs 8.8, 8.9)

1. The patient is supine.
2. The practitioner is seated at the head of the treatment table.
3. The practitioner slides his or her hands under the patient's thorax, with palms facing toward the ceiling, to the level of the restricted vertebra.
4. The pads of the index and middle fingers are placed on each side of the restricted vertebra, approximately 1.5 inches lateral to the spinous process.
5. The practitioner moves the pads of the index and middle fingers in an anterior and superior direction

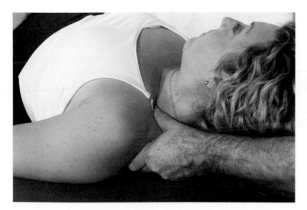

Figure 8.10 Treatment position for the first rib.

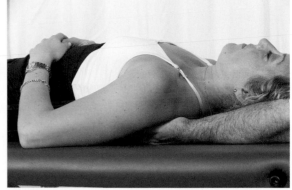

Figure 8.11 Treatment position for ribs 2–12.

bilaterally, until a point of BLT is achieved, and maintains this position.

6. The practitioner may add an activating force by having the patient hold his or her breath in either inhalation or exhalation, whichever phase facilitates the maintenance of the point of BLT.

7. Release of the ligamentous tension will be felt either prior to, or at the point when the patient can no longer hold his or her breathing.

Rib cage

First rib

(Fig. 8.10)

1. The patient may be seated or supine.

2. The practitioner contacts the superior surface of the first rib by placing his or her thumb just lateral to the costotransverse articulation.

3. While monitoring the first rib, the practitioner uses the opposite hand to induce any combination of flexion, extension, left or right rotation, or left or right side-bending until a point of BLT is achieved. The practitioner then maintains this position.

4. The practitioner may add an activating force by having the patient hold his or her breath in either inhalation or exhalation, whichever phase facilitates the maintenance of the point of BLT.

5. Release of the ligamentous tension will be felt either prior to, or at the point when the patient can no longer hold his or her breathing.

Ribs 2–12

(Figs 8.11–8.13)

1. The patient is supine.

2. The practitioner is seated at the head of the treatment table.

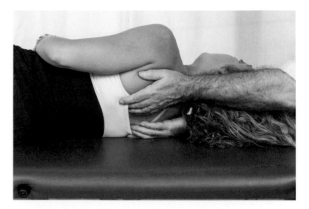

Figure 8.12 Lateral view showing hand placement for treatment of ribs 2–12.

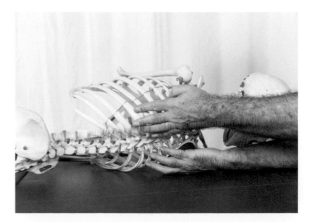

Figure 8.13 Skeletal view showing hand placement for treatment of ribs 2–12.

3. The practitioner slides his or her hands under the patient's thorax, with palms facing toward the ceiling, to the level of the restricted rib.
4. The practitioner places the index, middle and ring fingers of one hand on the angle of the restricted rib.
5. The practitioner then carries the restricted rib anteriorly, then superiorly and laterally, until a point of BLT is achieved. The practitioner then maintains this position.
6. The practitioner may add an activating force by having the patient hold his or her breath in either inhalation or exhalation, whichever phase facilitates the maintenance of the point of BLT.
7. Release of the ligamentous tension will be felt either prior to, or at the point when the patient can no longer hold his or her breathing.

Pelvis

Lumbosacral decompression

(Figs 8.14–8.16)

1. The patient is supine.
2. The practitioner sits at the side of the table at the level of the patient's pelvis.
3. The practitioner places one hand on the sacrum, with the fingertips at the lumbosacral junction and the sacrum resting comfortably in the palm of the hand.
4. The practitioner's other hand is placed transversely across the lumbar spine, with the ulnar side of the hand in contact with the fingertips of the hand on the sacrum, and the lower lumbar spinous processes resting on the palm of the hand.
5. The practitioner then applies either gentle traction to separate L5 from the sacrum, or gentle compression to bring L5 and the sacrum closer together

– whichever movement allows for the achievement of a point of BLT. The practitioner then maintains this position.

7. The practitioner may add an activating force by having the patient hold his or her breath in either inhalation or exhalation, whichever phase facilitates the maintenance of the point of BLT.
8. Release of the ligamentous tension will be felt either prior to, or at the point when the patient can no longer hold his or her breathing.

Sacroiliac decompression

(Figs 8.17–8.19)

1. The patient is supine.
2. The practitioner stands at the side of the table.

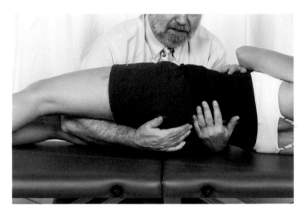

Figure 8.15 Lateral view showing hand position for treatment of lumbosacral decompression.

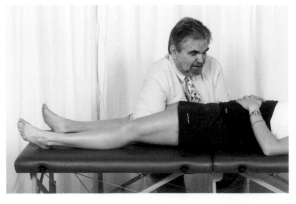

Figure 8.14 Physician and patient position for lumbosacral decompression.

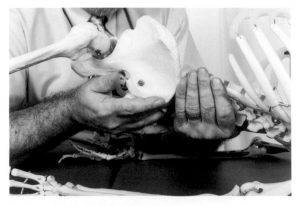

Figure 8.16 Skeletal view showing hand position for treatment of lumbosacral decompression.

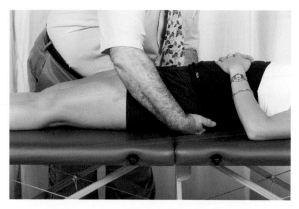

Figure 8.17 Physician and patient position for sacroiliac decompression.

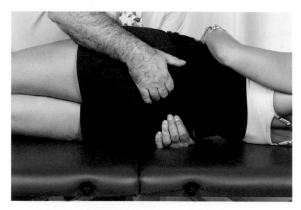

Figure 8.18 Lateral view showing hand placement for sacroiliac decompression.

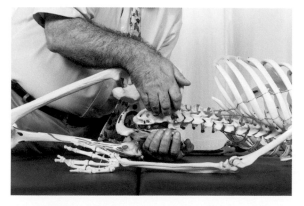

Figure 8.19 Skeletal view showing hand placement for sacroiliac decompression.

3. The patient is instructed to lift the buttocks off the table.
4. The practitioner reaches around the patient's pelvis, placing the finger pads of his or her hands in the sacral sulcus on each side. The patient then lowers the pelvis to the table, with the pelvis now resting comfortably in the practitioner's hands.
5. The practitioner applies gentle traction laterally and inferiorly with each hand, moving the innominates away from the sacrum until a point of BLT is achieved. The practitioner then maintains this position.
6. The practitioner may add an activating force by having the patient hold his or her breath in either inhalation or exhalation, whichever phase facilitates the maintenance of the point of BLT.
7. Release of the ligamentous tension will be felt either prior to, or at the point when the patient can no longer hold his or her breathing.

Innominate release

(Fig. 8.20)

1. The patient is supine.
2. The practitioner stands at the side of the table at the level of the patient's pelvis.
3. The practitioner places the palms of his or her hands on the patient's anterior superior iliac spines (ASISs).
4. The practitioner then gently compresses the ASISs medially.
5. The practitioner next determines in which directions the innominates prefer to move by simultaneously gently rotating one innominate anteriorly and the other one posteriorly, and then repeating this manoeuvre in the opposite directions.

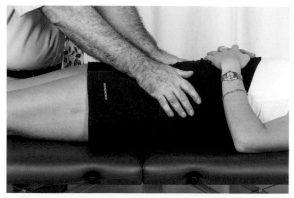

Figure 8.20 Treatment position for innominate release.

6. The practitioner then rotates the innominates in the direction of least resistance (direction of ease) until a point of BLT is achieved. The practitioner then maintains this position.

7. The practitioner may add an activating force by having the patient hold his or her breath in either inhalation or exhalation, whichever phase facilitates the maintenance of the point of BLT.

8. Release of the ligamentous tension will be felt either prior to, or at the point when the patient can no longer hold his or her breathing.

Upper extremity

Clavicle

(Fig. 8.21)

1. The patient is seated.

2. The practitioner can be seated or standing facing the patient.

3. The practitioner places the thumb of one hand on the inferomedial aspect of the clavicle immediately lateral to the sternoclavicular joint.

4. The practitioner's other thumb is placed on the inferomedial aspect of the lateral end of the clavicle just medial and inferior to the acromioclavicular joint.

5. The patient is instructed to lean forward slightly, while the practitioner applies gentle pressure with both thumbs, moving the clavicle laterally, superiorly and slightly posteriorly.

6. At the same time, the patient is asked to turn slowly toward the unaffected side, until the practitioner determines that a point of BLT has been achieved. The practitioner then maintains this position.

7. The practitioner may add an activating force by having the patient hold his or her breath in either inhalation or exhalation, whichever phase facilitates the maintenance of the point of BLT.

8. Release of the ligamentous tension will be felt either prior to, or at the point when the patient can no longer hold his or her breathing.

Glenohumeral joint

(Fig. 8.22)

1. The patient lies in the lateral recumbent position with the affected shoulder closer to the ceiling.

2. The practitioner stands at the side of the table and behind the patient.

3. The practitioner places one hand on the humeral head region. The patient's elbow is flexed and the arm relaxed, and the practitioner grasps the patient's elbow with his or her other hand.

4. With the hand on the elbow, the practitioner moves the humerus slightly laterally, and then applies gentle compression toward the glenohumeral joint. At the same time, with the other hand over the glenohumeral joint region, the practitioner applies gentle inferior compression toward the patient's elbow.

5. The practitioner then uses a combination of gentle anterior and posterior motions with each hand, until a point of BLT is achieved. The practitioner then maintains this position.

6. The practitioner may add an activating force by having the patient hold his or her breath in either inhalation or exhalation, whichever phase facilitates the maintenance of the point of BLT.

7. Release of the ligamentous tension will be felt either prior to, or at the point when the patient can no longer hold his or her breathing.

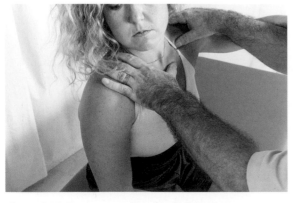

Figure 8.21 Treatment position for clavicle release.

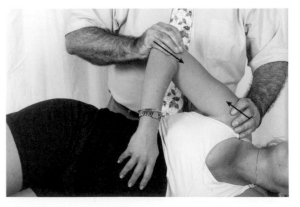

Figure 8.22 Positioning for treatment of the glenohumeral joint.

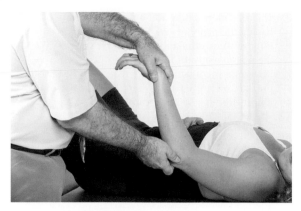

Figure 8.23 Positioning for treatment of the forearm and elbow.

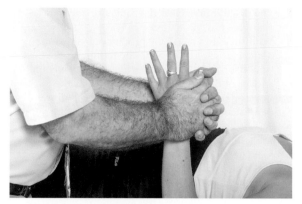

Figure 8.24 Treatment position for the carpals or metacarpals.

Forearm and elbow

(Fig. 8.23)

1. The patient is supine.
2. The practitioner sits or stands at the side of the table (the same side as the affected upper extremity).
3. The practitioner grasps the patient's olecranon process with the thumb and index finger of one hand. With the other hand, the practitioner grasps the patient's wrist, flexes the patient's elbow to 90° (or as close to 90° as possible, depending on the patient's condition) and flexes the patient's wrist as fully as possible.
4. The practitioner then pronates the patient's forearm and extends the elbow until a point of BLT is achieved. The practitioner then maintains this position.
5. The practitioner may add an activating force by having the patient hold his or her breath in either inhalation or exhalation, whichever phase facilitates the maintenance of the point of BLT.
6. Release of the ligamentous tension will be felt either prior to, or at the point when the patient can no longer hold his or her breathing.

Carpals and metacarpals

(Fig. 8.24)

1. The patient can be seated or supine.
2. The practitioner stands or sits facing the patient.
3. The practitioner interlaces his or her hands and places them over the patient's carpal or metacarpal region (depending on the exact joints to be treated), making contact with the thenar eminences on each side of the patient's hand.

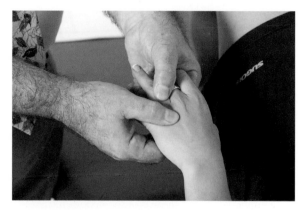

Figure 8.25 Treatment of the phalanges.

4. The practitioner then applies gently compression to the area with his or her thenar eminences, and instructs the patient to gently flex or extend the fingers, until a point of BLT is achieved.
5. The practitioner may add an activating force by having the patient hold his or her breath in either inhalation or exhalation, whichever phase facilitates the maintenance of the point of BLT.
6. Release of the ligamentous tension will be felt either prior to, or at the point when the patient can no longer hold his or her breathing.

Phalanges

(Fig. 8.25)

1. The patient can be seated or supine.
2. The practitioner stands or sits facing the patient.

3. The practitioner grasps the patient's hand and stabilizes it in pronation.
4. With the other hand, the practitioner grasps the phalanx to be treated, with the thumb on the dorsal surface and the index finger on the ventral surface of the phalanx, and just distal to the metacarpophalangeal or interphalangeal joint to be treated.
5. The practitioner applies gentle compression into the joint, and then gently moves the phalanx medially and laterally until a point of BLT is achieved.
6. The practitioner may add an activating force by having the patient hold his or her breath in either inhalation or exhalation, whichever phase facilitates the maintenance of the point of BLT.
7. Release of the ligamentous tension will be felt either prior to, or at the point when the patient can no longer hold his or her breathing.

Lower extremity

Hip

(Fig. 8.26)

1. The patient is in the lateral recumbent position with the affected hip closer to the ceiling.
2. The practitioner stands behind and facing the patient.
3. The practitioner uses one hand to stabilize the innominate.
4. With the other hand placed over the greater trochanter, the practitioner introduces gentle compression along the axis of the neck of the femur, in a medial and slightly superior direction.
5. At the same time, the practitioner introduces gentle compression medially and inferiorly with the hand that is stabilizing the innominate.
6. When a point of BLT is achieved, the practitioner maintains this position.

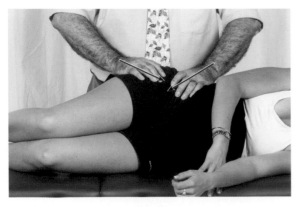

Figure 8.26 Treatment position for the hip joint.

7. The practitioner may add an activating force by having the patient hold his or her breath in either inhalation or exhalation, whichever phase facilitates the maintenance of the point of BLT.
8. Release of the ligamentous tension will be felt either prior to, or at the point when the patient can no longer hold his or her breathing.

Knee

(Figs 8.27, 8.28)

1. The patient is supine.
2. The practitioner stands at the side of the affected knee.
3. The practitioner contacts the anterior distal end of the femur with the palm of one hand, and the anterior proximal end of the tibia, over the tibial tuberosity, with the other hand.

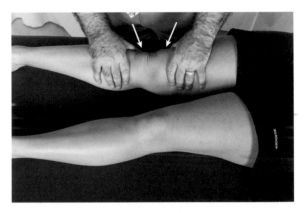

Figure 8.27 Treatment position for the knee joint, showing compression of the femur and tibia toward the table surface.

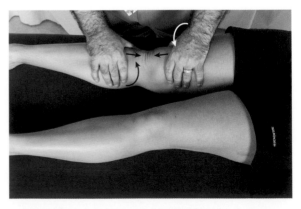

Figure 8.28 Treatment position for the knee joint, showing compression of the tibia and femur toward each other, and the use of external and internal rotation to achieve a final position of balanced ligamentous tension.

4. The practitioner then applies gentle pressure with both hands, moving the femur and tibia toward the table surface.
5. The practitioner then applies gentle compression with both hands, approximating the femur and tibia.
6. Stabilizing the femur in this position, the practitioner next introduces gentle internal and external rotation into the tibia, until a point of BLT is achieved, and then maintains this position.
7. The practitioner may add an activating force by having the patient hold his or her breath in either inhalation or exhalation, whichever phase facilitates the maintenance of the point of BLT.
8. Release of the ligamentous tension will be felt either prior to, or at the point when the patient can no longer hold his or her breathing.

Fibular head

(Fig. 8.29)

1. The patient is supine.
2. The practitioner is seated on the side of the affected lower extremity.
3. The practitioner flexes the patient's hip and knee to approximately 90° each.
4. The practitioner places one elbow on the table and the web of the hand in the patient's popliteal fossa to support the leg. The thumb of this hand rests on the superior aspect of the proximal fibular head. The practitioner applies gentle pressure with the thumb, to move the fibular head inferiorly.
5. With the other hand, the practitioner inverts and slightly internally rotates the foot.
6. This position is adjusted until a point of BLT is achieved, and the practitioner then maintains this position.
7. The practitioner may add an activating force by having the patient hold his or her breath in either

inhalation or exhalation, whichever phase facilitates the maintenance of the point of BLT.
8. Release of the ligamentous tension will be felt either prior to, or at the point when the patient can no longer hold his or her breathing.

Ankle

Anterior talus

(Figs 8.30, 8.31)

1. The patient is supine.
2. The practitioner stands on the side of the affected ankle.
3. The practitioner places the palm of one hand over the anterior distal tibia, and applies compression, carrying the tibia toward the table surface. The practitioner may use the other hand to add additional pressure as needed.

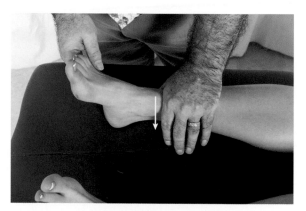

Figure 8.30 Treatment position for anterior talus, with compression of the tibia toward the table surface.

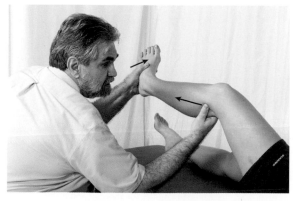

Figure 8.29 Positioning for treatment of the fibular head.

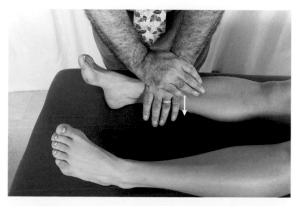

Figure 8.31 Treatment position for anterior talus, showing the use of both hands to apply compression of the tibia toward the table surface.

4. The practitioner then rolls the tibia into external and internal rotation, until a point of BLT is achieved, and then maintains this position.

5. The practitioner may add an activating force by having the patient hold his or her breath in either inhalation or exhalation, whichever phase facilitates the maintenance of the point of BLT.

6. Release of the ligamentous tension will be felt either prior to, or at the point when the patient can no longer hold his or her breathing.

Posterior talus

(Fig. 8.32)

1. The patient is supine, with the heel of the affected foot just beyond the edge of the table by approximately 1 inch.

2. The practitioner stands at the foot of the table, facing toward the head of the table.

3. The practitioner grasps the patient's foot by approximating the palms over the metatarsals and phalanges, with the thumbs approximated and resting on the dorsum of the foot. The practitioner's fingers wrap around the sides of the foot, with the finger pads approximated and in contact with the sole of the foot.

4. The practitioner brings the foot into slight plantar flexion.

5. The practitioner next applies gentle compression into the entire foot, and directed toward the floor, until a point of BLT is achieved. The practitioner then maintains this position.

6. The practitioner may add an activating force by having the patient hold his or her breath in either inhalation or exhalation, whichever phase facilitates the maintenance of the point of BLT.

7. Release of the ligamentous tension will be felt either prior to, or at the point when the patient can no longer hold his or her breathing.

Calcaneus

(Fig. 8.33)

1. The patient is supine.

2. The practitioner stands at the side of the affected foot, facing the foot of the table.

3. The practitioner flexes the patient's hip and knee, and places the elbow of his or her arm that is closest to the table just above the patient's popliteal fossa.

4. Using the same hand, the practitioner grasps the patient's calcaneus with the thumb and index finger.

5. With the other hand, the practitioner grasps the patient's foot at the distal metatarsal aspect, and slightly flexes the foot toward the calcaneus.

6. The practitioner then gently moves the calcaneus inferiorly until a point of BLT is achieved.

7. The practitioner may add an activating force by having the patient hold his or her breath in either inhalation or exhalation, whichever phase facilitates the maintenance of the point of BLT.

8. Release of the ligamentous tension will be felt either prior to, or at the point when the patient can no longer hold his or her breathing.

Tarsals, metatarsals and phalanges

(Fig. 8.34)

1. The patient is supine with the heels on the table.

2. The practitioner stands at the foot of the table, facing toward the patient.

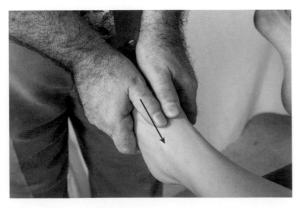

Figure 8.32 Treatment position for posterior talus, showing compression into the foot and toward the floor.

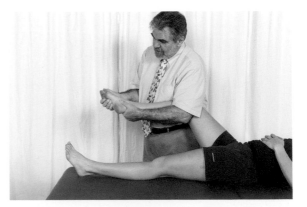

Figure 8.33 Treatment position for the calcaneus, showing the application of gentle traction directing the calcaneus inferiorly to achieve the point of balanced membranous tension.

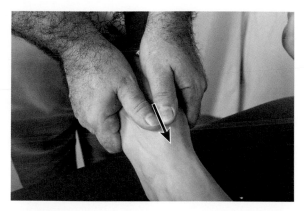

Figure 8.34 Treatment position for the tarsals, metatarsals or phalanges, showing the application of gentle compression of the foot toward the floor to achieve the point of balanced membranous tension.

3. The practitioner grasps the patient's foot with both hands over the area of the distal metatarsals and toes, with the thumbs approximated and resting on the dorsum of the foot, and the fingers wrapped around both sides of the foot with the finger pads approximated and in contact with the sole of the foot.

4. The practitioner places the foot into slight plantar flexion.

5. The practitioner then introduces gentle compression into the foot, directing the phalanges, metatarsals, and tarsals toward the table surface, until a point of BLT is achieved. The practitioner then maintains this position.

6. The practitioner may add an activating force by having the patient hold his or her breath in either inhalation or exhalation, whichever phase facilitates the maintenance of the point of BLT.

7. Release of the ligamentous tension will be felt either prior to, or at the point when the patient can no longer hold his or her breathing.

THIS CHAPTER

This chapter has described the principles of balanced ligamentous tension (BLT) and the techniques used to treat this type of somatic dysfunction. BLT is a concept based on the idea that, in a physiologically normal joint, as movement occurs, the relationships among the joint's ligaments change, but the overall tension within the ligamentous structures remains equally distributed.

NEXT CHAPTER

The next chapter by Edward Goering, DO, describes and gives detailed descriptions of the use of counterstrain when applied to visceral dysfunction.

REFERENCES

Carriero, J.E., 2003. Balanced ligamentous tension techniques. In: Ward, R.C. (Executive Ed.), Foundations of Osteopathic Medicine, second ed. Lippincott Williams & Wilkins, Philadelphia, PA.

Crow, W.T., 2011. Balanced ligamentous tension and ligamentous articular strain. In: Chila, A.G. (Executive Ed.), Foundations of Osteopathic Medicine, third ed. Lippincott Williams & Wilkins, Philadelphia, PA.

DiGiovanna, E.L., Schiowitz, S., Dowling, D.J., 2005. An Osteopathic Approach to Diagnosis and Treatment. Lippincott Williams & Wilkins, Philadelphia, PA.

Ehrenfeuchter, W.C., 2011. Screening osteopathic structural examination. In: Chila, A.G. (Executive Ed.), Foundations of Osteopathic Medicine, third ed. Lippincott Williams & Wilkins, Philadelphia, PA.

Lippincott, H.A., 1949. The Osteopathic Technique of Wm. G. Sutherland, DO. Yearbook of the Academy of Applied Osteopathy. Reprint. American Academy of Osteopathy, Indianapolis, IN.

Magoun, H.I. Sr., 1976. Osteopathy in the Cranial Field. The Journal Printing Company, Kirksville, MO.

Nicholas, A.S., Nicholas, E.A., 2012. Atlas of Osteopathic Techniques, second ed. Wolters Kluwer/ Lippincott Williams & Wilkins, Philadelphia, PA.

Seffinger, M.A., Hruby, R.J., 2007. Evidence-Based Manual Medicine: A Problem-Oriented Approach. Saunders Elsevier, Philadelphia.

Speece, C.A., Crow, W.T., 2001. Ligamentous Articular Strain: Osteopathic Manipulative Techniques for the Body. Eastland Press, Seattle, WA.

Van Buskirk, R., 1990. Nociceptive reflexes and somatic dysfunction. Journal of the American Osteopathic Association 90, 792–809.

Chapter | 9 |

Visceral positional release: the counterstrain model

Edward Goering

INTRODUCTION TO AND DEFINITION OF VISCERAL POSITIONAL RELEASE

Positional release treatment for the viscera has been developed following many different pathways. Manual practitioners who use positional release treatment to relieve tender points associated with somatic dysfunction, recognize the value of these findings. Somatic and visceral dysfunctions that have tender points as a manifestation are effectively treated with a variety of techniques. Understanding this premise allows us to apply this concept to musculoskeletal complaints as well as to visceral complaints.

First, recognize that tissue texture changes, asymmetries of anatomical landmarks, restriction of motion and tenderness (TART, see Chapter 2) are observable and palpable somatic manifestations. The tissue texture changes palpated in association with somatic dysfunction are manifest through the action of the sympathetic and parasympathetic (autonomic) nervous system. Local cytokine factors alter water content and blood flow to and from an area of dysfunction. Motion restriction and anatomical landmark asymmetries manifest through the action of the peripheral or somatic nervous system. Tenderness is due to increased sensitivity of the peripheral, autonomic and central nervous systems. The somatic dysfunctions will be reflected as tender points directly related to their primary disorder when we look at the anatomy.

Positional release techniques are usually indirect and passive techniques. The manipulative procedure places the tissues in a position of ease, removing the distortion created by the inciting dysfunction. A simple mesenteric lift applied to the painful abdomen, held until relaxation and return of normal functioning occurs, is an indirect manoeuvre that is therapeutic with or without appreciation of the associated region of tenderness generated by the dysfunctional tissue. On some occasions, a direct force may be applied. For example, a shearing force may be required in some visceral or vascular structures to activate restorative physiological mechanisms (Gashev 2002). Activation of these mechanisms results in a normal physiological functioning of the visceral or vascular structures. In the walls of visceral structures are the interstitial cells of Cajal that are believed to influence the contraction of many visceral and vascular organs (Huang & Xu 2010).

Providing the appropriate activating energy through manipulative procedures is the goal of the procedures.

HISTORY

Dr Still recognized that manipulation of the viscera was very effective (Still 1911). Although there are very few descriptions of the techniques used by Dr Still, some of his early students, McDonnell (1994) and Barber (1898) described some of his techniques, as did Riggs (1901), Hazzard (1905), Woodall (1926), Goetz (1909), Smith (1912), Gaddis (1922), Teal (1922), Murray (1925), Young (1947, 1948), Hoover (1947, 1948, 1950) and Sutherland (1990).

Hoover called it a *ventral technique*, and addressed only the abdomen. Sutherland had techniques for both the pelvis and the abdomen. Woodall's applications were gynaecological.

In the more recent past, as scientific understanding of the clinical practice of manual medicine has evolved and improved, growth of the visceral positional release approaches has expanded. Barral is perhaps the most prolific author, innovator and teacher of visceral manipulation, currently. Many of the techniques adopted by positional release treatment clinicians are based on Barral's teachings (Barral 1995). Combining these treatment techniques with a good history, examination and thoughtful treatment has resulted in the identification of many specific tender point locations (as in the counterstrain model, described in Chapter 3). These techniques have grown from clinical understanding to clinical results. As with strain/counterstrain, developed by Dr Lawrence Jones, the basic scientific understanding is still evolving. Other current authors and educators in visceral technique include: Bensky (1995), Barral (1988, 1989, 1993, 1996, 1991, 1999), Lossing (1997), Finet & Willame (2000), Davidson (1992) and Blackman (2001).

Many of these approaches are not related to tender point location and reduction of pain, but are more focussed on restoring natural motion characteristics of each viscus. The balanced ligamentous tension (BLT) approach is used most often. (See Chapter 8 on BLT for further discussion of this approach.) For the sake of simplicity and clarity, this chapter focusses on reduction of visceral dysfunction related to somatic tender point pain with somatic positional release (counterstrain) procedures.

Over the years of working with positional release as it relates to tender points, it has become apparent that, on occasion, tender points and somatic dysfunctions resolve more quickly than the 90 seconds of holding tissues in an 'ease' position, initially recommended by Jones et al. (1995). This was a quandary for many of the practicing clinicians using his methods. Over the last decade, leading educators in this field, have given much effort to the better understanding of this question, e.g. Edward Goering, DO, DVM; Brian Tuckey, PT; Tim Hodges, LMT and Randy Kusonose, PT. The resolution of the problem regarding timing, is considered to relate to the origin of the type of dysfunction, and to variations in the physiological processes involved. Musculoskeletal complaints, for the most part, appear to require a more extended period of time (90 seconds) in the treatment ('ease') position. However, visceral treatments commonly require substantially shorter treatment time. This is thought to be due to the anatomical structure and physiological aetiology of the nociceptive and proprioceptive input that causes/maintains the tender point (Baily & Dick 1992) – the manifestation of the visceral dysfunction, whether somatic or visceral. From a clinical perspective, it is relatively easy to explain the treatment time, resolution of symptoms and body system to which the tender point is related.

THEORY

Trauma, disease and postural/structural abnormalities result in the abnormal force vectors and energy that are stored in the visceral structures. Each visceral organ will manifest pathological effects differently. Treatment requires understanding of the different structures and functions involved with each organ. Treatment of the visceral organs specifically will help the clinician to recognize their unique effect on the body tissues.

With visceral manipulation, it is important to recognize which structure is actually being treated. Many of the solid organs are not specifically treated; rather the supportive and suspensory structures are the focus of treatment. Barral refers to treatment of the liver and states that the primary focus is often the suspensory ligament structure. In treatment of the kidneys, focus is on superior or inferior displacement; however, when treating the ureters, traction may be applied to the structure, resulting in resolution of symptoms.

A sound understanding of visceral somatic reflexes is required for the clinician to develop a good working knowledge of these techniques. The amount of time required for treatment of specific structures may vary from 15 to 90 seconds. This variation is dependent upon the structures being treated and the physiological mechanism being activated.

Indirect manipulative techniques are very effective and having a tender point to help direct the treatment technique increases efficacy. Applying the same process to other systems in the body has shown to improve effectiveness of the treatments (Jones et al. 1995).

The lymphatic system is known to be affected by the endothelial nitrous oxide synthetase (ENOS) system. Traction or stress over the valvular region of the lymphatic vessel causes an increased release of nitrous oxide that, in turn, induces increased relaxation of the muscular layer. This increased stretch will result in a strong contraction of the muscular wall of the vessel (Ribera et al. 2013). In the visceral system, the tubular structures are also affected by changes in the level of nitrous oxide synthetase activation, in the endothelium. This increased activation results in increased levels of nitrous oxide, which affect the interstitial cell of Cajal that, in turn, affects the tension and contractility of the visceral structure. The muscular component of the visceral wall is also directly affected by nitrous oxide (Huang & Xu 2010). This change reduces nociceptive activation, reducing sympathetic tone and manifestations of visceral dysfunction, resulting in reduction or removal of tender points and palpated TART changes (see Chapter 2).

The term 'referred pain' is used for pain localized not at the site of its origin, but in areas that may be adjacent or at a distance from that site, generally comprised in the same metameres. Pain can be referred by deep somatic or by visceral structures. Myofascial pain syndrome is a typical syndrome characterized by referred pain from deep somatic structures (see Chapter 7). Referred pain from visceral organs is most important from a clinical point of view. The patterns of referred pain originating from various viscera are important for a correct diagnosis. Different pathogenetic mechanisms may be involved in the onset of referred pain: convergence of impulses in the central nervous system and reflexes inducing muscle contraction, sympathetic activation and antidromic activation of afferent fibres, which induces so-called 'neurogenic inflammation' (Procacci & Maresca 1999).

Realizing that consistent pain patterns are generated by the various visceral structures is a well-accepted phenomenon. Discovering and utilizing this property of visceral pain helps improve the results of manipulative therapeutic procedure. Visceral pain patterns have demonstrated consistent patterns and characteristics (Gebhart & Bielefeldt 2008). Studies have demonstrated cutaneous pain patterns consistent with visceral organ hyperalgesia. For example Tozzi et al. (2012) have demonstrated that the manipulative treatment of the kidney has reduced low back pain. The recognition of TART changes in the tissues of the body is an accepted osteopathic concept and physiological process, the description of which is presented in more detail in Chapter 2. These changes lay the basic groundwork for the clinical utilization of tender points discovered for specific organ systems to be treated.

INDICATIONS, CONTRAINDICATIONS AND COMPLICATIONS

1. Visceral dysfunction can be associated with a known medical diagnosis. Almost all medical diagnoses of the viscera have a component that is functional within the visceral structure or its attachments. These changes are separate and often different from the somatic manifestations of the dysfunction.
2. Visceral dysfunction can manifest with secondary somatic dysfunction. This is treated in a more typical musculoskeletal way.

Contraindications

These include abdominal aneurysm, internal bleeding, uncontrolled infections, active inflammatory bowel disease and severe pain with evaluation or manipulation. Medical indications for acute emergency medical evaluation are also contraindications for visceral manipulation. Pregnancy is a relative contraindication.

PALPATION AND EVALUATION

Identification of the visceral dysfunctional component is obtained by careful history and physical evaluation, including palpatory examination. This includes the motility and mobility of the specific visceral structures to be evaluated, including attachment evaluation. Barral (1995) describes in detail the appropriate evaluations of mobility and motility of the organs and supportive structures. Findings may include oedema, temperature changes and associated musculoskeletal alterations. Careful evaluation of the body following the initial visceral diagnosis allows tender points to be identified. Over time, these have been shown to be consistently located.

Visceral dysfunctions generally present as deep multisegmental restrictions, and tender points related to these areas are often resistant to typical positional release treatment if directed towards somatic structures. Recognizing that such points may represent a manifestation of a visceral dysfunction is important, so that application of the correct viscerally oriented positional manoeuvres may be implemented.

Visceral tender points are consistently found in the same location, and often elicit a sharper response from the patient. They tend to resolve more quickly and completely than typical somatic tender points.

The case study that follows in Box 9.1 is followed by illustrated examples of the application of the counterstrain model of visceral positional release.

Bronchus

(Fig. 9.1)

These patients may have a history of reactive airway disease or recent pulmonary infection. They present with shortness of breath and reduced rib excursion; the tender

Box 9.1 **Case history: gastroesophageal reflux disease (GERD)**

A 36-year-old male presented to an outpatient ambulatory care clinic complaining of persistent mid-epigastric discomfort with a history of gastroesophageal reflux disease (GERD) diagnosed by his primary care physician 1 year ago. He also complained of a dull pain in the mid-posterior thoracic spine. He described persistent heartburn, a bitter taste in his mouth upon arising in the morning and occasional wakening in the night with coughing. His symptoms persisted, despite medication prescribed by his physician: a proton pump inhibitor (PPI) and a histamine receptor antagonist (H2 blocker), for more than 6 months. He had not had any weight loss, or bleeding from his stomach or intestines. He tried conservative measures, such as not eating after 6 pm in the evening, not drinking alcohol or caffeine or eating chocolate, all of which could lower the tone of the lower oesophageal sphincter muscle and exacerbate the GERD symptoms. He considered elevating the head of his bed next.

Physical examination

The patient's vital signs were normal. His heart and lung examinations were also normal and his abdomen was non-distended, non-obese, with active bowel sounds in all four quadrants. There was no hepatosplenomegaly or tenderness to percussion or palpation. Musculoskeletal and osteopathic structural examination was by observation and palpation: the patient sat with a forward bent posture. There was acute tenderness over the inferior surface of the anterior left sixth rib on the anterior axillary line (gastroesophageal sphincter counterstrain point), anterior inferior sternum (anterior sixth thoracic counterstrain point) and on the medial end of the seventh

rib as it attached to the sternum (left anterior seventh thoracic counterstrain point); there were also tender points on the posterior surface of the left second and third ribs (stomach counterstrain tender point) and diffuse TART (tissue texture changes, asymmetry, altered range of motion and tenderness) changes noted over the T5 through T8 left paravertebral region.

Assessment

1. Gastroesophageal reflux disease
2. Somatic dysfunction in the thoracic region, rib cage and abdomen.

Treatment plan

Osteopathic manipulative treatment using strain/counterstrain of the anterior seventh and sixth thoracic tender points reduced much of the somatic complaints. Treatment of the anterior sixth rib counterstrain point also resulted in partial treatment of the pain emanating from the oesophagus. Resolution of these secondary somatic dysfunctions (from visceral stimuli) resulted in reduced somatic pain; however, tenderness identified with specific organ structures remained.

Treatment of the organs suspected as involved with the indirect manoeuvre, described later in the text, e.g. the oesophagus, gastroesophageal sphincter and stomach, resulted in marked improvement of the patient. He noted that he was able to stand erect and his 'heartburn' was dramatically reduced. Over the next 6 weeks with intermittent treatment he had complete resolution of symptoms and was able to discontinue all medications.

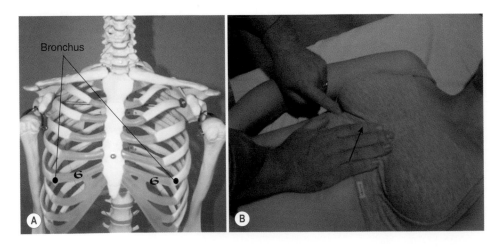

Figure 9.1
(A) Bronchus.
(B) Example of the strain/counterstrain visceral treatment technique.

point is found on the inferior aspect of the sixth rib on the anterior axillary line of the affected bronchi.

Treatment is performed by placing the patient in the supine position. Hand placement is over the lower one-third of the sternum with a gentle compression and fascial glide toward the ipsilateral shoulder compressing the pulmonary tissue in an indirect manner.

Oesophagus

(Fig. 9.2)

These patients may have a history of gastroesophageal reflux disease that is not responsive to medication. The tender points seen with these patients are typically at AT6 (on the midline at the xipho–sternal junction) and left AT7 (on the midline, or inferolateral to the tip of the xiphoid). However, they will also have a tender point over the manubriosternal junction.

Treatment of this dysfunction is accomplished with a seated patient in front of the operator in a slouched position and gentle fascial glide of the oesophagus superiorly from the left inferior aspect of the xyphoid process. This is an indirect positional release. There is also a second tender point for this distal oesophagus over the left second rib. Treatment is essentially the same, except the patient will be in a supine position as the fascial glide is performed.

Pancreas

(Fig. 9.3)

These patients may have a history of gastric upset, perhaps severe mechanical trauma. The tender point associated with this dysfunction is on the ninth rib just lateral to the medial edge of the scapula.

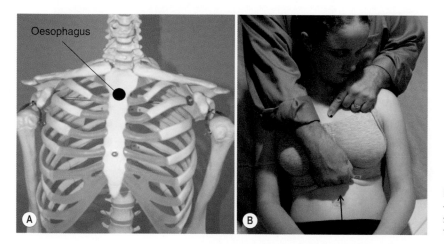

Figure 9.2 (A) Abdominal viscera – oesophagus. (B) Example of the strain/counterstrain visceral treatment technique.

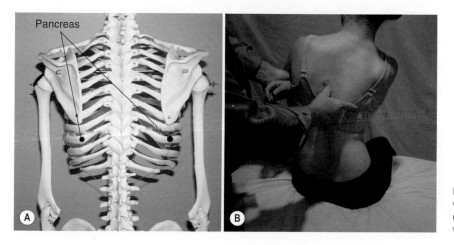

Figure 9.3 (A) Abdominal viscera – pancreas. (B) Example of the strain/counterstrain visceral treatment technique.

Treatment is performed with the patient seated; the arm on the affected side is adducted across the chest with the hand under the opposite arm. There is rotation of the upper body away from the side of the tender point and slight side-bending toward the side of the tender point. This positioning indirectly reduces tension on the posterior capsule. In a study utilizing myofascial release, soft tissue and strain/counterstrain treatment for 20 minutes/day resulted in a significant reduction in length of stay for patients with pancreatitis (Radjieski 1998).

Ureter

(Fig. 9.4)

Patients with this problem present with deep abdominal discomfort. They may have a history of renal infection, lithiasis or other urinary problem affecting the ureter. The tender point for this organ is located lateral to the PSIS, about 2 cm inferior and lateral, and it is bilateral.

Treatment for this problem is with a supine patient, lower trunk rotated away from the tender point side. The operator places an open hand over the kidney region on the ipsilateral side (superior and lateral to the umbilicus). A firm downward pressure is followed with a fascial glide in a caudad and slightly lateral direction.

Bladder

(Fig. 9.5)

These patients may have a history of recurrent sterile urinary tract problems. The tender points are often found adjacent to the low ilium sacroiliac tender point. These are over the posterior-superior aspect of the pubis.

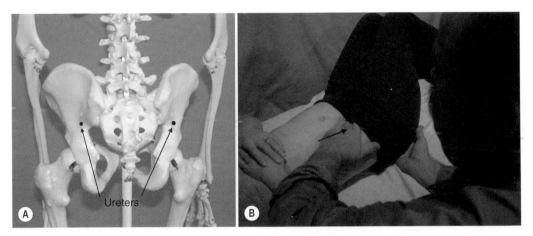

Figure 9.4 (A) Urogenital system – ureter. (B) Example of the strain/counterstrain visceral treatment technique.

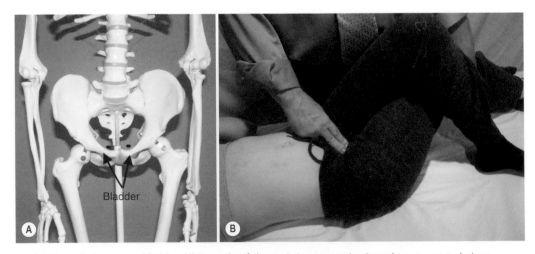

Figure 9.5 (A) Urogenital system – bladder. (B) Example of the strain/counterstrain visceral treatment technique.

The following case studies (Boxes 9.2 and 9.3) provide examples of therapeutic application of the technique in clinical practice.

They do not respond to low ilium sacroiliac treatment. This dysfunction is treated with the supine patient with the involved leg extended, with the uninvolved leg flexed and resting lateral to the knee on the involved side. The operator stands on the uninvolved side grasping the back of the involved-side knee in the popliteal fossa, lifting it gently inducing slight hip flexion and internal rotation of the involved-side leg. Adduction of the involved-side leg should be fairly marked.

THIS CHAPTER

This chapter has shown that visceral manipulation is a well-established modality in the treatment of many visceral complaints. The relationship between the body and viscera is well identified and documented. This approach utilizing the viscera-somatic relationship to identify a tender point, in the tradition of the strain-counterstrain model, becomes somewhat intuitive. Understanding the unique location of the specific tenderness developed as a result of the visceral disorder is helpful in the speed of correction and accuracy of treatment. Many of the manoeuvres are well known to practitioners of visceral manipulation. An understanding of the relationship between these separate manifestations will lead to more accurate and effective treatment, as well as a fuller understanding of the symptoms presented by the patient.

NEXT CHAPTER

The next chapter, by Anthony J. Lisi, DC, offers an overview as well as detailed protocols for assessment and rehabilitation as used in the McKenzie method.

REFERENCES

Baily, M., Dick, L., 1992. Nociceptive considerations in treating with counterstrain. Journal of the American Osteopathic Association 92, 334–341.

Barber, E., 1898. Osteopathy Complete. Hudson-Kimberly, Kansas City, MO.

Barral, J., 1989. Visceral Manipulation II. Eastland Press, Vista, CA.

Barral, J., 1991. The Thorax. Eastland Press, Vista, CA.

Barral, J., 1993. Urogenital Manipulation. Eastland Press, Vista, CA.

Barral, J., 1996. Manual Thermal Diagnosis. Eastland Press, Vista, CA.

Barral, J., Mercier, P., 1988. Viscera Manipulation. Eastland Press, Vista, CA.

Barral, J.P., 1995. Visceral Manipulation. Eastland Press, Vista, CA.

Barral, J.P., Croibier, A., 1999. Trauma: An Osteopathic Approach. Eastland Press, Vista, CA.

Bensky, D., 1995. Asthma treated by visceral manipulation. American Academy of Osteopathy Journal 5, 11–17.

Blackman, E., 2001. Posterior Midline. Port Richmond, CA.

Davidson, S.M., 1992. Vitalize the Viscera. Seminar, Phoenix, AZ, 12 January.

Finet, G., Willame, C., 2000. Treating Visceral Dysfunction. Stillness Press, Portland, OR.

Gaddis, C.J., 1922. Bedside technique. Journal of the American Osteopathic Association 21, 691.

Gashev, A., 2002. Physiologic aspects of lymphatic contractile function: current perspectives. Annals of the New York Academy of Sciences 979, 178–187.

Gebhart, G.F., Bielefeldt, K., 2008. Visceral pain. In: Bushnell, M.C., Basbaum, A.I. (Eds.), The Senses: A Comprehensive Reference. Academic Press, San Diego, CA, pp. 543–570. Online. Available: <http://rfi.fmrp.usp.br/pg/fisio/cursao2012/viscelpainp1.pdf>.

Goetz, E., 1909. A Manual of Osteopathy (with the

Application of Physical Culture, Baths and Diet), second ed. Nature's Cure Company, Cincinnati, OH.

Hazzard, C., 1905. The Practice and Applied Therapeutics of Osteopathy. Journal Printing Press, Kirksville, MO.

Hoover, H.V., 1947. Liver and Gall Bladder Technique. American Academy of Osteopathy Yearbook, Indianapolis, IN.

Hoover, H.V., 1948. A Consideration of an Osteopathic Lesion of the Whole Liver and Its Effects on Hepatic Dysfunction. American Academy of Osteopathy Yearbook, Indianapolis, IN.

Hoover, H.V., 1950. Technique for Removing Still Lesion Usually Found in Gall Bladder Disease. American Academy of Osteopathy Yearbook, Indianapolis, IN.

Huang, X., Xu, W.X., 2010. The pacemaker functions of visceral interstitial cells of Cajal. Acta Physiologica Sinica 62, 387–397.

Jones, L.H., Kusunose, R.S., Goering, E.K., 1995. Jones Strain-CounterStrain. Jones Strain Counterstrain Inc., Carlsbad, CA.

Lossing, K.J., 1997. An Osteopathic Approach to Gastroesophageal Reflux Disease. Residency Thesis, Ohio University, Athens, OH.

McDonnell, C.P., 1994. Selected Writings of Carl Philip McConnell, DO. Squirrel's Tail Press, Columbus, OH.

Murray, C., 1925. Practice of Osteopathy: Its Practical Application to the Various Diseases of the Human Body, sixth ed. Charles Henry Murray, Elgin, IL.

Procacci, P., Maresca, M., 1999. Referred pain from somatic and visceral structures. Current Review of Pain 3, 96–99.

Radjieski, J.M., Lumley, M.A., Cantieri, M.S., 1998. Effect of osteopathic manipulative treatment of length of stay for pancreatitis: a randomized pilot study. Journal of the American Osteopathic Association 98, 264–272.

Ribera, J., Paula, M., Melgar-Lesmes, P., et al., 2013. Increased nitric oxide production in lymphatic endothelial cells causes impairment of lymphatic drainage in cirrhotic rats. Gut 62, 138–145.

Riggs, W.L., 1901. A Manual of Osteopathic Manipulations and Treatment. New Science, Elkhart, IN.

Smith, R.K., 1912. Mechanical principles of the human body. Journal of the American Osteopathic Association 12, 210.

Still, A.T., 1911. Research and Practice of Osteopathy. Andrew Taylor Still, Kirksville, MO.

Sutherland, W.G., 1990. Teachings in the Science of Osteopathy. Rudra Press, Portland, OR.

Teal, C.C., 1922. Palpation of the colon with special reference to the cecum. Journal of the American Osteopathic Association 21, 492.

Tozzi, P., Bongiorno, D., Vitturini, C., 2012. Low back pain and kidney mobility: local osteopathic fascial manipulation decreases pain perception and improves renal mobility. Journal of Bodywork and Movement Therapies 16, 381–391.

Woodall, P.H., 1926. Intra-Pelvic Technic; or, Manipulative Surgery of the Pelvic Organs. Williams, Kansas City, MO.

Young, M.D., 1947. Head's Law and Its Relation to the Treatment of the Viscera. Year book. Academy of Applied Osteopathy, pp. 65–69.

Overview of the McKenzie method

Anthony J. Lisi

INTRODUCTION

Clinicians, who use manual means to treat musculoskeletal conditions, face the stark realization that many of our diagnostic and therapeutic methods are not supported by significant external evidence. Much of what is used in the field is an extension of one's clinical training, where the methods of one's mentors become the basis for ongoing practice. This is likely expanded by personal experience and collegial interaction. These manners of knowledge derivation are *integration* processes. Although useful in themselves, such processes require the parallel track of *synthesis* processes - systematic collection of data through clinical science and outcomes research (controlled clinical trials, systematic reviews, etc.). Indeed, the combination of both types of processes in the approach to clinical practice – termed *syntegration* – has been described as a more complete knowledge-based approach to patient care than either one alone (Errico 2005).

Although there are no shortage of manual practice approaches based on integration processes (such as mentoring and personal experience), there are few methods that are supported by data from synthesis processes. One notable exception is mechanical diagnosis and therapy of the spine, also known as the McKenzie method (1981). The McKenzie approach allows the clinician the rare opportunity to take methods supported by reasonable published data and integrate them with clinical experience, to improve patient care.

The McKenzie method is often incorrectly equated with spinal extension exercises alone. While these and other exercises are important components of the technique, McKenzie is more correctly understood as a system of diagnosis and treatment based upon predictable responses to mechanical examination. The diagnostic element of McKenzie is often overlooked by those who are not familiar with the system.

Perhaps the most defining element of the McKenzie diagnostic approach is the central role it gives to patient response. As a patient is put through a series of positions and repetitive movements, reactions are assessed. Does the range of motion increase or decrease? Does pain intensity rise or fall? Does the location of the pain change? These findings are considered more important than any palpatory assessment. Actually, in many cases, a successful McKenzie examination can be performed without the provider ever touching the patient!

At first, this approach may seem incongruous to the manual practitioner; and, indeed, those manual providers who would say, 'Palpation is all' may never reconcile with those McKenzie practitioners who would say, 'Palpation is anathema'. However, clinicians who are comfortable navigating the vast waters between these extreme positions can find a blend of approaches that works best for the particular patient's benefit.

This chapter provides an overview of the McKenzie method. It is aimed at introducing clinicians unfamiliar with this system to the principles and approaches used therein. After reading this chapter, providers should be able to incorporate elements of mechanical diagnosis and therapy into their clinical approach. For further education, the reader is directed to McKenzie's texts and to the McKenzie Institute (www.mckenziemdt.org).

EXAMINATION

The heart of the McKenzie assessment procedure is the mechanical examination (McKenzie 1981; Taylor 1996). While the full assessment also includes patient history and postural analysis, this chapter focusses exclusively on the mechanical examination. Furthermore, appropriate diagnosis of a patient with neck or back pain also requires a thorough physical examination, including orthopaedic and neurological assessment, and analysis of imaging, laboratory and/or other tests when indicated (Chou et al. 2007; Nordin et al. 2008). In a given patient, mechanical examination may not be indicated or may be contraindicated. Therefore, depending upon the reader's clinical training and licensure, before relying on mechanical examination he/she must first reach an appropriate diagnosis of mechanical neck or back pain, or ensure that the patient has been diagnosed by a suitable colleague.

This chapter presents information on mechanical assessment of the lumbar and cervical spine. The McKenzie methods have also been applied to management of extremity conditions, however that is beyond the scope of this text. Indeed the vast majority of published evidence supporting the use of McKenzie principles relates to the lumbar spine.

The mechanical examination is an assessment of the patient's response to end-range loading (the application of forces). The load can be applied singularly and sustained, or repetitively. This method is different from many other forms of musculoskeletal examination because it is patient-driven. That is, the patient performs much of the examination (via active range of motion) and the patient's responses to the examination manoeuvres are considered more important than what the provider may sense via palpation. During the course of the examination, the patient learns which positions and movements are beneficial, and which are harmful; thus the entire process interweaves patient education and active care. McKenzie advocates making the patient as independent as possible – to minimize the chances of becoming reliant on the provider – and this process begins during the examination.

Lumbar spine

The mechanical examination process of the lumbar spine is outlined in Box 10.1 and Figures 10.1–10.13.

Box 10.1   **Lumbar spine mechanical examination**

Static (sustained posture at end-range)
- Sitting slouched, sitting erect
- Standing slouched, standing erect
- Lying prone in extension, lying supine in flexion

Dynamic (repetitive end-range movements)
- Active:
  - Flexion standing, extension standing
  - Flexion supine (knee to chest); extension prone (prone press-up)
  - Side-gliding, right or left, standing or prone.
- Passive:
  - Mobilization (grades 3–4) in flexion, extension, right or left rotation.

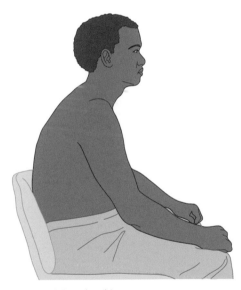

Figure 10.1 Sitting slouching.

At first the patient is instructed to assume a series of static sustained postures at end-range. The significance of the patient's response to these positions is discussed below; however, at this point, it is noteworthy to consider that each position attempts to elicit a change in patient symptomatology by varying the spinal configuration through a range of flexion to extension. This includes sitting slouched (Fig. 10.1), sitting erect (Fig. 10.2), standing slouched (Fig. 10.3) and standing erect (Fig. 10.4).

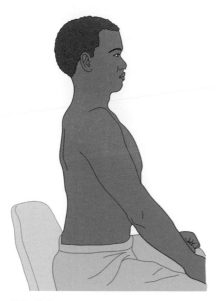

Figure 10.2 Sitting erect.

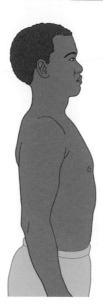

Figure 10.4 Standing erect.

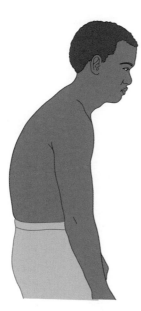

Figure 10.3 Standing slouched.

Note that the slouched positions put the lumbar spine in a position of relative flexion, while the erect postures introduce relative extension to the spine. Next, the patient will lie supine and then prone, so introducing relative flexion and extension, respectively. To increase extension the patient may lie propped up on the forearms (Fig. 10.5). To increase the amount of flexion, the patient may bring the knees to the chest (Fig. 10.6). If a patient's response (as explained below), is demonstrated at any point during the examination it is not necessary to further increase the given amount of flexion or extension. For instance, if symptoms change during supine lying, knees to chest would not be added.

The dynamic portion of the examination is the assessment of the effects of repetitive end-range movements. This includes both active and passive motions. The active movements are standing flexion (Fig. 10.7), standing extension (Fig. 10.8), prone extension (prone press-ups, as in Fig. 10.5) and supine flexion (knees to chest, as in Fig. 10.6). The patient is instructed to perform each of these movements up to 10 times in sequence, with the response assessed after each series of repetitions.

Note that up to this point, the entire mechanical examination can be performed without touching the patient, or with only minimal contact to guide the patient through the positions and movements. If the appropriate patient response has occurred (as explained below), the examination is complete. However, if a patient does not exhibit the desired clinical change, further assessment is needed, and the examiner moves on to passive dynamic movements, which are essentially grade 3–4 mobilizations. These are performed supine in flexion (Fig. 10.10), prone in extension (Fig. 10.11) and side-lying in rotation to the right and left (Fig. 10.13).

One variable not discussed above is side-gliding (Fig. 10.9) – or horizontal (x-axis) trunk translation. In the McKenzie system, a patient who initially presents with an antalgic list is also assessed for the response to side-gliding, both standing and prone, active and passive (Fig. 10.12). This assessment is typically reserved only for those patients with an initial tendency to list, with the transition movement performed in the direction that would neutralize the list.

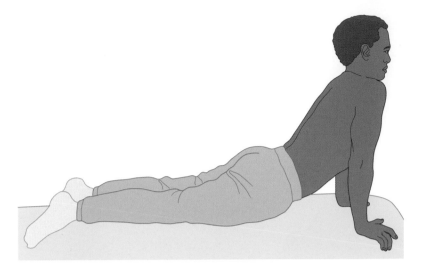

Figure 10.5 Lying prone in extension (press-ups).

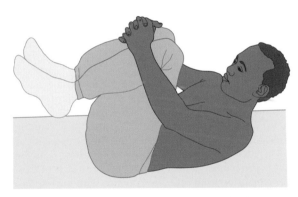

Figure 10.6 Lying supine in flexion (knees to chest).

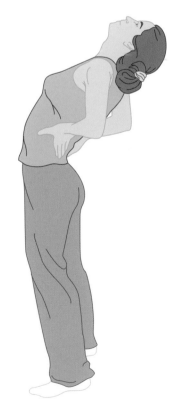

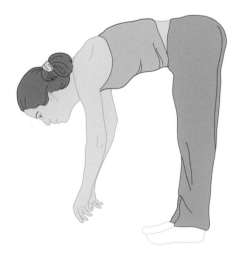

Figure 10.7 Standing in flexion.

Figure 10.8 Standing in extension.

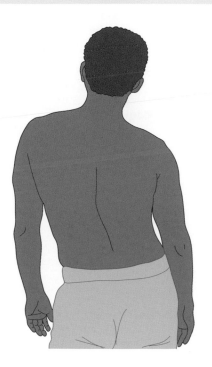

Figure 10.9 Side-gliding.

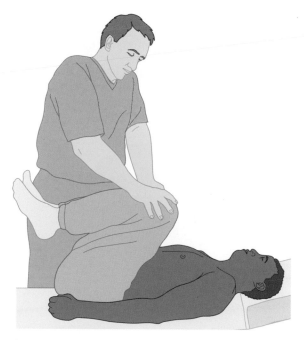

Figure 10.10 Supine flexion.

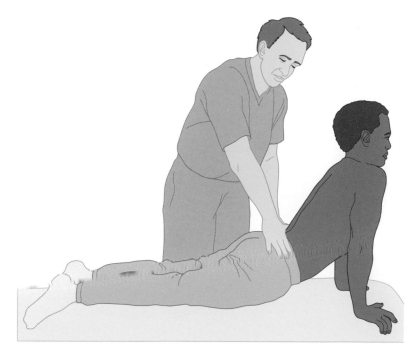

Figure 10.11 Prone extension.

Cervical spine

The mechanical examination process of the cervical spine is outlined in Box 10.2 and Figures 10.14–10.22. As with the lumbar spine, the examination proceeds first through a series of patient static sustained end-range postures, then repetitive active end-range motions, and finally, if needed, repetitive passive end-range motions (i.e. examiner manual assessment). The cervical spine examination has been subject to perhaps more revision than the lumbar spine examination, and consequently, greater variation seems to exist between seasoned McKenzie practitioners regarding the sequence and relevance of examination manoeuvres. As a baseline introduction for the novice, generally the

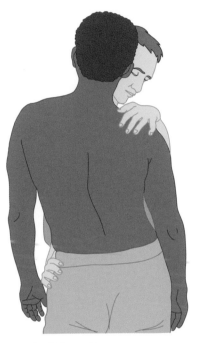

Figure 10.12 Side-gliding, with overpressure.

> Box 10.2   **Cervical spine mechanical examination**
>
> ### Static (sustained posture at end-range)
>
> - Protrusion, retraction
> - Flexion, retraction + extension
> - Retraction + left lateral flexion, retraction + right lateral flexion
> - Retraction + left rotation, retraction + right rotation
>
> ### Dynamic (repetitive end-range movements)
>
> - Active:
>   - Protrusion
>   - Retraction
>   - Retraction + extension
>   - Flexion
>   - Lateral flexion
>   - Rotation.
> - Passive:
>   - Mobilization (grades 3–4) in retraction plus either extension, right/left rotation or right/left lateral flexion.

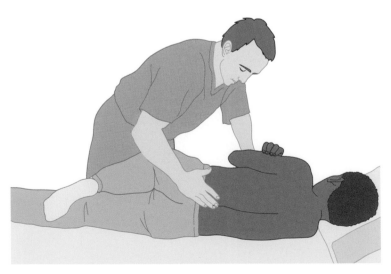

Figure 10.13 Side-lying rotation.

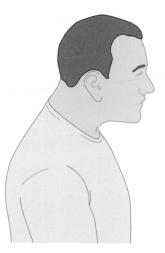

Figure 10.14 Protrusion.

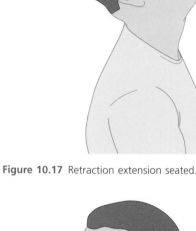

Figure 10.17 Retraction extension seated.

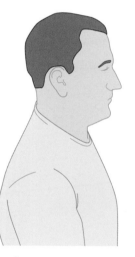

Figure 10.15 Retraction.

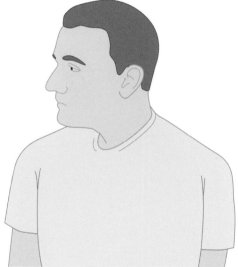

Figure 10.18 Right rotation.

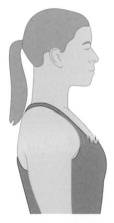 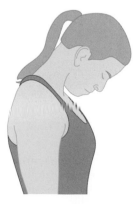

Figure 10.16 Flexion.

sagittal plane motions – protrusion, retraction, flexion and retraction plus extension – are performed first and have the greater weight (Figs 10.14–10.17). Rotation and/or lateral flexion movements (Figs 10.18–10.21) are typically reserved for cases in which the sagittal plan assessment has not revealed significant findings.

The examiner should consider the complex spinal mechanics associated with key examination movements. First, protrusion places the upper cervical region at the end-range of extension, while the lower cervical region is at the mid-range of flexion. Retraction places the upper cervical region at the end-range of flexion while the lower cervical region is at the mid-range of extension. Finally retraction plus extension places the upper cervical region

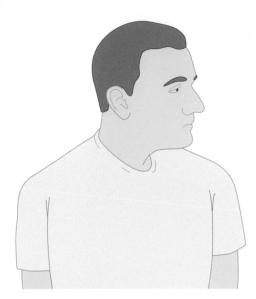

Figure 10.19 Left rotation.

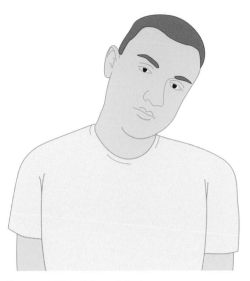

Figure 10.21 Left lateral flexion.

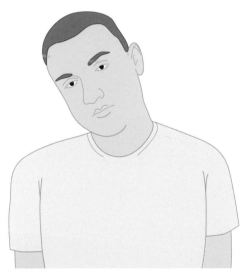

Figure 10.20 Right lateral flexion.

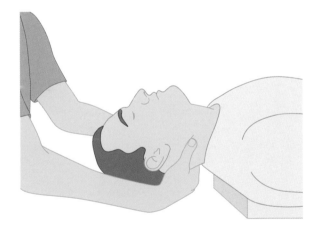

Figure 10.22 Retraction extension mobilization.

at the end-range of extension and the lower cervical region also at the end-range of extension. Analysis of findings associated with these movement tests can lead to treatment strategies targeting the involved regions.

Assessment of retraction, and/or retraction plus extension, is often performed with the patient supine and his/her head placed beyond the edge of the treatment table. This may be difficult for patients to achieve on their own, and is often guided by minimal hand contact of the examiner, which can be increased to full passive mobilization if needed (Fig. 10.22). This position can place certain patients at risk of injury and therefore must be employed with appropriate case selection. Relative contraindications can include cervical spinal stenosis, cervical instability, previous cervical spine surgery, cerebrovascular insufficiency, vertigo and general patient intolerance. However, with appropriate discretion, these manoeuvres can be performed safely and can yield important clinical information.

EXAMINATION FINDINGS

Whether evaluating the lumbar or cervical regions, while proceeding through the above mechanical examination, the clinician assesses the patient's response in terms of two main variables: range of motion and pain.

First, has the range of motion in any given direction increased, decreased or remained stable?

In this context, an improvement in antalgia is considered an increase in range of motion, such that the patient with an initial left list (shoulders left relative to the pelvis) who stands straighter after a manoeuvre is said to have gained right lateral flexion.

On the other hand, a patient who initially could flex the trunk forward 45° and after several repetitions of flexion can subsequently only flex 25°, clearly has a decrease in range of motion. As might be expected, an increase in range of motion that was initially restricted is considered a desirable finding; a decrease in range is undesirable.

Next, has the patient's pain complaint changed?

Pain is monitored in terms of intensity and location. The intensity of pain, simply, can increase, decrease or remain unchanged.

The location or distribution of pain may change independent of pain intensity. Thus, the pain may spread away from the lumbar region into the buttock, thigh and leg, becoming more distal in its distribution.

Alternatively, lower extremity pain may decrease or disappear, leaving a smaller distribution of lumbar pain only.

The former example, where pain moves distally, is called 'peripheralization'; the latter, where pain shrinks to a more proximal location, is called 'centralization' (Fig. 10.23). These terms are of great importance in the McKenzie system and will now be discussed in more detail.

Since McKenzie's original description, other authors have applied somewhat varied definitions to centralization, with the key concept remaining the abolition of distal pain in response to positions or repeated movements (Aina et al. 2004). Some studies have defined centralization as occurring as long as distal pain is eliminated during the course of treatment over days or weeks; whereas others require distal symptoms to be abolished during the examination. There has been some disagreement as to whether the distal pain must be abolished entirely or simply decreased. Apart from pain, reduction of distal paraesthesia has also been called centralization. These prior differences notwithstanding, it is important to clarify the following defining points. After the patient has assumed a particular position or performed a given repeated movement, centralization is said to have occurred in the following circumstances:

- The most distal symptoms (pain or paraesthesia) are eliminated or substantially decreased.
- If the patient presents with local low back pain only, that pain is eliminated.
- The change in distal pain is the defining element, and is often independent of proximal pain. That is, if a patient with low back pain and leg pain experiences relief of leg pain, yet an increase of low back pain, that patient is still said to have centralized. The converse of this is also true: the patient with relief of low back pain and an increase in leg pain has peripheralized.

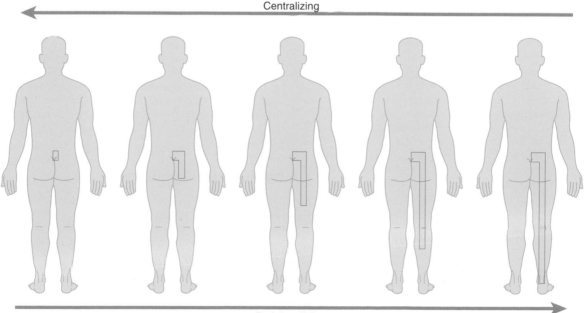

Figure 10.23 Representation of centralization and peripheralization. Moving from left to right depicts peripheralization; from right to left centralization.

- The reduction in symptoms is of some duration – seconds to minutes, perhaps hours in excellent responders. There must be some plasticity to the change. (This also applies to peripheralization; in contrast, for example to the palpation of a latent myofascial trigger point, which may cause distal pain while pressure is applied, but results in elimination of distal pain essentially instantly when pressure is removed. If a patient has peripheralized, the distal pain will linger for some time after the posture or repeated movements have ceased.)

As will be seen, achieving centralization is considered advantageous to the patient, and achieving peripheralization is considered disadvantageous (Donelson et al. 1991). For this reason, if centralization begins to occur during the course of a particular movement examination, that movement is continued. If peripheralization begins to occur, that movement is ceased. As an example, consider a patient with low back pain radiating to the right buttock. If after four repetitions of standing extension, the buttock pain has resolved and the back pain has decreased, additional repetitions of extension would be continued to see if the back pain would decrease further. However, if the back and buttock pain remained, and pain began to be felt in the posterior thigh also, extension would be halted and the examination would continue through the other motions.

THE SYNDROMES

McKenzie has classified mechanical low back and neck pain into three syndromes: postural, dysfunction and derangement. Each syndrome is defined by a theoretical model of the underlying pathology, plus patient history, postural assessment and mechanical examination findings (Table 10.1). The validity of the theoretical models remains largely undemonstrated, but as McKenzie has stated, the observed clinical phenomena in response to mechanical assessment are important, regardless of the proposed mechanisms, for these phenomena provide guidance for conservative management that has been shown to improve clinical outcome. In order to achieve that outcome, the McKenzie approach outlines treatment implications or strategies for each syndrome. These include strategies for educating patients on proper posture/ergonomics, patient self-care exercises and manual therapy.

Postural syndrome

The postural syndrome includes patients who are experiencing pain simply due to poor posture. The presumed pathology here is that there is no pathology: this is normal tissue being brought to pain by prolonged loading, for which it is not suited. Consider an index finger supporting a load while in a position of flexion. Normal joints, ligaments, capsules and muscles are able to resist this load without discomfort. Now consider that same load being applied with the finger in a position of hyperextension. That same normal anatomy will now be subjected to loading that is biomechanically disadvantageous, and discomfort will result.

During examination, postural syndrome patients will have a full range of motion. Repetitive end-range motions do not typically bring on or worsen their pain. This pain is intermittent and only initiated by prolonged (inappropriate) postural overload; thus the patient may be asymptomatic during the examination. The examination procedure likely to be positive is the sustained static posture. Some patients may experience the onset of pain when in a given position for under a minute, while others may take several minutes or more. The practicality of such a prolonged examination varies from one clinical setting to another; however, history findings will guide the examiner to the most likely culpable postures. For instance, the young computer programmer who experiences low back pain after working for many hours will most likely be found to be positive in prolonged seated flexion, rather than prone extension.

Treatment implications for the postural syndrome patient are straightforward – instruct the patient to avoid the problematic posture that is causing pain. Here, it is argued that this advice is the most important intervention and perhaps the only intervention a patient really needs. Giving the patient appropriate education on body mechanics and exercise aimed at strengthening supporting muscles empowers the individual to care for himself.

If the patient truly has full and painless range of motion, it is argued that manual treatment aimed at joints and or myofascial structures is unnecessary and may inappropriately contribute to patient dependence on the provider. To be sure, the patient without any articular or myofascial restriction may be very rare in given clinical populations. Nevertheless, if such a patient is encountered, it is likely that appropriate education and activation will be of greatest value.

Dysfunction syndrome

The dysfunction syndrome patient is characterized by chronic soft-tissue contracture or fibrosis. This may be facet joint capsular fibrosis, nerve root adhesions, etc. Such situations may arise in response to a major trauma or to cumulative microtrauma.

Upon examination, these patients will demonstrate a restriction in range of motion in one or more directions. Pain will be elicited at the inappropriately premature end-range. However, this pain will diminish essentially instantly when the patient returns to neutral. During the course of a repetitive motion examination, there may be a gradual increase in the restricted range of motion, as the

Table 10.1 A brief summary of the McKenzie syndromes

Syndrome	Mechanical examination findings	Pathology model	Treatment strategies
Postural	AROM is full and pain-free Repetitive motions are pain-free Sustained posture at normal end-range causes pain	Normal tissue being strained by prolonged inappropriate posture	Avoid painful positions; maintain correct posture
Dysfunction	AROM is restricted in one or more directions with local pain at end-range Repetitive motions are painful at end-range, but may increase range of motion	Chronic soft-tissue contracture or fibrosis (facet capsular fibrosis, nerve root adhesions)	Repetitive motions that increase pain are indicated to break adhesions and increase elasticity This applies to: Patient exercises Patient posture/ergonomics Manual treatment
Derangement	AROM is restricted in one or more directions; painful at end-range Repetitive motion reveals centralization (± peripheralization)	Discogenic pain with competent annulus (contained annular tear, internal disc disruption or herniated disc)	Motions that centralize are indicated Motions that peripheralize are contraindicated This applies to: Patient exercises Patient posture/ergonomics Manual treatment
	AROM is restricted in one or more directions; painful at end-range Repetitive motion reveals peripheralization only (no centralization)	Discogenic pain with incompetent annulus (non-contained annular tear, internal disc disruption or herniated disc)	Avoid peripheralization Often poor prognosis; often poor response to conservative treatment

AROM, active range of motion.

shortened soft tissue is repeatedly brought to tension. This can be thought of as the spinal analogue to the clinical presentation of chronic hamstring tightness. An initial simple stretch of hip flexion is painful. Removing the stretch relieves the pain. Repeating the stretch is painful, yet again; however, doing so, may start to increase the hip flexion range of motion.

In contrast to the postural syndrome, the therapeutic approach to the dysfunction syndrome patient is to strive for repeated motions that *increase* pain. It is postulated that these motions are required in order to break inappropriate adhesions and increase overall elasticity. These motions are indicated for patient home exercise as well as clinician manual therapy.

The point of clarification is that McKenzie stresses patient self-reliance as the primary goal of treatment. Thus, it would be preferred to have the patient perform the exercises alone if he can achieve the proper response. If the patient is unable to reach any lasting decrease in pain and increase in range of motion by exercise alone, only then would the clinician add manual therapeutic means (in accordance with pain reproduction). Furthermore, the clinician would keep these interventions to a minimum, with the intention of simply assisting the patient to become independent as quickly as possible.

Most contemporaries in spine care would certainly agree on the importance of patient independence and active care; however, the suggestion that *any* amount of passive care leads to patient dependence on the provider has not been demonstrated. Thus, the McKenzie stipulation that *all* passive care be omitted in patients who demonstrate success with self-care can be viewed as a guiding suggestion, rather than an admonition. Consequently, the clinician can find rich opportunity to blend manual therapies with repeated motion exercises that both attempt to stretch inappropriately shortened tissue, and educate the patient on the importance of self-sufficiency in the process.

Derangement syndrome

The portion of the McKenzie methods supported by the most significant evidence is the approach to the derangement syndrome patient. In short, derangement refers to lumbar intervertebral disc pathology. McKenzie originally described seven subcategories of derangement. However, in the 2003 revision of his text (McKenzie & May 2003) these have been collapsed into three subcategories. For the purposes of this chapter we will consider derangement to be divided into two subcategories only, corresponding with the relevant supporting evidence.

Lumbar intervertebral disc pathology includes both pathoanatomy (morphometric changes) and pathophysiology (changes in function, namely nociception). The pathoanatomy includes a wide spectrum of structural changes visible on advanced imaging: internal disc disruption, disc bulges and focal herniated discs, with or without nerve root compromise. In each of these cases, a distinction can be made between situations in which the outer annulus is fully intact, and those in which it is breached in one or multiple places. The former is called 'contained' pathology, where the outer annulus contains any distortion present; the latter is 'non-contained' pathology, where the hydrostatic mechanism of the disc is compromised (Fardon & Milette 2001).

As has been shown numerous times, the mere presence of disc pathology as seen on imaging does not correlate with symptoms (Boden et al. 1990; Boos et al. 1995). However, a very interesting relationship has been shown to exist regarding symptomatic, i.e. painful, lumbar discs. It has been demonstrated that patients with low back pain who exhibit centralization upon McKenzie examination are very likely to display a painful lumbar disc(s) with contained pathology, as evidenced by provocative discography (Donelson et al. 1997; Laslett et al. 2005). Conversely, those patients who exhibit peripheralization without centralization are very likely to display a painful lumbar disc(s) with non-contained pathology as evidenced by provocative discography. In other words, the presence of centralization and/or peripheralization upon mechanical examination is highly correlated with painful lumbar discs upon discography. Moreover, patients who centralize (whether or not they peripheralize also) are likely to demonstrate contained pathology, whereas those who peripheralize only (and do not centralize) are likely to demonstrate non-contained pathology.

During mechanical examination, derangement syndrome patients will display restriction in active range of motion in one or more directions. Pain will be produced at the premature end-range and perhaps during the range of motion prior to that point (this is in contrast to the pain of the dysfunction syndrome, which is only elicited at the restricted end-range). Repetitive motion examination will reveal centralization and/or peripheralization. When centralization occurs, it is typically in response to one given direction of motion only; the opposing direction very commonly, but not always, will cause peripheralization. The motion that results in centralization is called that patient's *directional preference*. In the lumbar spine, extension has been shown to be the most common directional preference (Donelson et al. 1991).

A number of studies have examined the frequency with which centralization occurs in patient populations. In one retrospective study, it was seen that 76 of 87 patients (87%) experienced centralization of symptoms in response to repeated end-range movements in a single direction (Donelson et al. 1990). In each case, movement in the opposite direction always exacerbated distal symptoms.

A prospective study examining only sagittal motions in 145 patients with low back pain, with or without lower extremity pain, demonstrated a frequency of 47% (Donelson et al. 1991). In a prospective descriptive analysis of the centralization phenomenon in 289 patients with low back pain or neck pain, with or without extremity symptoms, 30.8% of subjects were classified as centralizers, 23.2% as non-centralizers and 46% as partial reduction (Werneke et al. 1999). A systematic review of 62 previously published studies reported that in back and neck pain patients, the prevalence of centralization was 44.4% overall, and 74% in acute pain patients, whereas the prevalence of directional preference was 70% overall (May & Aina 2012). This review suggested that although more data are needed, currently the findings of centralization or directional preference appear to have utility in establishing treatment approaches and prognosis. A more recent study of 304 subjects found that centralization and directional preference are both associated with functional improvement in patients with neck pain (Edmond et al. 2014). Interestingly, this work provided more evidence that centralization and directional preference are individual diagnostic entities, each occurring in somewhat different patient subpopulations – centralization more likely in younger subjects and those with fewer comorbidities, and directional preference more likely in patients with acute pain.

Good reliability (kappa = 0.823; percentage agreement of 89.7%) has been shown among 40 physical therapists in deciding whether centralization, peripheralization or neither, had occurred (Fritz et al. 2000).

Another study also demonstrated good reliability between two physical therapists for classifying patients into McKenzie syndromes (kappa = 0.70; percentage agreement of 93%) (Razmjou et al. 2000). In this work, when centralization or peripheralization occurred, the reliability increased to excellent (kappa = 0.96; percentage agreement of 97%).

Other work has shown that patients who centralize achieve superior clinical outcomes compared with those who do not. Long (1995) investigated 223 subjects with chronic low back pain with or without lower extremity pain and found that the centralizer group had a significantly greater decrease in maximum pain intensity scores on the NRS-101 Pain Scale and a significantly higher return-to-work status. Improved return-to-work rates were also seen among centralizers in a study of 126 consecutive patients with low back pain, with or without leg pain

(Karas et al. 1997). The centralizers among 289 patients with low back or neck pain experienced a greater reduction in pain intensity on an 11-point pain scale, and increase in function as measured by the Oswestry Questionnaire or Neck Disability Index (Werneke et al. 1999).

For those patients who can be made to centralize, treatment is always aimed at achieving centralization and avoiding peripheralization. Thus, exercises, ergonomics and manual therapies are employed following the patient's directional preference. For instance, a patient who centralized upon repeated extension will be given extension exercise, advised to maintain lordotic postures and receive manual treatment favouring extension. As in the dysfunction syndrome, the McKenzie approach advocates refraining from passive treatment in cases where patients can achieve positive changes – in this instance centralization – by performing active exercises (Box 10.3).

Those patients who peripheralize only, and do not centralize upon any movement, present the clinician with a more challenging situation. In the absence of a clear directional preference, there is not one particular motion for which to strive. Avoiding peripheralization does remain a guiding principle for exercise, body mechanics and in-office care; however, this alone is not as valuable as having a particular direction/posture that results in positive change. In fact, it has been shown that these patients often have a poor response to conservative treatment, and may be more likely to require surgical intervention (Donelson et al. 1997).

Any discussion of managing patients with mechanical neck or low back pain would be remiss without considering the role that non-mechanical factors may have on a given patient's clinical presentation. Contemporary concepts describe a biopsychosocial model of the complex interaction between biological, psychological and social or cultural factors that influence physical health or illness (Suls et al. 2013). This is especially relevant to patients with spinal pain complaints, where pain-related fear has been shown to be positively associated with disability (Zale et al. 2013). In relation to the McKenzie assessment in particular, evidence suggests that mental (OR 1.16; 95% confidence interval (CI) 1.03–1.30) and depressive symptoms (OR 1.23; 95% CI 1.01–1.51) are associated with non-centralizers more so than centralizers (Christiansen et al. 2009). Thus, all clinicians treating patients with back or neck pain must account for and address the potential contribution of psychosocial factors.

In summary, remembering the following key points may be particularly helpful to the clinician. Centralization occurs with a frequency of 30.8–87%, and good to excellent inter-examiner reliability regarding assessment of centralization has been demonstrated.

A single preferred direction of motion typically results in centralization. When present, centralization and/or peripheralization indicate painful intervertebral disc pathology.

Box 10.3 General note on manual therapy

The McKenzie method emphasizes the primary importance of patient education and self-care. The technique includes a focussed role for manual therapy in the context of achieving desired mechanical outcomes.

As has been described in the text, centralization of symptoms and/or increase in restricted range of motion are advantageous for a patient. The goal of the McKenzie approach is to identify positions/movements that produce the advantageous results (diagnosis), and then apply these positions/movements to reach a positive outcome (treatment). Manual therapy is included in both diagnosis and treatment. However, in each case it is employed only as a second tier option for situations where active methods did not achieve the desired result.

In the McKenzie system, the mechanical methods can be thought of as existing on a continuum from active to passive means, as shown below.

ACTIVE ————————————————▶ PASSIVE

| Posture | Repeated active motions | Repeated active motions with clinician overpressure | Articular mobilization (grades 3–4) | Manipulation (grade 5) |

The guiding principle is to utilize active methods first, moving sequentially further to the right on the spectrum only when the preceding method has failed. In some patients, successful diagnosis and outcome can be obtained with active methods from the start. Other cases will initially require the use of mobilization or manipulation in order to achieve centralization and/or increased range of motion. Yet, during the course of care, the intent is to use less of the passive and more of the active methods as quickly as possible, while still maintaining positive outcome.

The manual therapies described within the McKenzie method are joint mobilization and manipulation, with the latter considered more aggressive than the former. However, the eclectic clinician may blend other forms of soft-tissue therapies into this approach. Since the principles of centralization and peripheralization in particular are supported by significant evidence for those patients who demonstrate either, it would behove the clinician to strive for centralization and avoid peripheralization during the application of any myofascial release technique.

Pain that centralizes probably arises from a disc with a competent annulus; pain that peripheralizes but does not centralize, probably arises from a disc with an incompetent annulus. For patients with intervertebral disc pathology, those whose symptoms can be made to centralize have a better prognosis for response to conservative care than those whose symptoms cannot.

THIS CHAPTER

This chapter has presented an overview of an evidence-based approach to mechanical diagnosis and treatment called the McKenzie method. This method includes an assessment of a patient's response to mechanical positioning in order to reach a diagnosis and identify a treatment strategy. The discussion focussed on three diagnostic categories: postural syndrome, dysfunction syndrome and derangement syndrome, of both the lumbar and cervical regions. This chapter covered the application of these principles to manual therapy treatment planning.

NEXT CHAPTER

The next chapter, by Dylan Morrissey PT, PhD, contains details of the use of 'unloading'/kinesio-taping as a form of positional release.

REFERENCES

Aina, A., May, S., Clare, H., 2004. The centralization phenomenon of spinal symptoms – a systematic review. Manual Therapy 9, 134–143.

Boden, S.D., Davis, D.O., Dina, T.S., et al., 1990. Abnormal magnetic-resonance scans of the lumbar spine in asymptomatic subjects. A prospective investigation. The Journal of Bone and Joint Surgery. American Volume 72, 403–408.

Boos, N., Rieder, R., Schade, V., et al., 1995. Volvo Award in Clinical Sciences. The diagnostic accuracy of magnetic resonance imaging, work perception and psychosocial factors in identifying symptomatic disc herniations. Spine 20, 2613–2625.

Chou, R., Qaseem, A., Snow, V., et al.; Clinical Efficacy Assessment Subcommittee of the American College of Physicians; American College of Physicians; American Pain Society Low Back Pain Guidelines Panel. 2007. Diagnosis and treatment of low back pain: a joint clinical practice guideline from the American College of Physicians and the American Pain Society. Annals of Internal Medicine 147, 478–491.

Christiansen, D., Larsen, K., Kudsk Jensen, O., et al., 2009. Pain responses in repeated end-range spinal movements and psychological factors in sick-listed patients with low back pain: is there an association? Journal of Rehabilitation Medicine 41, 545–549.

Donelson, R., Aprill, C., Medcalf, R., et al., 1997. A prospective study of centralization of lumbar and referred pain: a predictor of symptomatic discs and anular competence. Spine 22, 1115–1122.

Donelson, R., Grant, W., Kamps, C., et al., 1991. Pain response to sagittal end-range spinal motion. A prospective, randomized, multicentered trial. Spine 16, S206–S212.

Donelson, R., Silva, G., Murphy, K., 1990. Centralization phenomenon. Its usefulness in evaluating and treating referred pain. Spine 15, 211–213.

Edmond, S.L., Cutrone, G., Werneke, M., et al., 2014. Association between centralization and directional preference and functional and pain outcomes in patients with neck pain. Journal of Orthopaedic and Sports Physical Therapy 44, 68–75.

Errico, T.J., 2005. Syntegration: a 'more complete' knowledge-based approach to the practice of medicine – North American Spine Society Presidential Address, Chicago, IL. Spine Journal 5, 6–12.

Fardon, D.F., Milette, P.C., Combined Task Forces of the North American Spine Society, American Society of Spine Radiology, and American Society of Neuroradiology, 2001. Nomenclature and classification of lumbar disc pathology. Recommendations of the Combined Task Forces of the North American Spine Society, American Society of Spine Radiology, and American Society of Neuroradiology. Spine 26, E93–E113.

Fritz, J.M., Delitto, A., Vignovic, M., et al., 2000. Interrater reliability of judgments of the centralization phenomenon and status change during movement testing in patients with low back pain. Archives of Physical Medicine and Rehabilitation 81, 57–61.

Karas, R., McIntosh, G., Hall, H., et al., 1997. The relationship between nonorganic signs and centralization of symptoms in the prediction of return to work for patients with low back pain. Physical Therapy 77, 354–360.

Laslett, M., Oberg, B., Aprill, C.N., et al., 2005. Centralization as a predictor of provocation discography results in chronic low back pain, and the influence of disability and distress on diagnostic power. Spine Journal 5, 370–380.

Long, A.L., 1995. The centralization phenomenon. Its usefulness as a predictor or outcome in conservative treatment of chronic low back pain (a pilot study). Spine 20, 2513–2520.

McKenzie, R., 1981. The Lumbar Spine: Mechanical Diagnosis and Therapy. Spinal Publications, Waikanae, New Zealand.

McKenzie, R., May, S., 2003. The Lumbar Spine: Mechanical Diagnosis and Therapy. Spinal Publications, Waikanae, New Zealand, pp. 553–563.

May, S., Aina, A., 2012. Centralization and directional preference: a systematic review. Manual Therapy 17, 497–506.

Nordin, M., Carragee, E.J., Hogg-Johnson, S., et al., Bone and Joint Decade 2000–2010 Task Force on Neck Pain and Its Associated Disorders, 2008. Assessment of neck pain and its associated disorders: results of the Bone and Joint Decade 2000–2010. Task Force on Neck Pain and Its Associated Disorders. Spine (Phila PA 1976) 33 (4 Suppl.), S101–S122.

Razmjou, H., Kramer, J.F., Yamada, R., 2000. Intertester reliability of the McKenzie evaluation in assessing patients with mechanical low-back pain. Journal of Orthopaedic and Sports Physical Therapy 30, 368–389.

Suls, J., Krantz, D.S., Williams, G.C., 2013. Three strategies for bridging different levels of analysis and embracing the biopsychosocial model. Health Psychology 32, 597–601.

Taylor, M.D., 1996. The McKenzie method: a general practice interpretation: the lumbar spine. Australian Family Physician 25, 189–201.

Werneke, M., Hart, D.L., Cook, D., 1999. A descriptive study of the centralization phenomenon. A prospective analysis. Spine 24, 676–683.

Zale, E.L., Lange, K.L., Fields, S.A., et al., 2013. The relation between pain-related fear and disability: a meta-analysis. Journal of Pain 14, 1019–1030.

Chapter |11|

'Offloading' taping to reduce pain and facilitate movement

Dylan Morrissey

INTRODUCTION

These are exciting times for clinicians and researchers interested in taping for therapeutic effect. First, the emergence of Kinesio-taping ('K-taping') has made an impact in our clinics and on our sports fields. Second, the quantity and quality of research about taping in general has accelerated exponentially and research on K-taping is increasing (Fig. 11.1). What does this mean for the clinician? More importantly, what does this mean for patients?

The positive outputs are many and varied. First, patient outcomes should improve as therapeutic paradigms evolve and mature. Second, exploration of a diversity of mechanisms underlying observed effects should enhance understanding of presenting pathology, optimize clinical reasoning and enable further innovation. This chapter presents some taping techniques, and makes some observations about the available evidence. Some of these observations may challenge some emerging accepted truths, or perhaps re-state some clinically proven 'facts'. Hopefully they will stimulate thought, and be tested rigorously, as were some of the hypotheses presented in earlier editions.

There are ways to make sense of, and translate into clinical practice, the research explosion. Scientific method utilizes systematic review, which is powerful evidence when performed well, with clinical insight, drawing on and analysing high quality rigorous evidence. Alongside systematic review, a theoretical framework for finding ways to categorize emerging evidence is useful. We need to use both as befits maturing professions driving forward clinical and academic innovation in parallel.

A recent systematic review was carried out of patellar taping for patellofemoral pain (PFP) is an example of how much the evidence, and the resultant clinical translation has progressed (Barton et al. 2014). Jenny McConnell innovated with an empirical approach to taping to reduce PFP, which revolutionized conservative management of PFP and has withstood the quantification test. Time and again these approaches have been evaluated and both effects and mechanisms explored. We now have level 1 evidence that patellar taping has positive effects on

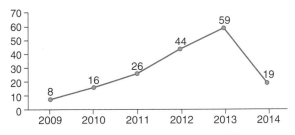

Figure 11.1 The frequency of K-taping research featured in *Web of Science. (Thanks to PhD student, Jack Shih-fan Tu for providing this graph and support with writing.)*

symptoms, and detailing the mechanisms underlying those effects, a number of studies have identified moderate evidence that:

- Tailored (customized to the patient to control lateral tilt, glide and spin) and untailored patellar taping provide immediate pain reduction of large and small effect, respectively, while tailored patellar taping promotes earlier onset of vastus medialis oblique (VMO) contraction (relative to vastus lateralis contraction).
- Tailored patellar taping promotes the capacity to tolerate increased internal knee extension moments (mechanisms). Further, and in-keeping with how taping is applied clinically, there is limited evidence that:
  - Tailored patellar taping combined with exercise provides superior pain reduction compared with exercise alone at 4 weeks
  - Untailored patellar taping added to exercise at 3–12 months has no benefit.

The value of 'offloading' soft tissue and articular structures has been proven. The clinical translation is therefore clear – although there is always room for further exploration.

What further categorization over and above effects and mechanisms could we apply? How can we make sense of new research without the benefit of systematic review?

First, we need to be clear about the aim of a given technique in a specific patient at a particular time.

- Can we produce an effect with our hands that could be reproduced with tape, thus extending the treatment window beyond immediate contact?
- How does the proposed technique fit with the rest of the multimodal treatment approach being applied?
- Never apply taping techniques 'off the shelf' – there is so much more to be gained from innovation, applied clinical reasoning, then proving effects immediately by testing and re-testing comparable signs.
- Clearly explain to the patient the rationale for the technique, how it fits with the rest of the treatment

programme and what they should expect (if possible, recording this as a video on the patient's mobile phone), so they have a verbatim record of what has been planned that they can review as required.

- Consider effects on both tissue and whole organism levels, therefore applying the full range of clinical reasoning in expert application of a biopsychosocial approach.
- Choose the type of tape according to its properties, and match these to specific goals, while also considering mechanisms.
- Finally, complete the loop – have we made best use of existing research? Keep up-to-date with conference proceedings, the literature and new reviews.

The situation with systematic reviews of K-taping is not clear and perhaps the field is a little young to facilitate clinically meaningful reviews. Five recent systematic reviews found little in the way of consistent effects except on short-term pain and range of movement (Kalron & Bar-Sela 2013; Morris et al. 2013; Mostafavifar et al. 2012; Taylor et al. 2014; Williams et al. 2012). This is valuable in itself, especially in the context of designing and delivering a treatment package, but a feature of the source materials is of taping techniques typically being applied in a standardized fashion, as was the case with early studies on patellar taping, perhaps because this approach seems consistent with typical research methods. Further, many studies are done in asymptomatic subjects rather than patients, thus limiting external validity. What is required, and has resulted in stronger evidence for patellar taping, is evaluation of tailored taping in relevant groups with carefully chosen outcome measures. Assessment of mechanisms alongside such effects studies would be even more useful. Until we have such studies, it is unlikely that evidence synthesis will be able to fully reveal the place of such approaches in our clinical armamentarium. At present, we have to, as it were, accept the null hypothesis of no effect, but keep on working to address the absence of evidence.

As a final observation, there is no reason in the literature to regard 'Kinesio-taping' as any different to any other taping techniques. This may sound controversial but the same effects can be delivered using different tape in the same situations.

Montalvo's review found little difference between K-taping and a McConnell type approach, suggesting therefore that the application and reasoning is more important than the actual tape used (Montalvo et al. 2013). Kinesio-tape itself is typically beautifully made, has a particular adhesive mass and costs more than most other common types of tape. One can probably do more with this type of tape than with any other due to its excellent qualities, but there is nothing intrinsically special or new about a particular weave or adhesive mass. It was Rose

MacDonald who opened the eyes of many therapists in the UK to the need for therapists to understand the synergy that could be achieved by a detailed understanding of tape properties alongside clear taping goals and detailed overt clinical reasoning, in order to maximize results. It is that evidence-informed synergy, applied with a good knowledge of the literature and explicit clinical reasoning, that is the real goal. That said, if one was allowed only one type of tape, it would be good quality K-tape, because of the versatility its excellent manufacture offers. We do simply need to regard it as one of the tools of the trade, and not be beguiled by extravagant claims of its effects.

APPLICATION

Unloading taping to reduce musculoskeletal pain, and proprioceptive taping to improve movement patterns, are useful empirical adjunctive treatment approaches. It is probable that they operate by similar mechanisms, the precise nature of which remain as yet unproven, despite an increasing evidence base. Particular attention has been paid to the effects of taping on muscle recruitment (Kuo & Huang 2013; Lumbroso et al. 2014); bone loading in people with medial tibial stress syndrome (Griebert et al. 2014); calf pain in endurance athletes (Merino-Marban et al. 2014); postural stability (Semple et al. 2012); pain scores during functional tasks; fascial and upper limb dystonia (Pelosin et al. 2013) and neuromuscular recruitment and movement patterns (An et al. 2012). Since the last edition, some progress has been made in understanding mechanisms by which taping effects are mediated. The particular effects of taping along the line of a muscle have been explored (Alexander et al. 2008; Kuo & Huang 2013). Hypotheses regarding mechanisms based on the available literature are revisited in this chapter. These concepts are accompanied by clinical guidelines for the application of taping in a variety of situations with illustrative case histories.

Taping can be used in a number of ways to reduce movement-associated pain. Based on a thorough assessment of presenting movement patterns and pain mechanisms, taping can be used as a useful treatment approach in itself, or as a means of maintaining treatment effects. It can be used to provide a physical effect on the tissues that lasts for hours or even days, supplementing the relatively brief therapist–patient contact. Taping can be used to affect pain directly by offloading irritable myofascial and/or neural tissues. Taping can also be indirectly used to alter the pain associated with identified faulty movement patterns (Table 11.1). These effects are both proprioceptively and mechanically mediated, depending on the approach used. This is easily demonstrated in the shoulder girdle, with this area therefore being particularly used to demonstrate taping approaches in the following text.

Table 11.1 Means of pain reduction by taping

Direct	Indirect (proprioceptively mediated)
Longitudinal offload (Box 11.1)	Inhibition or excitation of movement synergists dependent on direction and individually proven effects as shown by assessment
Transverse offload (Box 11.2)	Facilitation of underactive movement synergists Promotion of optimal interjoint coordination Direct optimization of joint alignment during static postures or movement

DIRECT METHODS

Longitudinal offload

Painful tissues that are held in tension either because of the unrelieved influence of gravity or because of chronically increased background muscle tone, e.g. due to habitual postures, can often be effectively helped by taping if the tissue can be passively supported in a shortened position. This is particularly useful when addressing symptoms associated with adverse neural dynamics (Fig. 11.2). It is suggested that free nerve endings and c-fibre end-organs, which intertwine with the tissues, are irritated by the mechanical and chemical effects of the tissue under tension. This is reduced by holding the tissue in a shortened position, therefore reducing pain fibre stimulation (Fig. 11.3). It is important to test this with a patient prior to taping application.

Transverse offload

A transverse offload approach can be used particularly for myofascial tissues that may be mediated either by similar means to that described above or by a more mechanical effect. This type of technique has been shown to be effective in reducing elbow pain associated with lateral epicondylalgia (Vicenzino et al. 2003). Transverse offloading of muscle structures effectively lengthens the muscle being used and may be inhibitory (Figs 11.4, 11.11) or may alter the free nerve endings position in connective tissue (Fig. 11.3).

A number of suggested techniques mix the two approaches effectively, and it may be that the combination of methods reduces the load on tissues within the taped area (Fig. 11.5).

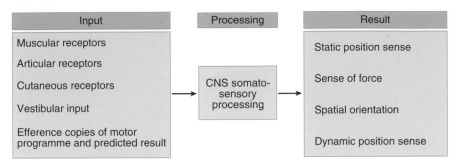

Figure 11.2 Proprioceptive summary. Input from a number of peripheral sources is integrated with expected movement patterns and the commands sent to the periphery with the result being a CNS representation of movement parameters.

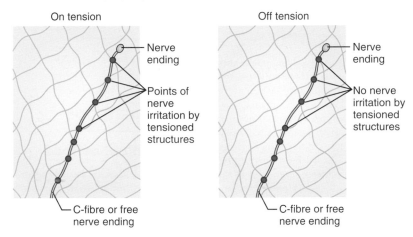

Figure 11.3 Free nerve endings piercing the multidirectional fascial planes may be irritated when there is sustained significant tension placed on the tissues. Taping that holds these tissues in a shortened position helps to reduce symptoms associated with movement.

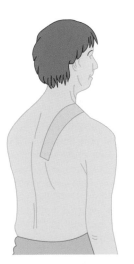

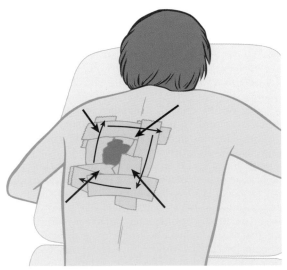

Figure 11.4 Upper trapezius inhibition. From anterior aspect of upper trapezius just above the clavicle over the muscle belly to approximately the level of rib 7 in a vertical line. Once partially attached a firm downward pull is applied and the tail of the tape attached.

Figure 11.5 The skin over the thoracic spine is gathered centrally in the direction of the large arrows and the skin taped in the direction of the small arrows (see Taping guidelines).

INDIRECT METHODS: WITH REFERENCE TO THE SHOULDER GIRDLE

Normal upper limb function is dependent on the ability to statically and dynamically position the shoulder girdle in an optimal coordinated fashion (Glousman et al. 1988; Kibler 1998).

Movement faults, for example of the scapulothoracic 'joint', have been shown to be strongly associated with common pathologies (Hébert et al. 2002; Ludewig & Cook 2000; Lukasiewicz et al. 1999; Michener et al. 2003).

Physiotherapy that aims to improve joint stability, optimal interjoint coordination and muscle function has been shown to be clinically effective in the management of a variety of shoulder presentations (Braun et al. 2013; Ginn et al. 1997). Proprioception is a critical component of coordinated shoulder girdle movement, with significant deficits having been identified in pathological and fatigued shoulders (Carpenter et al. 1998; Forwell & Carnahan 1996; Voight et al. 1996; Warner et al. 1996). It is an integral goal of rehabilitation programmes to attempt to minimize or reverse these proprioceptive deficits (Lephart et al. 1997; Magee & Reid 1996).

Taping is clinically seen to be a useful adjunct to a patient-specific integrated treatment approach aiming to restore full pain-free movement of the shoulder girdle, although the evidence that taping affects scapular muscle recruitment patterns is mixed – suggesting that the optimal techniques to use for given presentations remain to be fully established and evaluated (Ackermann et al. 2002; Alexander et al. 2003; Cools et al. 2002). It is very clear from the literature that shoulder taping must be fully integrated into the overall treatment approach, so that its effects can be realized.

Initial studies of the effects of taping on motoneuron pool excitability have shown physiological effects that conflict with clinical experience, but these are early days in the exploration of the pathophysiological effects of taping on musculoskeletal dysfunction, so little could be taken from this work (Alexander et al. 2003). Extensions of that work have shown that motoneuron pool excitability is likely reduced by rigid tape (Alexander et al. 2008) but there may be some post-removal facilitation following removal of loosely applied K-tape (Firth et al. 2010). This mechanistic work would seem to contradict the findings of Semple (2012), who found improved postural control with calf taping; Merino-Marban et al. (2014), who showed reduced calf pain in duathletes and Lumbroso (2014), who showed increased calf force.

Furthermore, it is likely that the lack of tailoring of taping to an individual, and a lack of clear rationale for a given taping approach in a given person explains the lack of consistent effects.

Taping is particularly useful in addressing movement faults at the scapulothoracic, glenohumeral and acromio-clavicular joints. Recent work has shown that scapular taping, of various kinds, can increase the scapular external, upward and posterior tilt rotations during elevation (e.g. Shaheen et al. 2013; Van Herzeele et al. 2013), precisely the movements associated with reversal of dyskinesia and improvement of symptoms in shoulder conditions (Worsley et al. 2013). Further, the acromiohumeral distance may be increased by simple taping procedures, described in previous editions but evaluated using K-tape by Luque-Suarez in 2013. The effects on pain tend to be short term (Thelen et al. 2008), with the clinical rationale therefore being of allowing a window of opportunity to rehabilitate dynamic function. The kinematic effects shown on acromiohumeral distance and scapular rotation are likely to improve shoulder impingement presentations.

Possible physiological mechanisms

Proprioception is a complex process that is difficult to define (Jerosch & Prymka 1996). Essentially, information from mechanoreceptors in the skin, muscles, fascia, tendons and articular structures is integrated with visual and vestibular input at all CNS levels in order to allow perception of:

- position sense (static)
- kinaesthesia (dynamic)
- force detection.

Proprioception is particularly important for upper limb interjoint coordination (Sainburg et al. 1993) due to the complexity of the kinetic chain, the relative lack of osseous stability and the precision of the tasks performed. The literature focusses on the role of articular and myofascial structures in contributing to shoulder girdle proprioception, while cutaneous input is regarded as having a lesser role (Carpenter et al. 1998; Jerosch & Prymka 1996; Lephart et al. 1997; Warner et al. 1996).

Proprioception has been shown to be compromised in upper limb pathologies, such as subacromial impingement (Machner et al. 2003) and glenohumeral instability (Barden et al. 2004). Full return to sport is dependent on reversal of these deficits. These deficits can be normalized after long periods of rehabilitation and recovery following surgery (Pötzl et al. 2004), while immediate improvements have been shown in pathological shoulders when cutaneously mediated proprioceptive feedback is augmented by compressive bracing (Ulkar et al. 2004).

Taping as a form of proprioceptive biofeedback

A potential mechanism by means of which proprioceptive shoulder taping may be effective is via augmented cutaneous input (Figs 11.5–11.7).

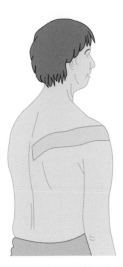

Figure 11.6 Retraction of the shoulder: from the anterior aspect of the shoulder, 2 cm medial to the joint line, around deltoid muscle just below acromial level to T6 area without crossing the midline. Tape pull is into retraction.

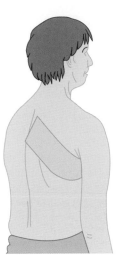

Figure 11.8 Serratus anterior facilitation and inferior angle abduction: from 2 cm medial to the scapula border, following the line of the ribs down to the mid-axillary line. Four one-third overlapping strips are applied with the origin and insertion pulled together and bunching the skin.

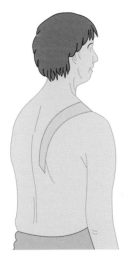

Figure 11.7 Retraction/upward rotation. From anterior shoulder just below the coracoid to low thoracic (T10) area. The initial pull on the tape is up and then back as the tape comes over the midline.

Tape is applied in such a way that there is little or no tension while the body part is held or moved in the desired direction or plane. The tissues will therefore develop more tension when movement occurs outside these parameters. This tension will be sensed consciously, thus giving a stimulus to the patient to correct the movement pattern. Over time and with sufficient repetition and feedback, these patterns can become learned components of the motor engrams for given movements. This process

therefore represents cutaneously mediated proprioceptive biofeedback.

Taping as a means of altering muscle function

Mechanically, if taping can be applied in such a fashion that a chronically inhibited (underactive) muscle is held in a shortened position (Fig. 11.8), there will be a shift of the length–tension curve to the left, and greater force development in the inner range through optimized actin–myosin overlap during the cross-bridge cycle (Fig. 11.9).

Similarly, if taping can be applied in such a fashion that a relatively short, overactive, muscle is held in a lengthened position, there will be a shift of the length–tension curve to the right, and lesser force development through decreased actin–myosin overlap during the cross-bridge cycle at the point in joint range at which the muscle is required to work (Fig. 11.4).

The taping method used to inhibit upper trapezius activity (as in Fig. 11.4) has been investigated in a pilot study (O'Donovan 1997) and shown to have a significant inhibitory effect on the degree of upper trapezius activity in relation to lower trapezius during elevation (Morin et al. 1997). Alexander (2003) has also shown inhibition of lower trapezius, by means of H-reflex latency and amplitude, with scapular taping albeit with a counter-intuitive procedure.

Inhibition is demonstrated as soon as the tape is applied. Clinical effects of taping the shoulder girdle can

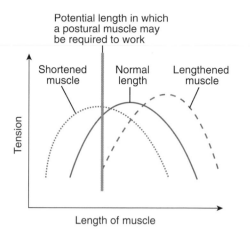

Figure 11.9 Length–tension curves. Although lengthened muscle has the capability to generate more force, postural muscles frequently need to be able to generate most force in inner range positions in which case it is often desirable that they are relatively short.

be significant and immediate, especially in promoting altered movement patterns and allowing earlier progression of rehabilitation. A recent study has shown that the pull involved in applying the second of the two tapes is critical to the electromyographical and mechanical positional changes observed during successful taping application (Brown 1999). The mechanisms by which the above study results, and the clinical effects seen during application, still merit further investigation.

Taping guidelines: shoulder as an example

It is essential to be clear about the aims of taping in order to ensure optimal results:

- In the case of the shoulder this would be assessed for its habitual resting position and for movement faults contributing to the symptom presentation.
- The skin would then be prepared by removal of surface oils and body hair.

Box 11.1 Case history: direct longitudinal offload

A 34-year-old woman presented with acute discogenic low back and long leg sciatic pain, due to an exacerbation of existing low back pain caused by sleeping awkwardly on a long-haul plane journey.

The presentation was both severe and irritable, to the extent that she had to be examined side-lying, in order to avoid exacerbation.

A key comparable sign was a 20° straight leg raise reproducing all her leg and back pain symptoms.

Application of longitudinal offload taping along the course of the sciatic nerve, and its common peroneal branches, reduced her symptoms on SLR and increased the pain-free range to 45° in conjunction with manual therapy techniques. The tissues had been supported in this way during assessment and the 'offload' was shown to be effective in terms of reduced pain and increased range of movement.

This allowed her to walk far more normally, with markedly reduced pain.

The V-shaped tapes were placed at the base of the fibula, at the head of the fibula, two-thirds of the way down the posterior aspect of the thigh and at the top of the posterior aspect of the thigh. These were applied in the order stated. Interestingly, an initial attempt to apply the tape in a reverse order was not successful (Fig. 11.10).

This taping was used throughout the first 2 weeks of her management, by which time she was significantly better and able to discontinue that aspect of her treatment.

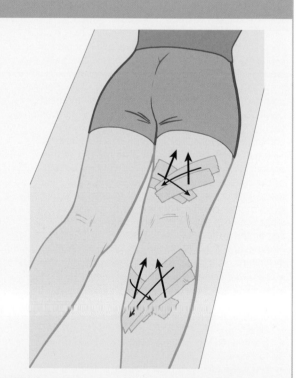

Figure 11.10 The tissues over the sciatic nerve are offloaded superiorly in the direction of the large arrows and the skin taped in the direction of the small arrows (see Taping guidelines).

Box 11.2 Case history: direct transverse offload

A recreational racquet sports player presented with lateral elbow pain with clear local soft tissue components, as well as a positive radial nerve tension test and low cervical facet joint stiffness.

Static resisted contraction (SRC) of the common extensor origin muscles and extensor carpi radialis brevis in particular was comparable (Fig. 11.11).

As part of the management, a transverse offload tape was applied to the common extensor origin with immediate reduction of symptoms from SRC and improved grip strength, through reduction of pain inhibition.

This remained part of her management until return to sport, when it was replaced with an 'Aircast' lateral epicondyle brace, which can be used to similar effect.

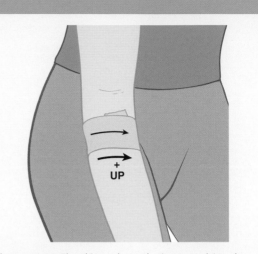

Figure 11.11 The skin and muscle tissue overlying the common extensor origin is lifted and pulled medially in the direction of the large arrows and the skin taped in the direction of the small arrows (see Taping guidelines).

Box 11.3 Case history: shoulder pain

This case represents a particular example of inhibition of overactive movement synergists and antagonists and facilitation of underactive movement synergists.

A 33-year-old cricketer presented complaining of persistent and progressive shoulder pain of nonspecific onset but particularly related to bowling and throwing. He had experienced episodes of pain towards the end of the previous season, which had not interfered with participation nor persisted after the end of the season. He had experienced problems from the start of the current season, which had progressed to the extent that he was no longer able to bowl or throw overarm, had pain persisting between games, while overhead activities of daily living were compromised.

Assessment showed clear impingement features, including:

- Localized pain to the front of the shoulder
- A painful arc on mid-range elevation that was associated with marked protraction and tipping of the scapula and accentuated on slow eccentric elevation
- Generalized loss of thoracic extension and rotation focussed at T5±T7
- A positive empty-can test (Magee & Reid 1996) (a static resisted contraction of abduction with the arm medially rotated and held at 90° of abduction in the scapular plane)
- General restriction of glenohumeral accessory joint glides

- Restricted medial rotation with scapulothoracic relative flexibility on the kinetic medial rotation test
- Painful, weak static resisted abduction and lateral rotation
- Tight overactive pectoralis minor as demonstrated by the shoulder girdle not being able to lower to the supporting surface when the patient was supine and gentle pressure was applied antero-posteriorly through the coracoid process.

An initial treatment plan was formulated, including: thoracic manipulation (HVLA thrust) to increase the available thoracic extension during elevation; pectoralis lengthening using trigger point treatment and specific soft-tissue mobilization to decrease the active scapula tipping; local soft-tissue deinflammation with ice; and scapula setting – initially in neutral but then incorporated into dynamic movement. It was decided to emphasize upward rotation and retraction as he demonstrated an excessively protracted, tipped scapula during elevation.

The scapula setting (Box 11.4) proved difficult for the patient to master, so the shoulder was taped (Figs 11.5, 11.7). This resulted in an immediate improvement in the patient's ability to set the scapula and an improved scapulohumeral rhythm associated with a marked decrease in the painful arc symptoms. The taping was reapplied for 3 weeks while his treatment and rehabilitation were progressed to the extent that he had achieved satisfactory control of scapula movement during functional activities and had begun to resume some of his sporting activities

Box 11.4 **Scapula setting**

Scapula setting has been defined as 'Dynamic orientation of the scapula in a position so as to optimize the position of the glenoid and so allow mobility and stability of the glenohumeral joint' (Mottram 1997).

- The shoulder would be actively positioned in the desired position by the patient with the guidance of the therapist, or passively if the patient is unable to maintain the desired position.
- A hypoallergenic mesh tape would be applied without tension (e.g. Mefix, Molnlycke, Sweden).
- A robust zinc oxide tape (Strappal, Smith and Nephew, UK) would then be applied.
- Further tapes may then be applied as necessary.

The taping is continued until the patient has learnt to actively control movement in the desired fashion, or the effects on symptoms are maintained when it is not worn.

An example of how taping can be used in the management of a patient with excessive tipping of the scapula is presented in the case history in Box 11.3 An example of how taping can be used to elevate a depressed scapula and stabilize a traumatically unstable acromioclavicular joint is presented in the case history in Box 11.5.

The case histories have been deliberately chosen to show a range of taping techniques that can be used either in conjunction with other modalities and methods, or in isolation.

Skin reactions

If the client develops a skin reaction, this can either be due to an allergic reaction, a 'heat rash' or because the tape is concentrating too much tension into one area. Tension concentrations usually occur around the front of the shoulder.

Heat rashes tend to be localized to the area under the tape and settle quickly. Allergic reactions are more irritating and widespread, and must be treated with great caution as reapplication is likely to lead to a more severe reaction due to immune sensitization.

Scapulohumeral function

The scapulothoracic joint gains some stability in relation to medially directed forces from the clavicular strut via the acromioclavicular joint. This still allows a large range and amplitude of translatory and rotary movement that is primarily produced, controlled and limited by the axioscapular myofascial structures (Kibler 1998).

Compromised thoraco-scapulohumeral rhythm results in the potential for impingement due to downward rotation of the glenoid associated with tipping or winging (Ludewig & Cook 2000; Lukasiewicz et al. 1999). An anterior tilt of the glenoid, resulting from adverse scapula positioning, is regarded as being a significant occult instability risk (Kibler 1998) (Box 11.6).

The scapulohumeral joint relies heavily on the passive stability provided by the capsulo-ligamentous structures and the dynamic stability provided by the rotator cuff (Glousman et al. 1988; Harryman et al. 1990, 1992; Payne et al. 1997; Terry et al. 1991). This stability is crucially dependent on intact proprioception (Nyland et al. 1998). Disruption by trauma or repetitive disadvantageous movement patterns is associated with impingement or instability (Barden et al. 2005; Machner et al. 2003).

CONCLUSION

Management of complex neuromusculoskeletal dysfunction and pathology and pain syndromes requires a multifactorial approach based on individual assessment. Strategies used to reduce pain, increase mobility, improve movement coordination and improve strength may be augmented by the use of taping used to offload tissues or to improve movement patterns by proprioceptive and mechanical means. The evidence for this approach is growing, both in terms of mechanisms and effects.

Taping is a particularly useful treatment adjunct, as it has the particular advantage of lasting well beyond the patient–therapist contact, thus extending the duration of therapeutic stimulus. Repetition and long duration experience of altered movement is essential in altering established motor engrams and overcoming the effects of established inhibition or pain presentations.

Box 11.5 Case history: shoulder injury

This case represents a particular example of promotion of optimal interjoint coordination as well as direct optimization of joint alignment during static postures or movement.

A 23-year-old rugby player presented 2 weeks after a shoulder pointer (fall onto the point of the shoulder causing an inferior blow to the acromion) and resultant acromioclavicular joint sprain.

Assessment showed a visible joint step with upper trapezius spasm accentuating this via its attachment to the lateral third of the clavicle. Range of movement was markedly reduced and the patient complained of constant pain aggravated by any movement. He was still using a sling. The scapula was noted to be in a downward rotated, depressed position, thus accentuating the step and resultant acromioclavicular joint pain.

The initial treatment therefore aimed to decrease the resting joint pain using large amplitude joint mobilizations and interferential therapy, which was partially successful.

In order to further reduce the resting pain and affect the pain on movement, it was necessary to improve the symmetry of the joint by decreasing upper trapezius activity and facilitating upward rotation and elevation of the scapula. This was done using tape (Figs 11.12, 11.13) and reinforced with soft-tissue techniques (trigger point massage and specific soft-tissue mobilization) to the upper trapezius (see Figs 11.4, 11.6, 11.12, 11.13).

An immediate improvement in symmetry was noted and a marked increase in pain-free ROM. He was able to discard the sling. Taping remained an integral part of the treatment until he was able to actively set the scapula independently.

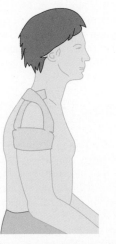

Figure 11.12 Elevation of the shoulder girdle. Apply tape in the following order: (1) Anchor strip applied at level of deltoid tuberosity, encircling two-thirds of the circumference of the arm; (2) elevatory strips applied from posterior arm/deltoid to the anterolateral aspect of the base of the neck; (3) elevatory strips applied from anterior arm/deltoid to the posterolateral aspect of the base of the neck; (4) locking strip over tape 1.

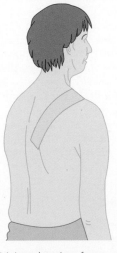

Figure 11.13 AC joint relocation; from coracoid process over the distal end of the clavicle with a downward pull applied just before the tail of the tape is attached to level of rib 6 in a vertical line. Only ever applied after successful application of elevatory taping (Fig. 11.12).

Box 11.6 Downward rotation and tipping

Downward rotation occurs about an axis located one-third of the length of the spine of the scapula lateral to the proximal end of the spine of the scapula. Tipping is when the inferior angle protrudes from the chest wall and the coracoid is pulled down and medially as compared to winging, where the entire medial border of the scapula lifts off the chest wall.

THIS CHAPTER

This chapter has contained details of the use of 'unloading'/Kinesio-taping as a form of positional release.

NEXT CHAPTER

The next chapter by Anthony Pusey, DO and Julia Brooks, DO, describes the application of positional release techniques in the treatment of animals.

REFERENCES

Ackermann, B., Adams, R., Marshall, E., 2002. The effect of scapula taping on electromyographic activity and musical performance in professional violinists. Australian Journal of Physiotherapy 48, 197–203.

Alexander, C., Stynes, S., Thomas, A., et al., 2003. Does tape facilitate or inhibit the lower fibres of trapezius? Manual Therapy 8, 37–41.

Alexander, C.M., McMullan, M., Harrison, P.J., 2008. What is the effect of taping along or across a muscle on motoneurone excitability? A study using triceps surae. Manual Therapy 13, 57–62.

An, H.M., Miller, C.G., McElveen, M., et al., 2012. The effect of kinesio tape® on lower extremity functional movement screen™ scores. International Journal of Exercise Science 5, 196–204.

Barden, J.M., Balyk, R., Raso, V., et al., 2005. Atypical shoulder muscle activation in multidirectional instability. Clinical Neurophysiology 116, 1846–1857.

Barden, J.M., Balyk, R., Raso, V.J., et al., 2004. Dynamic upper limb proprioception in multidirectional shoulder instability. Clinical Orthopaedics and Related Research 420, 181–189.

Barton, C., Balachandar, V., Lack, S., et al., 2014. Patellar taping for patellofemoral pain: a systematic review and meta-analysis to evaluate clinical outcomes and biomechanical mechanisms. British Journal of Sports Medicine 48, 417–424.

Braun, C., Bularczyk, M., Heintsch, J., et al., 2013. Manual therapy and exercises for shoulder impingement revisited. Physical Therapy Reviews 18, 263–284.

Brown, L., 1999. The Effect of Taping the Glenohumeral Joint on Scapulohumeral Resting Position and Trapezius Activity During Abduction. Unpublished MSc Thesis. University College London.

Carpenter, J.E., Blasier, R.B., Pellizzon, G., 1998. The effects of muscle fatigue on shoulder joint position sense. American Journal of Sports Medicine 26, 262–265.

Cools, A., Witvrouw, E., Danneels, L., et al., 2002. Does taping influence electromyographic muscle activity in the scapular rotators in healthy shoulders? Manual Therapy 7, 154–162.

Forwell, L.A., Carnahan, H., 1996. Proprioception during manual aiming in individuals with shoulder instability and controls. Journal of Orthopaedic and Sports Physical Therapy 23, 111–119.

Firth, B.L., Dingley, P., Davies, E.R., et al., 2010. The effect of kinesiotape on function, pain, and motoneuronal excitability in healthy people and people with Achilles tendinopathy. Clinical Journal of Sport Medicine 20, 416–421.

Ginn, K.A., Herbert, R.D., Khouw, W., et al., 1997. A randomized, controlled clinical trial of a treatment for shoulder pain. Physical Therapy 77, 802–809.

Glousman, R., Jobe, F., Tibone, J., et al., 1988. Dynamic electromyographic analysis of the throwing shoulder with glenohumeral instability. Journal of Bone and Joint Surgery 70, 220–226.

Griebert, M.C., Needle, A.R., McConnell, J., et al., 2014. Lower-leg Kinesio tape reduces rate of loading in participants with medial tibial stress syndrome. Physical Therapy in Sport [Epub ahead of print].

Harryman, D.T. 2nd, Sidles, J.A., Clark, J.M., et al., 1990. Translation of the humeral head on the glenoid with passive glenohumeral motion. Journal of Bone and Joint Surgery. American Volume 72, 1334–1343.

Harryman, D.T. 2nd, Sidles, J.A., Harris, S.L., et al., 1992. The role of the rotator interval capsule in passive motion and stability of the shoulder. Journal of Bone and Joint Surgery. American Volume 74, 53–66.

Hébert, L.J., Moffet, H., McFadyen, B.J., et al., 2002. Scapular behavior in shoulder impingement syndrome. Archives of Physical Medicine and Rehabilitation 83, 60–69.

Jerosch, J., Prymka, M., 1996. Proprioception and joint stability. Knee Surgery, Sports Traumatology, Arthroscopy 4, 171–179.

Kalron, A., Bar-Sela, S., 2013. A systematic review, of the effectiveness of Kinesio Taping® – Fact or fashion? European Journal of Physical and Rehabilitation Medicine 49, 699–709.

Kibler, W.B., 1998. The role of the scapula in athletic shoulder function. American Journal of Sports Medicine 26, 325–337.

Kuo, Y.L., Huang, Y.C., 2013. Effects of the application direction of kinesio taping on isometric muscle strength of the wrist and fingers of healthy adults – a pilot study. Journal of Physical Therapy Science 25, 287–291.

Lephart, S.M., Pincivero, D.M., Giraido, J.L., et al., 1997. The role of proprioception in the management and rehabilitation of athletic injuries. American Journal of Sports Medicine 25, 130–137.

Ludewig, P.M., Cook, T.M., 2000. Alterations in shoulder kinematics and associated muscle activity in people with symptoms of shoulder impingement. Physical Therapy 80, 276–291.

Lukasiewicz, A.C., McClure, P., Michener, L., et al., 1999. Comparison of 3-dimensional scapular position and orientation between subjects with and without shoulder impingement. Journal of Orthopaedic and Sports Physical Therapy 29, 574–586.

Lumbroso, D., Ziv, E., Vered, E., et al., 2014. The effect of kinesio tape application on hamstring and gastrocnemius muscles in healthy young adults. Journal of Bodywork and Movement Therapies 18, 130–138.

Luque-Suarez, A., Navarro-Ledesma, S., Petocz, P., et al., 2013. Short term effects of kinesiotaping on acromiohumeral distance in asymptomatic subjects: a randomised controlled trial. Manual Therapy 18, 573–577.

Machner, A., Merk, H., Becker, R., et al., 2003. Kinesthetic sense of the shoulder in patients with impingement syndrome. Acta Orthopaedica 74, 85–88.

Magee, D., Reid, D., 1996. Shoulder injuries. In: Zachazewski, J.E., Magee, D.J.Quillen, W.S. (Eds.), Athletic Injuries and Rehabilitation. Saunders, Philadelphia, PA, pp. 509–539.

Merino-Marban, R., Fernandez-Rodriguez, E., Mayorga-Vega, D., 2014. The effect of kinesio taping on calf pain and extensibility immediately after its application and after a duathlon competition. Research in Sports Medicine 22, 1–11.

Michener, L.A., McClure, P.W., Karduna, A.R., 2003. Anatomical and biomechanical mechanisms of subacromial impingement syndrome. Clinical Biomechanics 18, 369–379.

Montalvo, A.M., Buckley, W.E., Sebastianelli, W., et al., 2013. An evidence-based practice approach to the efficacy of kinesio taping for improving pain and quadriceps performance in physically-active patellofemoral pain syndrome patients. Journal of Novel Physiotherapies 3, 151.

Morin, G.E., Tiberio, D., Austin, G., 1997. The effect of upper trapezius taping on electromyographic activity in the upper and middle trapezius region. Journal of Sport Rehabilitation 6, 309–318.

Morris, D., Jones, D., Ryan, H., et al., 2013. The clinical effects of Kinesio® Tex taping: a systematic review. Physiotherapy Theory and Practice 29, 259–270.

Mostafavifar, M., Wertz, J., Borchers, J., 2012. A systematic review of the effectiveness of kinesio taping for musculoskeletal injury. Physician and Sports Medicine 40, 33–40.

Mottram, S., 1997. Dynamic stability of the scapula. Manual Therapy 2, 123–131.

Nyland, J.A., Caborn, D.N., Johnson, D.L., 1998. The human glenohumeral joint. A proprioceptive and stability alliance. Knee Surgery, Sports Traumatology, Arthroscopy 6, 50–61.

O'Donovan, N., 1997. Evaluation of the Effect of Inhibitory Taping on EMG Activity in Upper and Lower Trapezius During Concentric Isokinetic Elevation of the Upper Limb. Unpublished MSc Thesis. University College London.

Payne, L.Z., Deng, X.H., Craig, E.V., et al., 1997. The combined dynamic and static contributions to subacromial impingement. A biomechanical analysis. American Journal of Sports Medicine 25, 801–808.

Pelosin, E., Avanzino, L., Marchese, R., et al., 2013. Kinesiotaping reduces pain and modulates sensory function in patients with focal dystonia: a randomized crossover pilot study. Neurorehabilitation and Neural Repair 27, 722–731.

Pötzl, W., Thorwesten, L., Götze, C., et al., 2004. Proprioception of the shoulder joint after surgical repair for instability: a long-term follow-up study. American Journal of Sports Medicine 32, 425–430.

Sainburg, R.L., Poizner, H., Ghez, C., 1993. Loss of proprioception produces deficits in interjoint coordination. Journal of Neurophysiology 70, 2136–2147.

Semple, S., Esterhuysen, C., Grace, J., 2012. The effects of kinesio ankle taping on postural stability in semiprofessional rugby union players. Journal of Physical Therapy Science 24, 1239–1242.

Shaheen, A.F., Villa, C., Lee, Y.N., et al., 2013. Scapular taping alters kinematics in asymptomatic subjects. Journal of Electromyography and Kinesiology 23, 326–333.

Taylor, R.L., O'Brien, L., Brown, T., 2014. A scoping review of the use of elastic therapeutic tape for neck or upper extremity conditions. Journal of Hand Therapy 27, 235–246.

Terry, G.C., Hammon, D., France, P., et al., 1991. The stabilizing function of passive shoulder restraints. American Journal of Sports Medicine 19, 26–34.

Thelen, M.D., Dauber, J.A., Stoneman, P.D., 2008. The clinical efficacy of kinesio tape for shoulder pain: a randomized, double-blinded, clinical trial. Journal of Orthopaedic and Sports Physical Therapy 38, 389.

Ulkar, B., Kunduracioglu, B., Cetin, C., et al., 2004. Effect of positioning and bracing on passive position sense of shoulder joint. British Journal of Sports Medicine 38, 549–552.

Van Herzeele, M., Van Cingel, R., Maenhout, A., et al., 2013. Does the Application of Kinesiotape Change Scapular Kinematics in Healthy Female Handball Players? International Journal of Sports Medicine 34, 950–955.

Vicenzino, B., Brooksbank, J., Minto, J., et al., 2003. Initial effects of elbow taping on pain-free grip strength and pressure pain threshold. Journal of Orthopaedic and Sports Physical Therapy 33, 400–407.

Voight, M.L., Hardin, J.A., Blackburn, T.A., et al., 1996. The effects of muscle fatigue on and the relationship of arm dominance to shoulder proprioception. Journal of Orthopaedic and Sports Physical Therapy 23, 348–352.

Warner, J.J., Lephart, S., Fu, F., 1996. Role of proprioception in pathoetiology of shoulder instability. Clinical Orthopaedics and Related Research 330, 35–39.

Williams, S., Whatman, C., Hume, P.A., et al., 2012. Kinesio taping in treatment and prevention of sports injuries a meta-analysis of the evidence for its effectiveness. Sports Medicine 42, 153–164.

Worsley, P., Warner, M., Mottram, S., et al., 2013. Motor control retraining exercises for shoulder impingement: effects on function, muscle activation, and biomechanics in young adults. Journal of Shoulder and Elbow Surgery 22, e11–e19.

Chapter 12

Application of positional techniques in the treatment of animals

J. Brooks and †A. G. Pusey

INTRODUCTION

One of the myths in musculoskeletal medicine is that humans are uniquely susceptible to back pain because they have risen onto their hind legs by adapting a structure designed for four legs. A chat with any veterinary surgeon will dispel this impression, as they frequently encounter animals presenting with physical problems involving the spine and associated structures (Fig. 12.1) (Jeffcott 1979).

On further consideration, this is unsurprising. The forces of gravity and the potential effects of injury are common stressors for humans and animals alike. Animals have the added complication of interacting with people, and may be subjected to dietary changes, specialized exercise regimes and unnatural breeding programmes.

The clinical challenge for those working with animals is to make a diagnosis without the benefit of direct verbal communication. Veterinary surgeons use their clinical expertise and use of special investigations, such as imaging techniques and blood tests, to identify pathology. However, difficulties arise for vets confronted with cases where there is obviously discomfort and dysfunction, despite there being no identifiable pathology. Such cases are likely to be the product of an altered physiological state, rather than of frank pathology (Williams 1997). Osteopathy adds another dimension to addressing such problems, by using observation and palpatory skills to identify areas of disordered function, along with a range of physical treatments to influence possible disturbances in the integration of the peripheral and central nervous systems.

HISTORY OF ANIMAL TREATMENT

The early years of animal osteopathy were distinguished by isolated pockets of activity, where individuals experimented with techniques. In the 1970s, Arthur Smith in Leicestershire pioneered an approach for treating horses under general anaesthetic, encouraged by a veterinary surgeon whose back he had successfully treated. Elsewhere, racehorse trainers looking for optimum performance recruited osteopaths, such as Gregg Currie in Epsom,

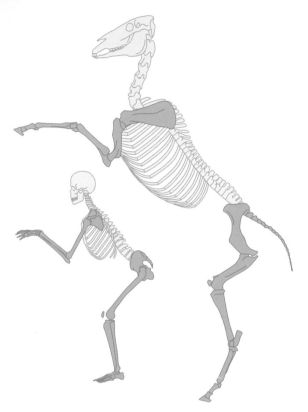

Figure 12.1 Animals and humans are similar in structure.

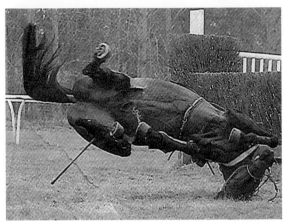

Figure 12.2 A horse may suffer compression rotation injuries that affect the whole spine (with permission from Ed Byrne).

and those working in rural areas were approached by local farmers. Latterly, special interest groups have provided a forum for disseminating information and formal studies leading to postgraduate qualifications are available in this field. At the present time, osteopaths in the UK work alongside many forward thinking veterinary surgeons wishing to offer another approach to musculoskeletal problems, and their services extend to organizations such as the Household Cavalry and zoos.

MECHANISMS OF INJURY

Causes of injury are many and varied. A horse may fall at 30 mph driving its half a ton of bodyweight into the ground (Fig. 12.2), or an elderly dog may relive its boisterous youth by playing with a new puppy. A cat may try to cross the road at an inopportune moment or a hunting owl might be swiped by a car aerial as it makes a low night flight. None can communicate verbally what they are feeling but the pathophysiological effects of injury provide a means of identifying the nature of musculoskeletal injury.

NEUROPHYSIOLOGICAL EFFECTS OF INJURY

These effects are widespread but may be divided for convenience into peripheral responses at the site of the injury (Bevan 1999), and central responses occurring within the central nervous system (Doubell et al. 1999).

Peripheral responses

An injury will result in local tissue changes to give the classic signs of inflammation, pain, heat, erythema and swelling. This site is usually fairly easy to identify clinically by eliciting a pain response by direct pressure over the area and feeling for swelling and increases in temperature. At this juncture, the animal may be treated successfully with anti-inflammatory drugs. However, the injury will also stimulate the small nerve fibres of the nociceptive system, which send warning signals to the dorsal horn of the spinal cord. Here the fibres arborize within the network of the spinal cord, to form a multitude of interconnections.

It is in this central network where changes can occur, that may not respond to first-line drug treatment, but which are accessible to physical treatments, such as osteopathy (Colles & Pusey 2003).

Central responses

On reaching the spinal cord, if the stimulus is of sufficient intensity, it will be relayed to the brain to register as pain. It will also interconnect with motor neurones of the ventral horn to increase muscle tone (He et al. 1988) and, via the lateral horn, increase sympathetic nervous system

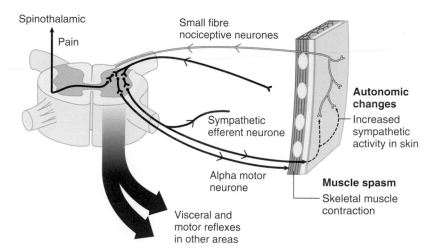

Figure 12.3 Neurophysiological responses to injury.

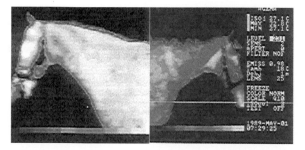

Figure 12.4 Infrared thermography showing reduced blood flow at surface in long-term response to injury. 'Normal' neck (left) and upper cervical dysfunction (right). *Note*: Temperature colour scale runs from left (lower temps) to right. Intervals ≈0.6°C (Colles et al. 1994).

activity to drive blood from the surface to the muscles (Figs 12.3, 12.4) (Sato & Schmidt 1973).

In the short term, this has a protective function by preventing further damage to the injured area. However, the long-term effect may be to leave a neurological footprint of abnormal patterning where the pain circuits maintain their activity after the initial injury has resolved (Patterson & Wurster 1997).

Retaining this abnormal patterning has a number of undesirable consequences. One effect is that the threshold at which the pain circuit fires is lowered, so that a relatively mild subsequent stimulus will fire an inappropriately large pain response. It will also alter the way an animal moves as a result of increased, possibly asymmetrical, tone in the some muscles. This is particularly significant in animals, as there are strong interconnections between spinal segments to support integrated movement between all four limbs. In fact, unlike the human system, these connections are so strong that in experiments on cats, it was found that

crude gait patterns could be generated, even when the connection between the spinal cord and brain had been severed (Pearson & Gordon 2000). This integration becomes compromised in the presence of altered patterns of muscular activity.

Another key aspect of muscle function, which is often overlooked, is its role in proprioception. In an unpublished study by Charlotte Frigast and Professor Joe Mayhew at the University of Edinburgh Veterinary School, temporary denervation of upper cervical roots was induced, and when these horses were subsequently turned in a circle, they lost balance or fell, suggesting a close link between neck muscles and other elements of the balance mechanism. Certainly, in horses presenting with upper cervical problems, a common observation is that they are not as coordinated as they were prior to injury.

Such changes may be quite subtle, but they leave the animal vulnerable to a recurrence of symptoms or cause other problems by virtue of the altered mechanics of movement.

This combination of neurophysiological responses to injury may be reflected in the natural history of a presenting problem, which can be summarized in what may be described as the 'traffic light' effect (Fig. 12.5).

These cases are more difficult to identify clinically, as it requires careful observation and palpation of the whole biomechanical structure to detect altered function, as opposed to the more obvious changes noted when acute inflammation exists.

DIAGNOSTIC PROCESS

This is a multistage process structured very much along the lines of the human approach but with particular emphasis

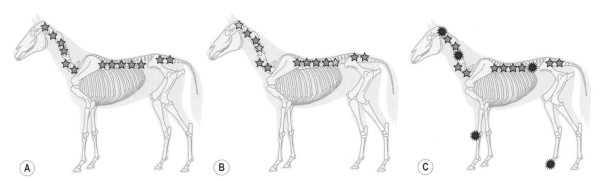

Figure 12.5 The 'traffic light' effect. (A) Green: In the normal horse appropriate screening of sensory input takes place at the level of the spinal cord. (B) Amber: Old injuries have left neurological footprints – regions of spinal cord which, despite being asymptomatic, have retained elements of abnormal patterning, with lowered threshold to external stimuli and altered muscular activity. (C) Red: Minor stresses on the system, such as a slight injury or increasing the amount or level of work, may result in acute symptoms at levels of abnormal patterning.

on the dynamic function of the animal observed in active movements.

Case history

The case history is the starting point of this process. It will often require an open mind and critical thinking, as this is obtained second-hand through the medium of the owner.

Demographics, such as age, breed and work of the animal, are important in building up a picture of the injuries that the animal may have sustained and the problems to which a particular breed may be susceptible.

With this background knowledge in mind, details of the presenting problem are elicited. This may give a picture of a sudden onset acute problem as a result of a specific trauma, such as a dog leaping awkwardly from a stile. More often, there is a history of increasing impairment of movement without a specific date of onset and no reported injury as a cause. However, in such cases, the owner will often mention minor alterations in activity and behaviour, such as a dog which prefers to be lifted from a car rather than jumping, or a horse that is sensitive to grooming on the neck.

Armed with this information, examination is the next phase.

Examination

Examination of the animal at rest and in movement is used to identify alterations in whole movement patterns and specific levels of dysfunction.

Static examination

This looks at the animal's weight-bearing and muscle development, which provides a visual record as to how the body is being used. For example, wasted muscle in the hip region of a Labrador may suggest stiffness in this area with the result that it tends to favour other limbs in weight-bearing. A horse with apparently well-developed shoulders and neck, but rather weak hind-quarters, may be compensating for poor hind limb and lumber spine function by overuse of the front half.

Active examination

In order to establish how the animal is using its body, it is observed in active movement from a number of viewpoints and at different speeds. For most domestic animals, a routine can be developed for observing movement from behind, in front and from the side at walk and trot. The osteopath is looking for fluidity and symmetry of motion, as activity is transmitted from one part of the body to another. Where dysfunction occurs, there can be very obvious breaks in the transmission of movement, identified by observations, such as a puckering of the skin or short, stubby action of the limbs.

Balance, coordination and flexibility can be assessed by observing more complex movements, such as tight turns and backing up.

Palpatory examination

Passive motion testing and palpation of the soft tissue are used to detect specific regions of dysfunction. Skin drag, where the fingers are pulled slowly along the paravertebral muscles, will pick up alterations in tissue texture, and regions of muscle spasm (Fig. 12.6). Joints at each level can be tested for the expected range of movement and asymmetries and reduced ranges may be identified.

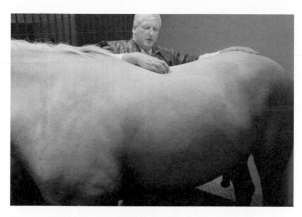

Figure 12.6 Skin drag test identifies areas of altered tissue texture and muscle tone.

TREATMENT

Once a full diagnostic routine has been completed and a biomechanical diagnosis proposed, treatment can begin.

General considerations

Treatment can take many forms. Some are adapted from human techniques, and others have been developed for a particular species of animal (Brooks et al. 2001). As in the approach to children, for treatment to be effective a degree of cooperation is necessary.

By spending a little time with the owner and animal, a relationship built on trust can be developed. Domestic pets, particularly dogs, are very accepting of treatment and, having assured themselves that you intend to do them no harm, may sink into a trance-like state during the course of treatment. However, herbivores, such as horses tend to be more suspicious and vigilant. Indeed, this characteristic in the wild may be the very key to their survival. In these cases, treatment may be facilitated by giving a light sedative, particularly where refined changes in joint complex movement are required, with a position needing to be held for some time. An effective agent, which allows the horse to remain standing while giving a good level of sedation, is a mixture of opioid and an alpha-2 adrenoceptor agonist. The latter reduces the sympathetic drive so reducing overlying muscle tone, while making the deeper structures of the joint complex accessible to examination and treatment. The opioid works through the central pain inhibiting pathways, which in combination with inhibitory input from the peripheral large fibre system (Melzack & Wall 1965), provided by osteopathic treatment, gives a dual beneficial effect.

Another consideration when choosing techniques is the complexity of the problem. Unless the problem is very short term and localized, treatment will have to address dysfunction of the animal as a whole, rather than being directed merely to the area that appears to be symptomatic. Positional techniques are particularly useful in complex strain patterns where there is involvement at multiple levels.

Positional release techniques

Positional release techniques in animals employ the idea of 'ease' and 'bind'. A normal joint has a point, usually at the middle of its range of movement, where there is minimum tension on the capsular ligaments and the overlying muscles, i.e. a point of 'ease'. Movement away from this point will increase tension or 'bind'. This information is processed in the central nervous system to map joint position and to generate an appropriate pattern of motor activity. Where abnormal neural patterning is retained following an injury, the relationship between joint structures is disturbed, and this 'point of ease' will be offset. Sensory information from that joint is subsequently changed at rest, as well as for any given movement. Difficulties arise with imposing new reference points on well-established networks, and the joint complex is likely to be less able to react appropriately, or to coordinate movement with other joints.

This new abnormal resting position may be isolated by testing each range of movement – flexion/extension, side-bending, rotation, translocation from side to side, traction/compression. These vectors are combined together at the point of ease (see notes on 'stacking' in Chapter 5). With the joint held in the position of minimum tension, there is minimum sensory input into the spinal cord. This appears to reduce conflicting information entering the network and allows the normal pattern to reassert itself. A change in neural activity is signalled by a relaxation of the muscles surrounding the joint complex, often accompanied by a deep sigh and altered breathing pattern.

This technique of finding the point of balanced 'ease' can be used on whole body parts, such as a limb, or on specific joint complexes, at strategic points of the skeleton.

Regional approaches

Certain regions are more susceptible to injury and have a greater impact on the function of the animal.

Cervical spine

The head and neck are vulnerable, particularly in horses. Huge forces are generated during a fall and occipitoatlantal-axial dysfunction is common.

One way of starting the technique is by lifting the head onto the shoulder and moving along the line of the jaw to find a point of balance. The jaw can then be used as a

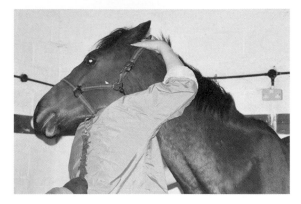

Figure 12.7 Using the mandible as a lever, the point of minimum tension in the upper cervical complex can be isolated.

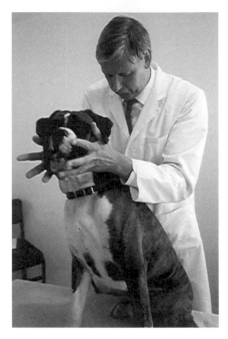

Figure 12.8 The temporomandibular joint is an important site of dysfunction.

lever to take the cervical joints through their ranges of movement. Often, upper cervical joint complexes are dealt with together by introducing elements of flexion and extension, the main movement of the occipitoatlantal articulation, alongside rotation at the atlantoaxial level. In this way, the point of ease can be isolated. This can be refined further by placing the hands onto the subocciput, in order to introduce secondary vectors of compression, traction and translocation (also described as translation or shunting) (Fig. 12.7).

Temporomandibular joint

Intimately associated with the top of the neck, not only mechanically but neurologically by virtue of trigeminal innervation, is the jaw. Dogs are particularly susceptible to strains in this region resulting perhaps from their predilection for carrying over-large sticks. Using fingers on the medial surface of the mandible, trigger point inhibition can be used while introducing traction or compression through the ramus into the jaw itself (Fig. 12.8). (See notes on Facilitated positional release in Chapter 5.)

The limbs

The limbs are also susceptible to alterations in normal relationships. Dogs move with rapid changes in direction, and strain patterns which reflect these forces may be transmitted up the leg, starting with the phalanges and working up through the limb into the thorax.

Another important area is where the scapula and forelimb connect with the thorax. Unlike humans, there is no actual bony connection between forelimb and rib cage. Instead the muscles of the thorax, notably the pectorals, form a muscular sling in which the thoracic cage can rotate to allow much of the lateral movement occurring in horses and dogs. Fascial binding in this region clamps the scapula

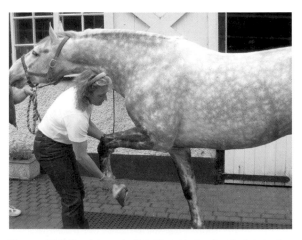

Figure 12.9 Fascial unwinding through the forelimb into the thorax. *(Photograph courtesy of Annabel Jenks DO.)*

to the thorax and restricts limb motion and lateral flexibility. A combination of stretch and fascial unwinding through the foreleg is an arduous, but rewarding, way of improving mobility (Fig. 12.9).

A similar procedure can be used for the hind limb. Problems here are often associated with lumbosacral and sacroiliac dysfunction.

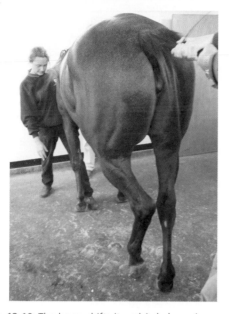

Figure 12.10 The horse shifts its pelvic balance in response to functional traction through the tail. *(Photograph courtesy of Jonathan Cohen BSc (Hons) Osteopathy.)*

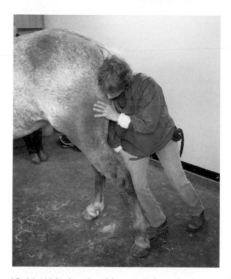

Figure 12.11 With the shoulder medial to the horse's ischial tuberosity, the fascia, muscles and joints of the sacrum and pelvis can be influenced. *(Photograph courtesy of Jonathan Cohen.)*

Lumbosacral and pelvic region

A method of accessing the lumbosacral and pelvic complex that is not available in human osteopathy involves the tail. The tail is formed by approximately 20 caudal vertebrae which, after the first three, start to lose shape and articulations, to form simple rods joined with cartilaginous discs. The muscles of the tail, particularly the sacrocaudalis dorsalis, link with the multifidus muscles of the lumbar spine and sacrum, which play an important role in the segmental stabilization of the spine (Geisler et al. 1996), as well as provision of proprioceptive information. As these muscles have been implicated in recurrent back pain, the tail provides a good 'handle' on these structures.

By gently holding the root of the tail and taking it through all its possible ranges of movement, an idea of the fascial tension, from the tail into the pelvis can be determined. This can be observed quite clearly, particularly in horses, where the tail may be held to one side of the midline. When a point of ease has been established, traction can be increased, and this is often accompanied by quite dramatic manoeuvring of the pelvic girdle by the animal itself, as it shifts its weight from one hind limb to the other (Fig. 12.10).

The pelvis may also be accessed via the pelvic diaphragm. By using a shoulder, placed medial to the ischial tuberosity in the horse, or fingers in the dog, trigger points can be identified. The animal will often lean into the pressure being applied, and this can be used to introduce ranges of movement in the sacroiliac articulation, using the ischial tuberosity as a lever (Fig. 12.11).

TREATMENT UNDER GENERAL ANAESTHETIC

In a number of cases, the complexity and longstanding nature of the problem may require treatment to be carried out under a general anaesthetic. This is particularly relevant in horses where the speed and weight of the animal means that huge forces are often involved in injury.

The horse is anaesthetized, intubated and supported on its back. In this position, examination and treatment resembles even more closely the procedure used in human practice. It is interesting to note that under these conditions, it is often possible to detect marked restrictions in joint function that were not apparent on examination of the conscious horse. This emphasizes the effectiveness of compensatory mechanisms that may develop over time.

Another point of interest is that some of these horses are unable to lie squarely on their back. The fascial and muscular patterns developed as a result of injury and subsequent compensation, may produce a functional scoliosis that is maintained even under full anaesthetic.

Such cases are ideal candidates for the 'whole body unwinding' technique. With a practitioner holding each leg, the limbs are put through all ranges of movement to reach a point of minimum tension (Fig. 12.12). This position often reflects the directional forces involved in the

Table 12.1 Duration of symptoms where known in cases presenting to an osteopathic clinic

Duration (months)	<6	6–11	12–17	18–23	24–29	30–35	≥36
Frequency	32	16	21	9	9	0	24
Percentage	29	14	19	8	8	0	22

Note: Three cases were lost to follow-up.

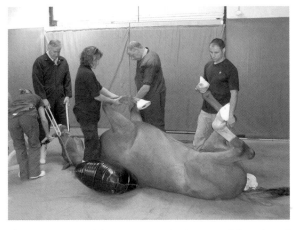

Figure 12.12 Fascial patterns may be 'unwound' by using all four limbs. *(Photograph courtesy of Jonathan Cohen.)*

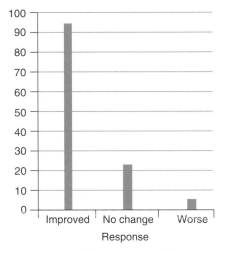

Figure 12.13 Outcome following osteopathic treatment at least 12 months after the last treatment.

original trauma. This is maintained until there is a sense of relaxation often accompanied by a change in breathing pattern.

IS EQUINE OSTEOPATHY (POSITIONAL RELEASE) EFFECTIVE?

While osteopathic treatment of horses appeared to be successful, based on anecdotal evidence, studies were required to establish the effect and effectiveness of the treatment. A clinical audit, carried out in 1995, defined the caseload referred to the clinic in terms of demographics and symptom presentation, as well as whether owners and veterinary surgeons felt that osteopathic intervention had been of long-term benefit to their animals. This retrospective study of 127 cases showed that horses presented to the clinic principally with back pain, nonspecific and shifting lameness and back stiffness, and those who were unable to perform the work expected of them. These problems had been present for over 2 years in 30%, and over 6 months in 71% of cases (Table 12.1). A follow-up at least 12 months after the final osteopathic treatment, showed

that 95 (75%) had maintained improvement and were working at the expected level, or above, according to owners and veterinary surgeon reports (Fig. 12.13).

The next step was to consider physiological markers which could be used to identify changes resulting from osteopathic treatment.

One response to injury and pain is muscle hypertonia (He et al. 1988) and this may be expressed as shortened stride length.

A pilot study showed that horses presenting to the clinic had a significantly reduced step length, by a mean of 11.4 cm ($p < 0.001$) in trot, compared with controls (Woodleigh 2003). After osteopathic treatment, there was a significant increase of mean 12.5 cm ($p < 0.05$) in step length in the clinical cases (Fig. 12.14).

Another useful physiological marker is the change in sympathetic nervous system activity in response to a painful stimulus (Sato & Schmidt 1973).

This is manifested by alterations in surface temperature, which can be detected by infrared thermography. In horses, there is general agreement regarding normal patterns of cutaneous heat distribution, with surface temperatures throughout the body remaining consistent to within

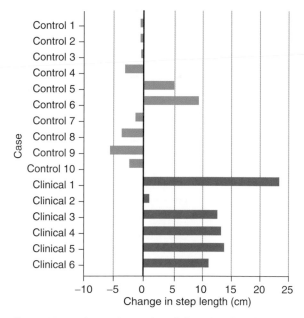

Figure 12.14 Change in step length from initial reading to follow-up for controls and clinical cases.

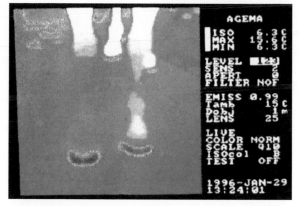

Figure 12.15 Cooling of distal forelimb: abnormal patterns of sympathetic nervous system activity may cause cooling along almost dermatomal distribution.

1°C. Although acute injuries are detected as 'hot spots' by virtue of local inflammatory changes, increased activity of the sympathetic network in response to pain will act on the arteriovenous shunts to move blood away from the surface to the muscles, that show up as cooler regions (Fig. 12.4). Where this pattern of activity is retained in the network, after the initial injury has resolved, areas of cooling almost along dermatomal distribution, may be detected (Fig. 12.15) (Colles et al. 1994).

A further study of 46 horses looked at thermal patterns in the gluteal region. These were found to be significantly cooler ($p < 0.02$) than expected in cases presenting to the osteopathic clinic. These regions showed a significant increase in temperature following treatment (Brooks 2003).

CONCLUSION

The treatment of animals is a rewarding field for those wishing to extend the boundaries of practice. There are the challenges of working where verbal communication is not possible, and where techniques must be adapted to the highly variable body sizes and shapes existing between species.

There is considerable overlap between human and animal practice and both have something to offer in the areas of clinical reasoning, palpatory skills and technique development – a case of the whole being greater than the sum of the parts.

THIS CHAPTER

This chapter has discussed the application of positional release techniques in the treatment of animals.

REFERENCES

Bevan, S., 1999. Nociceptive peripheral neurones: cellular properties. In: Wall, P.D., Melzack, R. (Eds.), Textbook of Pain, fourth ed. Harcourt, Edinburgh, pp. 85–103.

Brooks, J., 2003. Osteopathy in horses using infra-red thermography as a tool to monitor the effect of osteopathic treatment. In: 4th International Conference on Advances in Osteopathic Research. Royal Society of Medicine, London.

Brooks, J., Colles, C., Pusey, A., 2001. The role of osteopathy in the treatment of the horse. In: Rossdale, P.D., Green, G. (Eds.), Guardians of the Horse II. Newmarket, Romney.

Colles, C.M., Pusey, A.G., 2003. Osteopathic treatment of the axial skeleton of the horse. In: Ross, M.W., Dyson, S.J. (Eds.), Diagnosis and Management of Lameness in the Horse. Saunders, London, pp. 819–824.

Colles, C., Holah, G., Pusey, A., 1994. Thermal imaging as an aid to the diagnosis of back pain in the horse. Proceedings of the 6th European Congress of Thermography, Bath.

Doubell, T.P., Manion, R.J., Woolf, C.J., 1999. The dorsal horn: state dependant sensory processing, plasticity and the generation of pain. In: Wall, P.D., Melzack, R. (Eds.), Textbook of Pain, fourth ed. Harcourt, Edinburgh, pp. 165–181.

Geisler, H.C., Westerga, J., Gramsbergen, A., 1996. The function of the long back muscles; an EMG study in the rat. Behavioural Brain Research 80, 211–215.

He, X., Proske, U., Schaible, H.G., et al., 1988. Acute inflammation of the knee joint in the cat alters responses of flexor motoneurones to leg movements. Journal of Neurophysiology 59, 326–340.

Jeffcott, L.B., 1979. Back problems in the horse – a look at past, present and future. Equine Veterinary Journal 11, 129–136.

Melzack, R., Wall, P.D., 1965. Pain mechanisms: a new theory. Science 150, 971–979.

Patterson, M., Wurster, R.D., 1997. Neurophysiologic system: integration and disintegration. In: Ward, R.C. (Ed.), Foundations of Osteopathic Medicine. Williams and Wilkins, Baltimore, MD, pp. 137–151.

Pearson, K., Gordon, J., 2000. Locomotion. In: Kandel, E., Schwartz, J., Jessell, T. (Eds.), Principles of Neuroscience, fourth ed. McGraw-Hill, New York, pp. 740–747.

Sato, A., Schmidt, R.F., 1973. Somatosympathetic reflexes: afferent fibres, central pathways, discharge characteristics. Physiological Reviews 53, 916–947.

Williams, N., 1997. Managing back pain in general practice – is osteopathy the new paradigm? British Journal of General Practice 47, 653–655.

Woodleigh, M., 2003. Can osteopathic treatment under general anaesthetic increase stride length in horses? In: 4th International Conference on Advances in Osteopathic Research. Royal Society of Medicine, London.

Index

Page numbers followed by 'f' indicate figures, 't' indicate tables, and 'b' indicate boxes.